AF581754

Coronary Syndrome: Clinical Treatment, Prevention and Management for Better Outcomes

Coronary Syndrome: Clinical Treatment, Prevention and Management for Better Outcomes

Editors

Koichi Node
Atsushi Tanaka

MDPI • Basel • Beijing • Wuhan • Barcelona • Belgrade • Manchester • Tokyo • Cluj • Tianjin

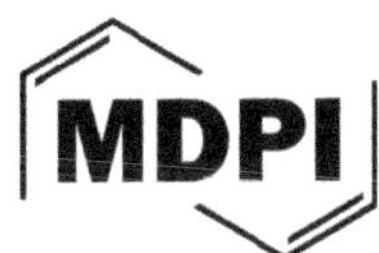

Editors
Koichi Node
Saga University
Saga
Japan

Atsushi Tanaka
Saga University
Saga
Japan

Editorial Office
MDPI
St. Alban-Anlage 66
4052 Basel, Switzerland

This is a reprint of articles from the Special Issue published online in the open access journal *Journal of Clinical Medicine* (ISSN 2077-0383) (available at: https://www.mdpi.com/journal/jcm/special_issues/cardiology_coronary_syndrome).

For citation purposes, cite each article independently as indicated on the article page online and as indicated below:

LastName, A.A.; LastName, B.B.; LastName, C.C. Article Title. *Journal Name* **Year**, *Volume Number*, Page Range.

ISBN 978-3-0365-7912-2 (Hbk)
ISBN 978-3-0365-7913-9 (PDF)

Contents

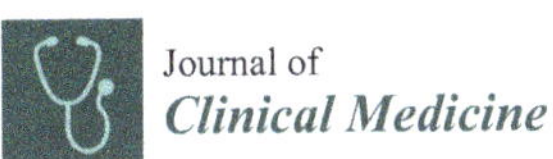
Journal of
Clinical Medicine

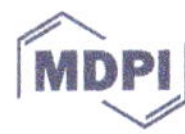

Editorial

What More Can Be Delivered to Future Patients with Coronary Syndromes?

Atsushi Tanaka * and Koichi Node *

Department of Cardiovascular Medicine, Saga University, Saga 849-8501, Japan
* Correspondence: tanakaa2@cc.saga-u.ac.jp (A.T.); node@cc.saga-u.ac.jp (K.N.)

Citation: Tanaka, A.; Node, K. What More Can Be Delivered to Future Patients with Coronary Syndromes? *J. Clin. Med.* **2022**, *11*, 5704. https://doi.org/10.3390/jcm11195704

Received: 19 September 2022
Accepted: 26 September 2022
Published: 27 September 2022

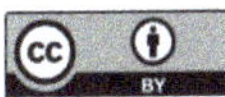

Coronary artery disease (CAD) is a major cardiovascular disease that imposes substantial clinical and socioeconomic burdens worldwide. To date, many studies have been conducted to address this issue, leading to innovations and advances in various medical technologies and treatments. Recently, based on its dynamic nature in clinical settings, the clinical concept of CAD has been subdivided into "acute coronary syndrome (ACS)" and "chronic coronary syndrome (CCS)" [1]. In this context, invasive and multidisciplinary therapies in the acute setting have been the mainstay of ACS treatment and have significantly contributed to improving patient survival rates. Simultaneously, the appropriate practice of optimal drug therapy has been recommended in relevant guidelines for the chronic management of CCS, which has contributed to the prevention of CAD recurrence and improved prognosis. However, CAD remains a problem worldwide, and the reality is that many patients still develop CAD. This raises the question: what is needed in the future to further overcome CAD? We aimed to answer this question in this study.

To begin with, we believe that there is a strong need to accumulate novel scientific and clinical knowledge in this field to develop seamless treatment and preventive strategies for acute and chronic coronary syndrome. Furthermore, accumulated data indicate that there are some residual risk factors for coronary syndrome combined with ACS and CCS. Moreover, the clinical management of cardiovascular/non-cardiovascular complications associated with coronary syndrome to achieve better outcomes is a critical issue. Therefore, we need to gather potential papers to solve these unmet needs in the clinical management of coronary syndrome in contemporary medical care settings. With the indispensable help of excellent authors and reviewers, our group was able to collate 13 papers on this topic that were published in the past two years. In this editorial, we would like to express our gratitude to those contributors and provide a very concise introduction to each of these papers (please refer to each publication for details).

Two papers on ischemia imaging have been published by Japanese researchers. Kamo et al. [2] reported that the subtraction computed tomography (CT) fractional flow reserve method was useful for improving the diagnostic performance of hemodynamically significant coronary stenosis in patients with severe calcification. Kouchi et al. [3] found that the myocardial perfusion ratio to the aorta derived from myocardial CT perfusion analysis had a higher diagnostic accuracy for detecting impaired myocardial perfusion than conventional semi-quantitative parameters, such as myocardial CT attenuation and transmural perfusion ratio.

Two papers on percutaneous coronary intervention (PCI) were published in Korea and Japan. Kim et al. [4] revealed that differences in reperfusion strategies did not significantly affect prognosis in patients with multivessel non-ST-elevation myocardial infarction and chronic kidney disease, emphasizing the need for further investigation of the optimal perfusion strategy. Noma et al. [5] reported that adjunctive catheter-derived thrombolysis with intracoronary monteplase delivery resulted in favorable outcomes in patients with ST-elevation myocardial infarction, especially in those with a high thrombus burden who were refractory to primary PCI procedures.

Two studies on coronary spasm were conducted in Japan and Korea. Teragawa et al. [6] identified active smoking as a possible risk factor associated with the increase in the index of microcirculatory resistance (IMR) for patients who underwent an invasive microvascular vasodilatory function test, showing that IMR differed according to the coronary artery branches and types of coronary spasm. Kim et al. [7] documented that the chronic use of nitrates in patients with vasospastic angina, relative to other types of vasodilators, such as nicorandil, was associated with an increased risk of adverse clinical outcomes in a prospective nationwide registry database.

Three studies on pharmacotherapy were also conducted in Korea and Japan. Kim et al. [8] reported that the prognostic benefit of statin therapy following PCI for acute myocardial infarction (AMI) was significant even in patients with advanced renal impairment, compared to non-statin users. However, since the incidence rate of adverse events in patients with chronic kidney disease is still high, further therapeutic approaches are needed, especially in these patient populations. Jo et al. [9] performed a multicenter, double-blind, randomized trial and found that a single pill of olmesartan/amlodipine plus rosuvastatin therapy was more effective and safe for the management of both hypertension and dyslipidemia than either olmesartan plus rosuvastatin or olmesartan plus amlodipine therapy. Mori et al. [10] further provided real-world evidence for the use of a modified Japanese dose of prasugrel (loading/maintenance: 20/3.75 mg) with a similar efficacy and safety to the standard dose of clopidogrel in patients with AMI.

Three papers investigating uric acid as a residual risk factor for coronary syndrome were published by Japanese and Italian researchers. Hiraga et al. demonstrated that serum uric acid (SUA) level was an independent factor inversely associated with systemic endothelial function in patients with a broad spectrum of CAD, including ischemia with non-obstructive CAD [11]. Watanabe et al. found that plasma xanthine oxidoreductase activity was an independent predictor of coronary spasm in both sexes and that this effect was especially pronounced in female patients [12]. Maloberti et al. [13] reviewed recent evidence to clarify the role of SUA in the care of coronary syndrome and concluded that further studies are warranted to determine the pathological and therapeutic relationship between SUA and CAD.

Finally, Goriki et al. [14] sought to create a laboratory-only risk score model to predict post-discharge mortality in survivors following AMI, revealing that a model comprising hemoglobin, renal function, albumin, and troponin I levels obtained prior to primary PCI could be clinically useful for the early risk stratification of one-year mortality.

However, patients are still developing coronary syndromes. We hope that what we have elucidated in this Topical Collection will help to better manage future patients with these diseases; however, we also understand that significant research is still required to overcome coronary syndromes. It is also our strong hope that this collection will promote further research to enable a better understanding and clinical management of coronary syndromes in the near future. Once again, we would like to express our gratitude to the authors and reviewers for their dedicated contributions to our Topical Collection "Coronary Syndrome: Clinical Treatment, Prevention and Management for Better Outcomes" in *the Journal of Clinical Medicine*.

Funding: This work was partly supported by the Japan Society for the Promotion of Science KAKENHI Grant Number JP21K08130 and the Takeda Science Foundation.

Acknowledgments: The authors are grateful to Aya Yamada (Saga University) for her assistance.

Conflicts of Interest: The authors declare no conflict of interest related to this work.

References

1. Knuuti, J.; Wijns, W.; Saraste, A.; Capodanno, D.; Barbato, E.; Funck-Brentano, C.; Prescott, E.; Storey, R.F.; Deaton, C.; Cuisset, T.; et al. 2019 ESC Guidelines for the Diagnosis and Management of Chronic Coronary Syndromes. *Eur. Heart J.* **2020**, *41*, 407–477. [CrossRef]
2. Kamo, Y.; Fujimoto, S.; Nozaki, Y.O.; Aoshima, C.; Kawaguchi, Y.O.; Dohi, T.; Kudo, A.; Takahashi, D.; Takamura, K.; Hiki, M.; et al. Incremental Diagnostic Value of CT Fractional Flow Reserve Using Subtraction Method in Patients with Severe Calcification: A Pilot Study. *J. Clin. Med.* **2021**, *10*, 4398. [CrossRef] [PubMed]
3. Kouchi, T.; Tanabe, Y.; Takemoto, T.; Yoshida, K.; Yamamoto, Y.; Miyazaki, S.; Fukuyama, N.; Nishiyama, H.; Inaba, S.; Kawaguchi, N.; et al. A Novel Quantitative Parameter for Static Myocardial Computed Tomography: Myocardial Perfusion Ratio to the Aorta. *J. Clin. Med.* **2022**, *11*, 1816. [CrossRef] [PubMed]
4. Kim, Y.H.; Her, A.Y.; Jeong, M.H.; Kim, B.K.; Hong, S.J.; Lee, S.J.; Ahn, C.M.; Kim, J.S.; Ko, Y.G.; Choi, D.; et al. Outcomes of different reperfusion strategies of multivessel disease undergoing new-generation drug-eluting stent implantation in patients with non-ST-elevation myocardial infarction and chronic kidney disease. *J. Clin. Med.* **2021**, *10*, 4629. [CrossRef] [PubMed]
5. Noma, S.; Miyachi, H.; Fukuizumi, I.; Matsuda, J.; Sangen, H.; Kubota, Y.; Imori, Y.; Saiki, Y.; Hosokawa, Y.; Tara, S.; et al. Adjunctive Catheter-Directed Thrombolysis during Primary PCI for ST-Segment Elevation Myocardial Infarction with High Thrombus Burden. *J. Clin. Med.* **2022**, *11*, 262. [CrossRef]
6. Teragawa, H.; Oshita, C.; Uchimura, Y.; Akazawa, R.; Orita, Y. Coronary Microvascular Vasodilatory Function: Related Clinical Features and Differences According to the Different Coronary Arteries and Types of Coronary Spasm. *J. Clin. Med.* **2021**, *11*, 130. [CrossRef]
7. Kim, H.J.; Jo, S.H.; Lee, M.H.; Seo, W.W.; Kim, H.L.; Lee, K.Y.; Yang, T.H.; Her, S.H.; Lee, B.K.; Park, K.H.; et al. Nitrates vs. other types of vasodilators and clinical outcomes in patients with vasospastic angina: A propensity score-matched analysis. *J. Clin. Med.* **2022**, *11*, 3250. [CrossRef] [PubMed]
8. Kim, Y.H.; Her, A.Y.; Jeong, M.H.; Kim, B.K.; Hong, S.J.; Kim, S.; Ahn, C.M.; Kim, J.S.; Ko, Y.G.; Choi, D.; et al. Efficacy of Statin Treatment According to Baseline Renal Function in Korean Patients with Acute Myocardial Infarction Not Requiring Dialysis Undergoing Newer-Generation Drug-Eluting Stent Implantation. *J. Clin. Med.* **2021**, *10*, 3504. [CrossRef] [PubMed]
9. Jo, S.H.; Kang, S.M.; Yoo, B.S.; Lee, Y.S., Youn, H.J.; Min, K.; Yu, J.M.; Yoon, H.J.; Kim, W.S.; Kim, G.H.; et al. A prospective randomized, double-blind, Multi-Center, phase III clinical trial evaluating the efficacy and safety of olmesartan/amlodipine plus rosuvastatin combination treatment in patients with concomitant hypertension and dyslipidemia: A leisure study. *J. Clin. Med.* **2022**, *11*, 350. [CrossRef] [PubMed]
10. Mori, H.; Mizukami, T.; Maeda, A.; Fukui, K.; Akashi, Y.; Ako, J.; Ikari, Y.; Ebina, T.; Tamura, K.; Namiki, A.; et al. A Japanese Dose of Prasugrel versus a Standard Dose of Clopidogrel in Patients with Acute Myocardial Infarction from the K-ACTIVE Registry. *J. Clin. Med.* **2022**, *11*, 2016. [CrossRef]
11. Hiraga, T.; Saito, Y.; Mori, N.; Tateishi, K.; Kitahara, H.; Kobayashi, Y. Impact of Serum Uric Acid Level on Systemic Endothelial Dysfunction in Patients with a Broad Spectrum of Ischemic Heart Disease. *J. Clin. Med.* **2021**, *10*, 4530. [CrossRef] [PubMed]
12. Watanabe, K.; Watanabe, T.; Otaki, Y.; Murase, T.; Nakamura, T.; Kato, S.; Tamura, H.; Nishiyama, S.; Takahashi, H.; Arimoto, T.; et al. Gender Differences in the Impact of Plasma Xanthine Oxidoreductase Activity on Coronary Artery Spasm. *J. Clin. Med.* **2021**, *10*, 5550. [CrossRef] [PubMed]
13. Maloberti, A.; Biolcati, M.; Ruzzenenti, G.; Giani, V.; Leidi, F.; Monticelli, M.; Algeri, M.; Scarpellini, S.; Nava, S.; Soriano, F.; et al. The Role of Uric Acid in Acute and Chronic Coronary Syndromes. *J. Clin. Med.* **2021**, *10*, 4750. [CrossRef] [PubMed]
14. Goriki, Y.; Tanaka, A.; Yoshioka, G.; Nishihira, K.; Kuriyama, N.; Shibata, Y.; Node, K. Development of a Laboratory Risk-Score Model to Predict One-Year Mortality in Acute Myocardial Infarction Survivors. *J. Clin. Med.* **2022**, *11*, 3497. [CrossRef]

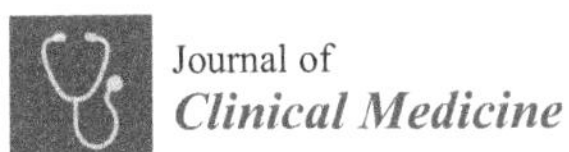
Journal of
Clinical Medicine
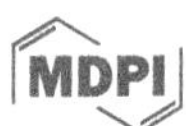

Article

Efficacy of Statin Treatment According to Baseline Renal Function in Korean Patients with Acute Myocardial Infarction Not Requiring Dialysis Undergoing Newer-Generation Drug-Eluting Stent Implantation

Yong Hoon Kim [1,*,†], Ae-Young Her [1,†], Myung Ho Jeong [2], Byeong-Keuk Kim [3], Sung-Jin Hong [3], Seunghwan Kim [4], Chul-Min Ahn [3], Jung-Sun Kim [3], Young-Guk Ko [3], Donghoon Choi [3], Myeong-Ki Hong [3] and Yangsoo Jang [3]

1 Division of Cardiology, Department of Internal Medicine, Kangwon National University School of Medicine, Chuncheon 24289, Korea; hermartha1@gmail.com
2 Department of Cardiology, Cardiovascular Center, Chonnam National University Hospital, Gwangju 61469, Korea; myungho@chollian.net
3 Division of Cardiology, Severance Cardiovascular Hospital, Yonsei University College of Medicine, Seoul 03722, Korea; kimbk@yuhs.ac (B.-K.K.); HONGS@yuhs.ac (S.-J.H.); DRCELLO@yuhs.ac (C.-M.A.); kjs1218@yuhs.ac (J.-S.K.); ygko@yuhs.ac (Y.-G.K.); cdhlyj@yuhs.ac (D.C.); mkhong61@yuhs.ac (M.-K.H.); jangys1212@yuhs.ac (Y.J.)
4 Division of Cardiology, Inje University College of Medicine, Haeundae Paik Hospital, Busan 48108, Korea; cloudksh@gmail.com
* Correspondence: yhkim02@kangwon.ac.kr
† Yong Hoon Kim and Ae-Young Her contributed equally to this work as the first authors.

Citation: Kim, Y.H.; Her, A.-Y.; Jeong, M.H.; Kim, B.-K.; Hong, S.-J.; Kim, S.; Ahn, C.-M.; Kim, J.-S.; Ko, Y.-G.; Choi, D.; et al. Efficacy of Statin Treatment According to Baseline Renal Function in Korean Patients with Acute Myocardial Infarction Not Requiring Dialysis Undergoing Newer-Generation Drug-Eluting Stent Implantation. *J. Clin. Med.* **2021**, *10*, 3504. https://doi.org/10.3390/jcm10163504

Academic Editors: Atsushi Tanaka and Koichi Node

Received: 20 July 2021
Accepted: 6 August 2021
Published: 9 August 2021

Abstract: We investigated the 2-year efficacy of statin treatment according to baseline renal function in patients with acute myocardial infarction (AMI) not requiring dialysis undergoing newer-generation drug-eluting stent (DES) implantation. A total of 18,875 AMI patients were classified into group A (statin users, n = 16,055) and group B (statin nonusers, n = 2820). According to the baseline estimated glomerular filtration rate (eGFR; ≥90, 60–89, 30–59 and <30 mL/min/1.73 m^2), these two groups were sub-classified into groups A1, A2, A3 and A4 and groups B1, B2, B3 and B4. The major adverse cardiac events (MACE), defined as all-cause death, recurrent MI (re-MI) and any repeat revascularization, were evaluated. The MACE (group A1 vs. B1, p = 0.002; group A2 vs. B2, p = 0.007; group A3 vs. B3, p < 0.001; group A4 vs. B4, p < 0.001), all-cause death (p = 0.006, p < 0.001, p < 0.001, p < 0.001, respectively) and cardiac death (p = 0.004, p < 0.001, p < 0.001, p < 0.001, respectively) rates were significantly higher in statin nonusers than those in statin users. Despite the beneficial effects of statin treatment, the MACE (group A1 vs. A2 vs. A3 vs. A4: 5.2%, 6.4%, 10.1% and 18.5%, respectively), all-cause mortality (0.9%, 1.8%, 4.6% and 12.9%, respectively) and cardiac death (0.4%, 1.0%, 2.6% and 6.8%, respectively) rates were significantly increased as eGFR decreased in group A. These results may be related to the peculiar characteristics of chronic kidney disease, including increased vascular calcification and traditional or nontraditional cardiovascular risk factors. In the era of newer-generation DESs, although statin treatment was effective in reducing mortality, this beneficial effect was diminished in accordance with the deterioration of baseline renal function.

Keywords: statin; myocardial infarction; renal function

1. Introduction

During the past two decades, rapid coronary reperfusion and revascularization with newer antiplatelet and anticoagulation therapies have improved the survival of patients with acute myocardial infarction (AMI) [1,2]. Ischemic heart disease accounts for almost 1.8 million annual deaths, or 20% of all deaths in Europe [3]. Similar to Western countries, AMI continues to be a major cause of mortality in the Asia-Pacific population [4]. Statin, an inhibitor of 3-hydroxy-3-methylglutaryl-coenzyme A (HMG-CoA) reductase activity, has both fundamental lipid-lowering capacity and additional pleiotropic effects on reducing morbidity and mortality [5,6]. The current guidelines recommend that statin therapy should be initiated or continued in all patients with AMI if there are no contraindications to its use [7,8]. Every 30% decrease in glomerular filtration rate (GFR) was associated with a 29% increase in the risk of a major vascular event (MVE) [9]. Hence, individuals with chronic kidney disease (CKD) grade 3a to 4 (GFR: 15–59 mL/min/1.73 m^2) have a 2- or 3-fold increased risk of cardiovascular mortality compared with those without CKD [10]. Some suggested mechanisms for the progression of CKD in patients with cardiovascular and renal diseases include endothelial dysfunction, oxidative stress and systemic inflammation of the glomerular capillary wall [11]. Statins alleviate many adverse effects of reduced nitric oxide availability in the inflammatory environment and improve endothelial function [12]. Moreover, statin treatment has been considered a mainstay strategy for CKD patients with respect to reducing the all-cause mortality [13]. Although previous reports [14–16] showed that statin treatment reduced the risk of major adverse events in patients with CKD, there are some debates [17]. Additionally, their study population [14–17] was not confined to patients with AMI. Kim et al. [18,19] showed that stent generation could be regarded as an important determinant of major adverse cardiac events (MACE) in patients with ST-segment elevation myocardial infarction (STEMI) and AMI. Therefore, we believe that the presence or absence of beneficial effects of statin treatment on major adverse events should be re-estimated in patients with AMI according to renal function under the current newer-generation drug-eluting stent (DES) era to provide more accurate real-world information to interventional cardiologists. Hence, in this study, we evaluated the 2-year efficacy of statin treatment according to baseline renal function in patients with AMI undergoing newer-generation DES implantation.

2. Method

2.1. Study Population

The study population was recruited from the Korea AMI Registry (KAMIR) [4]. Details of this registry can be found on the KAMIR website (http://www.kamir.or.kr (accessed on 15 April 2021). All patients aged ≥18 years at the time of hospital admission were included. The KAMIR was established in November 2005 and involved more than 50 communities and teaching hospitals in South Korea. A total of 45,555 patients with AMI who underwent successful stent implantation and who were not receiving continuous renal replacement therapy including hemodialysis or peritoneal dialysis between January 2006 and June 2015 were eligible for inclusion in this study. Patients with the following were also excluded: deployed bare-metal stents (n = 2362, 5.2%) and first-generation DES (n = 11,166, 24.5%), incomplete laboratory results (n = 8330, 18.3%), loss to follow-up (n = 2247, 4.9%), post-percutaneous coronary intervention (PCI) thrombolysis in myocardial infarction (TIMI) flow grade <3 (n = 2089, 4.6%), in-hospital death (n = 447, 1.0%) and treatment with other kinds of statins, except for atorvastatin, rosuvastatin, simvastatin, pitavastatin, pravastatin and fluvastatin (n = 39, 0.09%). Thus, a total of 18,875 AMI patients who underwent successful PCI with a newer-generation DES were included. The types of new-generation DESs used are listed in Table 1. Among the AMI patients, 16,055 (85.1%) were classified into group A (statin users) and 2820 (15.0%) into group B (statin nonusers). Thereafter, groups A and B were further subclassified into groups A1 and B1 (eGFR ≥ 90 mL/min/1.73 m^2, n = 6847 (42.6%) and n = 889 (31.5%), respectively), groups A2 and B2 (eGFR 60–89 mL/min/1.73 m^2, n = 6557 (40.8%) and n = 1227 (43.5%), respectively), groups A3 and B3 (eGFR 30–59 mL/min/1.73 m^2, n = 2144 (13.4%) and n = 537 (19.0%), respectively) and groups A4 and B4 (eGFR < 30 mL/min/1.73 m^2, n = 507 (3.2%) and n = 167 (5.9%), respectively) according to their baseline renal function and strata used to define CKD stages (Figure 1) [20]. However, because the number of patients included in stages 4 and 5 was small, they were grouped into one group (A4 or B4) in our study. The detailed reasons for not using statins in group B were as follows: (1) expected risk was higher than the benefit due to several etiologic factors such as end-stage renal failure, advanced age ≥75 years or severe heart failure (HF) (n = 1213, 43.0%), (2) abnormal liver function (aspartate aminotransferase or alanine aminotransferase was higher than 3-fold the upper normal limit) (n = 689, 24.4%), (3) multi-organ failure (n = 121, 4.3%), (4) statin-induced myopathy or arthralgia (n = 110, 3.9%) and (5) unknown (n = 687, 24.4%). All data were collected using a web-based case report form at each participating center. The study was conducted in accordance with the ethical guidelines of the 2004 Declaration of Helsinki and was approved by the ethics committee at each participating center and the Chonnam National University Hospital Institutional Review Board ethics committee (CNUH-2011-172). All 18,875 patients included in the study provided written informed consent prior to enrollment. They also completed a 2-year clinical follow-up through face-to-face interviews, phone calls or chart reviews. All clinical events were evaluated by an independent event adjudication committee. The event adjudication process was previously described by the KAMIR investigators. [21].

Table 1. Baseline characteristics of statin users.

Variables	Total (n = 16,055)	Group A1 eGFR ≥ 90 mL/min/1.73 m^2 (n = 6847)	Group A2 eGFR 60–89 mL/min/1.73 m^2 (n = 6557)	Group A3 eGFR 30–59 mL/min/1.73 m^2 (n = 2144)	Group A4 eGFR < 30 mL/min/1.73 m^2 (n = 507)	p Value
Male, n (%)	12,053 (75.1)	5536 (80.9)	4988 (76.1)	1225 (57.1)	304 (60.0)	<0.001
Age (years)	63.0 ± 12.3	58.9 ± 11.5	64.3 ± 12.1	70.8 ± 10.4	68.9 ± 10.9	<0.001
LVEF (%)	52.8 ± 10.8	54.0 ± 10.0	52.8 ± 10.7	50.0 ± 12.3	48.1 ± 11.9	<0.001
BMI (kg/m^2)	24.2 ± 3.2	24.3 ± 3.2	24.2 ± 3.2	23.9 ± 3.2	23.5 ±3.4	<0.001
SBP (mmHg)	131.6 ± 27.2	133.4 ± 25.0	131.4 ± 27.7	126.6 ± 30.2	132.2 ± 33.3	<0.001
DBP (mmHg)	79.9 ± 16.2	81.7 ± 15.3	79.6 ± 16.4	75.7 ± 17.1	77.4 ± 18.0	<0.001
Cardiogenic shock, n (%)	575 (3.6)	124 (1.8)	247 (3.8)	160 (7.5)	44 (8.7)	<0.001
CPR on admission, n (%)	557 (3.5)	186 (2.7)	218 (3.3)	129 (6.0)	24 (4.7)	<0.001
Killip class III/IV, n (%)	1454 (9.1)	322 (4.7)	578 (8.8)	416 (19.4)	138 (27.2)	<0.001
STEMI, n (%)	8737 (54.4)	3640 (53.2)	3764 (57.4)	1160 (54.1)	173 (34.1)	<0.001
Primary PCI, n (%)	8424 (96.4)	3511 (96.5)	3633 (96.5)	1115 (96.1)	165 (95.4)	0.809
NSTEMI, n (%)	7318 (45.6)	3207 (46.8)	2793 (42.6)	984 (45.9)	334 (65.9)	<0.001
PCI within 24 h, n (%)	6303 (86.1)	2865 (89.3)	2384 (85.4)	791 (80.4)	263 (78.7)	<0.001
Hypertension, n (%)	7761 (48.3)	2622 (38.3)	3238 (49.4)	1489 (69.4)	412 (81.3)	<0.001
Diabetes mellitus, n (%)	4201 (26.2)	1446 (21.1)	1534 (23.4)	903 (42.1)	318 (62.7)	<0.001
Dyslipidemia, n (%)	1936 (12.1)	792 (11.6)	815 (12.4)	271 (12.6)	58 (11.4)	0.351
Previous MI, n (%)	661 (4.1)	214 (3.1)	261 (4.0)	140 (6.5)	46 (9.1)	<0.001
Previous PCI, n (%)	1008 (6.3)	327 (4.8)	394 (6.0)	215 (10.0)	72 (14.2)	<0.001
Previous CABG, n (%)	72 (0.4)	18 (0.3)	23 (0.4)	23 (1.1)	8 (1.6)	<0.001
Previous HF, n (%)	150 (0.9)	24 (0.4)	52 (0.8)	54 (2.5)	20 (3.9)	<0.001
Previous CVA, n (%)	947 (5.9)	252 (3.7)	390 (5.9)	241 (11.2)	64 (12.6)	<0.001
Current smokers, n (%)	6957 (43.3)	3560 (52.0)	2721 (41.5)	566 (26.4)	110 (21.7)	<0.001
Peak CK-MB (mg/dL)	121.2 ± 186.0	123.9 ± 178.0	128.1 ± 206.3	103.5 ± 151.0	70.8 ± 127.9	<0.001
Peak troponin-I (ng/mL)	47.0 ± 128.3	41.9 ± 69.5	48.6 ± 138.4	46.4 ± 94.5	97.1 ± 204.6	<0.001
NT-ProBNP (pg/mL)	1935.2 ± 4876.9	1258.8 ± 1542.6	1543.0 ± 2163.7	3188.7 ± 5091.2	9248.5 ± 8231.4	<0.001
High-sensitivity CRP (mg/dL)	7.5 ± 37.5	6.1 ± 31.8	8.3 ± 42.5	8.9 ± 38.6	10.1 ± 32.4	<0.001

Table 1. *Cont.*

Variables	Total (*n* = 16,055)	Group A1 eGFR ≥ 90 mL/min/1.73 m^2 (*n* = 6847)	Group A2 eGFR 60–89 mL/min/1.73 m^2 (*n* = 6557)	Group A3 eGFR 30–59 mL/min/1.73 m^2 (*n* = 2144)	Group A4 eGFR < 30 mL/min/1.73 m^2 (*n* = 507)	*p* Value
Serum creatinine (mg/L)	1.1 ± 1.1	0.7 ± 0.1	1.0 ± 0.2	1.4 ± 0.3	5.1 ± 4.6	<0.001
eGFR (mL/min/1.73 m^2)	87.5 ± 35.5	115.3 ± 33.7	76.3 ± 8.5	49.2 ± 8.0	16.5 ± 8.5	<0.001
Blood glucose (mg/L)	165.8 ± 76.7	155.2 ± 63.4	163.2 ± 70.4	197.3 ± 101.1	209.0 ± 129.7	<0.001
Total cholesterol (mg/dL)	184.3 ± 45.4	186.4 ± 43.1	186.0 ± 45.6	177.1 ± 47.9	162.4 ± 52.3	<0.001
Triglyceride (mg/L)	137.0 ± 114.0	140.0 ± 118.0	137.6 ± 114.9	128.3 ± 96.9	125.7 ± 111.3	<0.001
HDL cholesterol (mg/L)	43.3 ± 14.7	43.3 ± 13.3	43.8 ± 15.5	42.7 ± 16.5	39.3 ± 12.7	<0.001
LDL cholesterol (mg/L)	116.4 ± 40.7	119.4 ± 41.2	116.9 ± 37.5	109.5 ± 46.5	95.9 ± 38.8	<0.001
Discharge medications, *n* (%)						
Aspirin, *n* (%)	15,954 (99.4)	6814 (99.5)	6515 (99.4)	2127 (99.2)	498 (98.2)	0.003
Clopidogrel, *n* (%)	13,600 (84.7)	5528 (80.7)	5674 (86.5)	1941 (90.5)	457 (90.1)	<0.001
Ticagrelor, *n* (%)	1565 (9.7)	786 (11.5)	599 (9.1)	145 (6.8)	35 (6.9)	<0.001
Prasugrel, *n* (%)	890 (5.5)	533 (7.8)	284 (4.3)	58 (2.7)	15 (3.0)	<0.001
Cilostazole, *n* (%)	2903 (18.1)	1146 (16.7)	1226 (18.7)	434 (20.2)	97 (19.1)	0.001
ACEIs, *n* (%)	8977 (55.9)	3784 (55.3)	3893 (59.4)	1122 (52.3)	178 (35.1)	<0.001
ARBs, *n* (%)	4580 (28.5)	2023 (29.5)	1665 (25.4)	677 (31.6)	215 (42.4)	<0.001
BBs, *n* (%)	13,856 (86.3)	5984 (87.4)	5666 (86.4)	1775 (82.8)	431 (85.0)	<0.001
CCBs, *n* (%)	960 (6.0)	313 (4.6)	389 (5.9)	177 (8.3)	81 (16.0)	<0.001
Statin, *n* (%)						
Atorvastatin, *n* (%)	8636 (53.8)	3556 (51.9)	3552 (54.2)	1202 (56.1)	326 (64.3)	<0.001
Rosuvastatin, *n* (%)	5003 (31.2)	2254 (32.9)	2025 (30.9)	608 (28.4)	116 (22.9)	<0.001
Simvastatin, *n* (%)	949 (5.9)	378 (5.5)	412 (6.3)	133 (6.2)	26 (5.1)	0.222
Pitavastatin, *n* (%)	1211 (7.5)	559 (8.1)	478 (7.3)	154 (7.2)	20 (3.9)	0.003
Pravastatin, *n* (%)	214 (1.3)	86 (1.3)	76 (1.2)	40 (1.9)	12 (2.4)	0.014
Fluvastatin, *n* (%)	42 (0.3)	14 (0.2)	14 (0.2)	7 (0.3)	7 (1.4)	<0.001
Infarct-related artery						
Left main, *n* (%)	294 (1.8)	111 (1.6)	106 (1.6)	51 (2.4)	26 (5.1)	<0.001
LAD, *n* (%)	7704 (48.0)	3440 (50.2)	3126 (47.7)	917 (42.8)	221 (43.6)	<0.001
LCx, *n* (%)	2713 (16.9)	1232 (18.0)	1085 (16.5)	324 (15.1)	72 (14.2)	0.003
RCA, *n* (%)	5344 (33.3)	2064 (30.1)	2240 (34.2)	852 (39.7)	188 (37.1)	<0.001
Treated vessel						
Left main, *n* (%)	468 (2.9)	175 (2.6)	179 (2.7)	82 (3.8)	32 (6.3)	<0.001
LAD, *n* (%)	9348 (58.2)	4105 (60.0)	3770 (57.5)	1175 (54.8)	298 (58.8)	<0.001
LCx, *n* (%)	4239 (26.4)	1875 (27.4)	1675 (25.5)	568 (26.5)	121 (23.9)	0.056
RCA, *n* (%)	6401 (39.9)	2509 (36.6)	2672 (40.8)	997 (46.5)	223 (44.0)	<0.001
ACC/AHA lesion type						
Type B1, *n* (%)	2180 (13.6)	827 (12.1)	978 (14.9)	303 (14.1)	72 (14.2)	<0.001

Table 1. *Cont.*

Variables	Total (n = 16,055)	Group A1 eGFR ≥ 90 mL/min/1.73 m^2 (n = 6847)	Group A2 eGFR 60–89 mL/min/1.73 m^2 (n = 6557)	Group A3 eGFR 30–59 mL/min/1.73 m^2 (n = 2144)	Group A4 eGFR < 30 mL/min/1.73 m^2 (n = 507)	p Value
Type B2, n (%)	5677 (35.4)	2643 (38.6)	2140 (32.6)	720 (33.6)	174 (34.3)	<0.001
Type C, n (%)	7249 (45.2)	3026 (44.2)	3002 (45.8)	983 (45.8)	238 (46.9)	0.198
Extent of CAD						
Single-vessel, n (%)	8150 (50.8)	3827 (55.9)	3250 (49.6)	875 (40.8)	198 (39.1)	<0.001
2-vessel, n (%)	4712 (29.3)	1925 (28.1)	1968 (30.0)	671 (31.3)	148 (29.2)	0.016
≥3-vessel, n (%)	3193 (19.9)	1095 (16.0)	1339 (20.4)	598 (27.9)	161 (31.8)	<0.001
Pre-PCI TIMI 0/1, n (%)	9308 (58.0)	3857 (56.3)	3966 (60.5)	1258 (58.7)	227 (44.8)	<0.001
Type of stent						
ZES, n (%)	5591 (34.8)	2219 (32.4)	2404 (36.7)	801 (37.4)	167 (32.9)	<0.001
EES, n (%)	7888 (49.1)	3335 (48.7)	3187 (48.6)	1092 (50.9)	274 (54.0)	0.031
BES, n (%)	2418 (15.1)	1161 (17.0)	944 (14.4)	249 (11.6)	64 (12.6)	<0.001
Others, n (%)	475 (3.0)	264 (3.9)	160 (2.4)	43 (2.0)	8 (1.6)	<0.001
IVUS, n (%)	3619 (19.7)	1358 (19.8)	1321 (20.1)	401 (18.7)	89 (17.6)	0.295
OCT, n (%)	113 (0.7)	61 (0.9)	47 (0.7)	4 (0.2)	1 (0.2)	0.004
FFR, n (%)	211 (1.3)	135 (2.0)	69 (1.0)	5 (0.2)	2 (0.4)	<0.001
Stent diameter (mm)	3.15 ± 0.42	3.16 ± 0.42	3.16 ± 0.43	3.11 ± 0.42	3.09 ± 0.43	<0.001
Stent length (mm)	27.1 ± 11.7	26.9 ± 11.6	26.9 ± 11.5	27.8 ± 12.3	29.0 ± 13.7	<0.001
Number of stents	1.48 ± 0.79	1.45 ± 0.77	1.48 ± 0.79	1.54 ± 0.82	1.60 ± 0.87	<0.001

Values are means ± SDs or numbers and percentages. The p values for continuous data were obtained from the analysis of variance. The p values for categorical data were obtained from the chi-square or Fisher's exact test. eGFR, estimated glomerular filtration rate; LVEF, left ventricular ejection fraction; BMI, body mass index; SBP, systolic blood pressure; DBP, diastolic blood pressure; CPR, cardiopulmonary resuscitation; STEMI, ST-segment elevation myocardial infarction; PCI, percutaneous coronary intervention; NSTEMI, non-STEMI; MI, myocardial infarction; CABG, coronary artery bypass graft; HF, heart failure; CVA, cerebrovascular accidents; CK-MB, creatine kinase myocardial band; NT-ProBNP, N-terminal pro-brain natriuretic peptide; CRP, C-reactive protein; HDL, high-density lipoprotein; LDL, low-density lipoprotein; ACEIs, angiotensin-converting enzyme inhibitors; ARBs, angiotensin receptor blockers; BBs, beta blockers; CCBs, calcium channel blockers; LAD, left anterior descending coronary artery; LCx, left circumflex coronary artery; RCA, right coronary artery; ACC/AHA, American College of Cardiology/American Heart Association; CAD, coronary artery disease; TIMI, thrombolysis in myocardial infarction; ZES, zotarolimus-eluting stent; EES, everolimus-eluting stent; BES, biolimus-eluting stent; IVUS, intravascular ultrasound; OCT, optical coherence tomography; FFR, fractional flow reserve.

2.2. Percutaneous Coronary Intervention (PCI) Procedure and Medical Treatment

Coronary angiography and PCI were performed via a transfemoral or transradial approach in accordance with the general guidelines [22]. Aspirin (200–300 mg) and clopidogrel (300–600 mg) when available, or alternatively, ticagrelor (180 mg) or prasugrel (60 mg), were prescribed as the loading doses to the individuals before PCI. After PCI, dual antiplatelet therapy (DAPT; a combination of aspirin (100 mg/day) with clopidogrel (75 mg/day) or ticagrelor (90 mg twice a day) or prasugrel (5–10 mg/day)) was recommended for more than 12 months. Based on previous reports [23,24], triple antiplatelet therapy was administered (TAPT; 100 mg of cilostazol administered twice a day in addition to DAPT) at the discretion of the individual operator. In this study, the patients who received atorvastatin, rosuvastatin, simvastatin, pitavastatin, pravastatin and fluvastatin were included (Table 1) and the type and dose of statins to be used were left to the physicians' discretion.

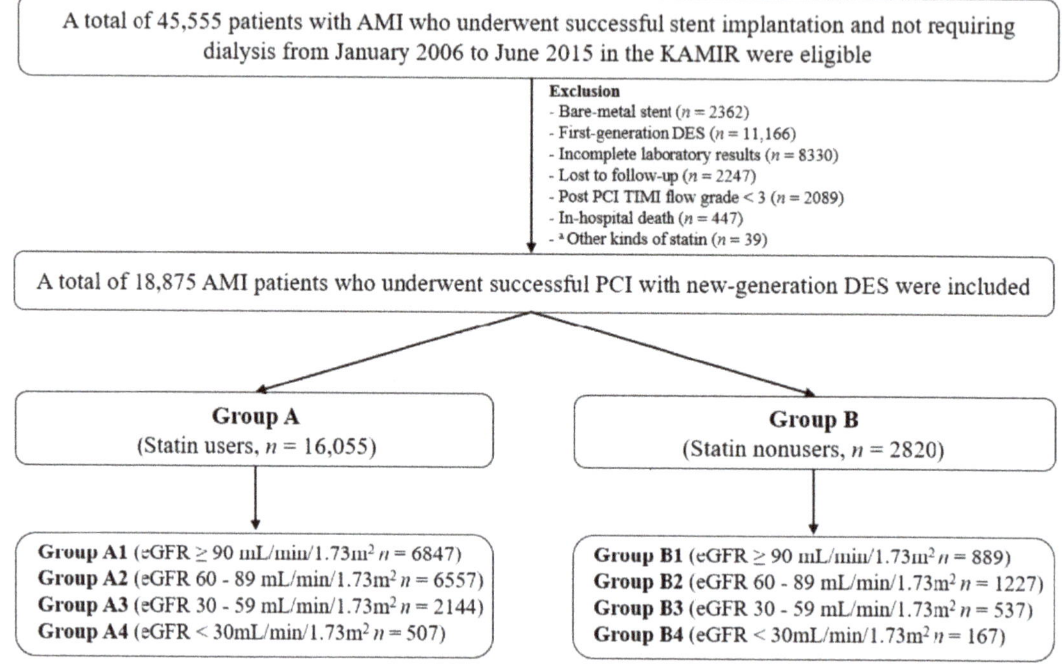

Figure 1. Flowchart. AMI, acute myocardial infarction; KAMIR, Korea AMI Registry; PCI, percutaneous coronary intervention; DES, drug-eluting stent; eGFR, estimated glomerular filtration rate. [a] Statins except for atorvastatin, rosuvastatin, simvastatin, pitavastatin, pravastatin and fluvastatin.

2.3. Study Definitions and Clinical Outcomes

AMI was defined according to the current guidelines [7,8]. A successful PCI was defined as a residual stenosis of <30% and TIMI flow grade 3 in the infarct-related artery (IRA). Glomerular function was calculated using the Chronic Kidney Disease Epidemiology Collaboration (CKD-EPI) equation for eGFR [25]. The major clinical endpoint was the occurrence of MACE, defined as all-cause mortality, recurrent myocardial infarction (re-MI) or any repeat coronary revascularization, including target lesion revascularization (TLR), target vessel revascularization (TVR) and non-TVR during the follow-up period. All-cause mortality was considered cardiac death (CD) unless an undisputed noncardiac cause was present [26].

2.4. Statistical Analysis

Differences in the continuous variables among the four groups were evaluated using analysis of variance or the Jonckheere–Terpstra test, and a post hoc analysis was performed using the Hochberg test or Dunnett's T3 test; data are presented as means ± standard deviations. For discrete variables, differences between two of the four or eight groups were analyzed using the chi-square or Fisher's exact test, as deemed appropriate, and data are presented as counts and percentages. We tested all variables in the univariate analysis ($p < 0.05$) (Table S1). After univariate analysis, we tested all variables with $p < 0.001$ in the multivariate Cox regression analysis, which are listed as follows: male sex, age, left ventricular ejection fraction (LVEF), body mass index (BMI), systolic blood pressure (SBP), diastolic blood pressure (DBP), cardiogenic shock, cardiopulmonary resuscitation (CPR) on admission, Killip class III/IV, STEMI, hypertension, diabetes mellitus (DM), previous MI, previous PCI, previous HF, previous cerebrovascular accident (CVA), current smoker, N-terminal pro-brain natriuretic peptide (NT-ProBNP), blood glucose level, total cholesterol level, triglyceride level, low-density lipoprotein (LDL) cholesterol level, high-density lipoprotein (HDL) cholesterol level, use of aspirin, use of angiotensin-converting enzyme inhibitor (ACEI), use of beta blockers (BBs), left main coronary artery (LM) infarct-related artery (IRA) and treated vessel, single-vessel disease, ≥3-vessel disease, stent diameter, stent length and number of stents. Various clinical outcomes were estimated using Kaplan–Meier curve analysis, and group differences were compared using the log-rank test. A two-tailed p value < 0.05 was considered statistically significant. All statistical analyses were performed using SPSS software v20 (IBM; Armonk, NY, USA).

3. Results

3.1. Baseline Characteristics

Tables 1–4 show the baseline, laboratory, angiographic and procedural characteristics of the study population.

Table 2. Baseline characteristics in statin nonusers.

Variables	Total (n = 2820)	Group B1 eGFR ≥ 90 mL/min/1.73 m^2 (n = 889)	Group B2 eGFR 60–89 mL/min/1.73 m^2 (n = 1227)	Group B3 eGFR 30–59 mL/min/1.73 m^2 (n = 537)	Group B4 eGFR < 30 mL/min/1.73 m^2 (n = 167)	p Value
Male, n (%)	2067 (73.3)	730 (82.1)	921 (75.1)	317 (59.0)	99 (59.3)	<0.001
Age (years)	64.1 ± 12.4	58.8 ± 11.6	64.3 ± 12.2	70.8 ± 10.5	69.8 ± 10.4	<0.001
LVEF (%)	50.9 ± 12.2	52.9 ± 11.5	51.5 ± 11.7	48.4 ± 13.1	44.2 ± 12.8	<0.001
BMI (kg/m^2)	23.8 ± 3.3	23.9 ± 3.4	23.8 ± 3.2	23.7 ± 3.5	23.1 ±3.4	0.055
SBP (mmHg)	128.6 ± 29.1	132.2 ± 26.7	129.7 ± 27.6	120.0 ± 32.1	128.0 ± 25.8	<0.001
DBP (mmHg)	77.9 ± 16.8	80.7 ± 15.3	78.9 ± 16.4	72.0 ± 17.5	73.7 ± 19.6	<0.001
Cardiogenic shock, n (%)	153 (5.4)	22 (2.5)	48 (3.9)	58 (10.8)	25 (15.0)	<0.001
CPR on admission, n (%)	151 (5.4)	30 (3.4)	59 (4.8)	51 (9.5)	11 (6.6)	<0.001
Killip class III/IV, n (%)	393 (13.9)	53 (6.0)	140 (11.4)	146 (27.2)	54 (32.3)	<0.001
STEMI, n (%)	1630 (57.8)	512 (57.6)	744 (60.6)	309 (57.5)	65 (38.9)	<0.001
Primary PCI, n (%)	1551 (95.2)	485 (94.7)	705 (94.8)	297 (96.1)	64 (98.5)	0.454
NSTEMI, n (%)	1190 (42.2)	377 (42.4)	483(39.4)	228 (42.5)	102 (61.1)	<0.001
PCI within 24 h	912 (76.6)	299 (79.3)	366 (75.8)	170 (74.6)	77 (75.5)	0.507
Hypertension, n (%)	1391 (49.3)	318 (35.8)	598 (48.7)	340 (63.3)	135 (80.8)	<0.001
Diabetes mellitus, n (%)	867 (30.7)	233 (26.2)	309 (25.2)	216 (40.2)	109 (65.3)	<0.001
Dyslipidemia, n (%)	249 (8.8)	75 (8.4)	108 (8.8)	48 (8.9)	18 (10.8)	0.809
Previous MI, n (%)	96 (3.4)	21 (2.4)	33 (2.7)	27 (5.0)	15 (9.0)	<0.001
Previous PCI, n (%)	186 (6.6)	44 (4.9)	73 (8.9)	52 (9.7)	17 (10.2)	0.001
Previous CABG, n (%)	12 (0.4)	2 (0.2)	3 (0.2)	6 (1.0)	1 (0.6)	0.047
Previous HF, n (%)	58 (2.1)	9 (1.0)	19 (1.5)	19 (3.5)	11 (6.6)	<0.001
Previous CVA, n (%)	193 (6.8)	36 (4.0)	75 (6.1)	57 (10.6)	25 (15.0)	<0.001
Current smokers, n (%)	1157 (41.0)	471 (53.0)	498 (40.6)	158 (29.4)	30 (18.0)	<0.001
Peak CK-MB (mg/dL)	144.5 ± 319.5	127.7 ± 154.2	168.6 ± 442.3	133.8 ± 201.7	91.7 ± 144.5	0.002
Peak troponin-I (ng/mL)	46.8 ± 85.9	42.4 ± 61.2	48.2 ± 87.5	48.2 ± 92.3	55.3 ± 145.3	0.215
NT-ProBNP (pg/mL)	2487.6 ± 4085.6	1499.8 ± 2460.2	1599.3 ± 2089.5	3802.2 ± 5998.2	9948.8 ± 9432.6	<0.001
High-sensitivity CRP (mg/dL)	9.8 ± 38.1	9.1 ± 34.5	8.3 ± 33.9	12.7 ± 47.9	15.2 ± 48.2	<0.001
Serum creatinine (mg/L)	1.2 ± 1.4	0.7 ± 0.1	1.0 ± 1.2	1.4 ± 0.3	5.1 ± 3.7	<0.001
eGFR (mL/min/1.73 m^2)	76.8 ± 38.3	114.7 ± 44.3	75.6 ± 8.5	48.6 ± 8.2	15.8 ± 8.2	<0.001
Blood glucose (mg/L)	177.7 ± 85.5	163.4 ± 65.7	169.6 ± 75.1	207.9 ± 108.3	217.0 ± 124.4	<0.001
Total cholesterol (mg/dL)	174.4 ± 43.5	180.4 ± 44.1	178.1 ± 41.5	163.9 ± 41.6	148.2 ± 45.6	<0.001
Triglyceride (mg/L)	132.4 ± 114.0	142.0 ± 122.3	135.5 ± 125.1	113.2 ± 73.0	117.5 ± 68.7	<0.001
HDL cholesterol (mg/L)	43.0 ± 15.6	43.1 ± 11.7	43.8 ± 17.1	42.5 ± 17.6	37.9 ± 14.8	<0.001
LDL cholesterol (mg/L)	108.2 ± 39.2	112.5 ± 37.6	111.3 ± 38.1	100.7 ± 41.8	83.9 ± 36.4	<0.001
Discharge medications, n (%)						
Aspirin, n (%)	2714 (96.2)	848 (95.5)	1192 (97.1)	518 (96.5)	156 (93.4)	0.040
Clopidogrel, n (%)	2726 (96.6)	843 (94.8)	1200 (97.8)	523 (91.1)	160 (95.8)	<0.001
Ticagrelor, n (%)	53 (1.9)	22 (2.5)	16 (1.3)	10 (1.9)	5 (3.0)	0.169
Prasugrel, n (%)	41 (1.5)	24 (2.7)	11 (0.9)	4 (0.7)	2 (1.2)	0.003
Cilostazole, n (%)	483 (17.1)	139 (15.6)	241 (19.6)	82 (15.3)	21 (12.6)	0.014
ACEIs, n (%)	1127 (40.0)	356 (40.0)	539 (43.9)	189 (35.2)	43 (25.7)	<0.001
ARBs, n (%)	677 (24.0)	238 (26.8)	280 (22.8)	124 (23.1)	35 (21.0)	0.123
BBs, n (%)	1838 (65.2)	605 (68.1)	839 (68.4)	315 (58.7)	79 (47.3)	<0.001
CCBs, n (%)	176 (6.2)	44 (4.9)	70 (5.7)	41 (7.6)	21 (12.6)	0.001
Infarct-related artery						
Left main, n (%)	58 (2.1)	20 (2.2)	14 (1.1)	16 (3.0)	8 (4.8)	0.003
LAD, n (%)	1324 (47.0)	434 (48.8)	593 (48.3)	228 (42.4)	69 (41.3)	0.037
LCx, n (%)	451 (16.0)	163 (18.3)	190 (15.5)	69 (12.8)	29 (17.4)	0.045
RCA, n (%)	987 (35.0)	272 (30.6)	430 (35.0)	224 (41.7)	61 (36.5)	<0.001
Treated vessel						
Left main, n (%)	77 (2.7)	26 (2.9)	21 (1.7)	17 (3.2)	13 (7.8)	<0.001
LAD, n (%)	1552 (55.0)	508 (57.1)	676 (55.1)	278 (51.8)	90 (53.9)	0.261
LCx, n (%)	670 (23.8)	228 (25.6)	274 (22.3)	127 (23.6)	41 (24.6)	0.363
RCA, n (%)	1132 (40.1)	318 (35.8)	492 (40.1)	253 (47.1)	99 (41.3)	<0.001

Table 2. *Cont.*

Variables	Total (n = 2820)	Group B1 eGFR ≥ 90 mL/min/1.73 m^2 (n = 889)	Group B2 eGFR 60–89 mL/min/1.73 m^2 (n = 1227)	Group B3 eGFR 30–59 mL/min/1.73 m^2 (n = 537)	Group B4 eGFR < 30 mL/min/1.73 m^2 (n = 167)	p Value
ACC/AHA lesion type						
Type B1, n (%)	509 (18.0)	161 (18.1)	223 (18.2)	109 (20.3)	16 (9.6)	0.019
Type B2, n (%)	857 (30.4)	296 (33.3)	371 (30.2)	133 (24.8)	57 (34.1)	0.005
Type C, n (%)	1141 (40.5)	340 (38.2)	494 (40.3)	224 (41.7)	83 (49.7)	0.044
Extent of CAD						
Single-vessel, n (%)	1369 (48.5)	481 (54.1)	614 (50.0)	211 (39.3)	63 (37.7)	<0.001
2-vessel, n (%)	818 (29.0)	242 (27.2)	352 (28.7)	172 (32.0)	52 (31.1)	0.242
≥3-vessel, n (%)	633 (22.4)	166 (18.7)	261 (21.3)	154 (28.7)	52 (31.1)	<0.001
Pre-PCI TIMI 0/1, n (%)	1745 (61.9)	544 (61.2)	788 (64.2)	330 (61.5)	83 (49.7)	0.004
Type of stent						
ZES, n (%)	1171 (41.5)	347 (39.0)	526 (42.9)	233 (43.4)	65 (38.9)	0.219
EES, n (%)	1269 (45.0)	389 (43.8)	556 (45.3)	245 (45.9)	79 (47.3)	0.790
BES, n (%)	315 (11.2)	123 (13.8)	122 (9.9)	52 (9.7)	18 (10.8)	0.024
Others, n (%)	84 (3.0)	34 (3.8)	31 (2.5)	12 (2.2)	7 (4.2)	0.176
IVUS, n (%)	502 (17.8)	169 (19.0)	218 (17.8)	85 (15.8)	30 (18.0)	0.509
OCT, n (%)	17 (0.6)	7 (0.8)	7 (0.6)	3 (0.6)	0	0.669
FFR, n (%)	7 (0.2)	3 (0.3)	0	3 (0.6)	1 (0.6)	0.100
Stent diameter (mm)	3.16 ± 0.44	3.18 ± 0.43	3.17 ± 0.43	3.11 ± 0.44	3.11 ± 0.44	0.019
Stent length (mm)	25.0 ± 9.4	24.1 ± 8.1	24.7 ± 8.5	26.0 ± 11.1	28.1 ± 14.4	<0.001
Number of stents	1.43 ± 0.76	1.40 ± 0.72	1.40 ± 0.75	1.53 ± 0.82	1.51 ± 0.76	0.004

Values are means ± SDs or numbers and percentages. The p values for continuous data were obtained from the analysis of variance. The p values for categorical data were obtained from the chi-square or Fisher's exact test. eGFR, estimated glomerular filtration rate; LVEF, left ventricular ejection fraction; BMI, body mass index; SBP, systolic blood pressure; DBP, diastolic blood pressure; CPR, cardiopulmonary resuscitation; STEMI, ST-segment elevation myocardial infarction; PCI, percutaneous coronary intervention; NSTEMI, non-STEMI; MI, myocardial infarction; CABG, coronary artery bypass graft; HF, heart failure; CVA, cerebrovascular accidents; CK-MB, creatine kinase myocardial band; NT-ProBNP, N-terminal pro-brain natriuretic peptide; CRP, C-reactive protein; HDL, high-density lipoprotein; LDL, low-density lipoprotein; ACEIs, angiotensin-converting enzyme inhibitors; ARBs, angiotensin receptor blockers; BBs, beta blockers; CCBs, calcium channel blockers; LAD, left anterior descending coronary artery; LCx, left circumflex coronary artery; RCA, right coronary artery; ACC/AHA, American College of Cardiology/American Heart Association; CAD, coronary artery disease; TIMI, thrombolysis in myocardial infarction; ZES, zotarolimus-eluting stent; EES, everolimus-eluting stent; BES, biolimus-eluting stent; IVUS, intravascular ultrasound; OCT, optical coherence tomography; FFR, fractional flow reserve.

Table 3. Baseline characteristics between statin users and nonusers 1.

Variables	Group A1 eGFR ≥ 90 mL/min/1.73 m^2 (n = 6847)	Group B1 eGFR ≥ 90 mL/min/1.73 m^2 (n = 889)	p Value	Group A2 eGFR 60–89 mL/min/1.73 m^2 (n = 6557)	Group B2 eGFR 60–89 mL/min/1.73 m^2 (n = 1227)	p Value
Male, n (%)	5536 (80.9)	730 (82.1)	0.367	4988 (76.1)	921 (75.1)	0.448
Age (years)	58.9 ± 11.5	58.8 ± 11.6	0.848	64.3 ± 12.1	64.3 ± 12.2	0.915
LVEF (%)	54.0 ± 10.0	52.9 ± 11.5	0.007	52.8 ± 10.7	51.5 ± 11.7	0.001
BMI (kg/m^2)	24.2 ± 3.2	23.9 ± 3.4	0.009	24.2 ± 3.2	23.8 ± 3.2	<0.001
SBP (mmHg)	133.4 ± 25.0	132.2 ± 26.7	0.221	131.4 ± 27.7	129.7 ± 27.6	0.051
DBP (mmHg)	81.7 ± 15.3	80.7 ± 15.3	0.074	79.6 ± 16.4	78.9 ± 16.4	0.220
Cardiogenic shock, n (%)	124 (1.8)	22 (2.5)	0.171	247 (3.8)	48 (3.9)	0.807
CPR on admission, n (%)	186 (2.7)	30 (3.4)	0.263	218 (3.3)	59 (4.8)	0.010
Killip class III/IV, n (%)	322 (4.7)	53 (6.0)	0.100	578 (8.8)	140 (11.4)	0.004
STEMI, n (%)	3640 (53.2)	512 (57.6)	0.013	3764 (57.4)	744 (60.6)	0.035
Primary PCI, n (%)	3511 (96.5)	485 (94.7)	0.054	3633 (96.5)	705 (94.8)	0.021
NSTEMI, n (%)	3207 (46.8)	377 (42.4)	0.013	2793 (42.6)	483(39.4)	0.035
PCI within 24 h	2865 (89.3)	299 (79.3)	<0.001	2384 (85.4)	366 (75.8)	<0.001
Hypertension, n (%)	2622 (38.3)	318 (35.8)	0.145	3238 (49.4)	598 (48.7)	0.678
Diabetes mellitus, n (%)	1446 (21.1)	233 (26.2)	0.001	1534 (23.4)	309 (25.2)	0.176
Dyslipidemia, n (%)	792 (11.6)	75 (8.4)	0.005	815 (12.4)	108 (8.8)	<0.001
Previous MI, n (%)	214 (3.1)	21 (2.4)	0.212	261 (4.0)	33 (2.7)	0.029
Previous PCI, n (%)	327 (4.8)	44 (4.9)	0.820	394 (6.0)	73 (8.9)	0.936
Previous CABG, n (%)	18 (0.3)	2 (0.2)	0.834	23 (0.4)	3 (0.2)	0.788
Previous HF, n (%)	24 (0.4)	9 (1.0)	0.004	52 (0.8)	19 (1.5)	0.011
Previous CVA, n (%)	252 (3.7)	36 (4.0)	0.585	390 (5.9)	75 (6.1)	0.823
Current smokers, n (%)	3560 (52.0)	471 (53.0)	0.579	2721 (41.5)	498 (40.6)	0.552
Peak CK-MB (mg/dL)	123.9 ± 178.0	127.7 ± 154.2	0.538	128.1 ± 206.3	168.6 ± 442.3	0.002
Peak troponin-I (ng/mL)	41.9 ± 69.5	42.4 ± 61.2	0.823	48.6 ± 138.4	48.2 ± 87.5	0.905
NT-ProBNP (pg/mL)	1258.8 ± 1542.6	1499.8 ± 2460.2	0.004	1543.0 ± 2163.7	1599.3 ± 2089.5	0.389
High-sensitivity CRP (mg/dL)	6.1 ± 31.8	9.1 ± 34.5	0.012	8.3 ± 42.5	8.3 ± 33.9	0.972
Serum creatinine (mg/L)	0.7 ± 0.1	0.7 ± 0.1	0.062	1.0 ± 0.2	1.0 ± 1.2	0.245
eGFR (mL/min/1.73 m^2)	115.3 ± 33.7	114.7 ± 44.3	0.725	76.3 ± 8.5	75.6 ± 8.5	0.060
Blood glucose (mg/L)	155.2 ± 63.4	163.4 ± 65.7	0.001	163.2 ± 70.4	169.6 ± 75.1	0.007
Total cholesterol (mg/dL)	186.4 ± 43.1	180.4 ± 44.1	<0.001	186.0 ± 45.6	178.1 ± 41.5	<0.001
Triglyceride (mg/L)	140.0 ± 118.0	142.0 ± 122.3	0.639	137.6 ± 114.9	135.5 ± 125.1	0.592
HDL cholesterol (mg/L)	43.3 ± 13.3	43.1 ± 11.7	0.676	43.8 ± 15.5	43.8 ± 17.1	0.943
LDL cholesterol (mg/L)	119.4 ± 41.2	112.5 ± 37.6	<0.001	116.9 ± 37.5	111.3 ± 38.1	<0.001

Table 3. *Cont.*

Variables	Group A1 eGFR ≥ 90 mL/min/1.73 m^2 (n = 6847)	Group B1 eGFR ≥ 90 mL/min/1.73 m^2 (n = 889)	p Value	Group A2 eGFR 60–89 mL/min/1.73 m^2 (n = 6557)	Group B2 eGFR 60–89 mL/min/1.73 m^2 (n = 1227)	p Value
Discharge medications, n (%)						
Aspirin, n (%)	6814 (99.5)	848 (95.5)	<0.001	6515 (99.4)	1192 (97.1)	<0.001
Clopidogrel, n (%)	5528 (80.7)	843 (94.8)	<0.001	5674 (86.5)	1200 (97.8)	<0.001
Ticagrelor, n (%)	786 (11.5)	22 (2.5)	<0.001	599 (9.1)	16 (1.3)	<0.001
Prasugrel, n (%)	533 (7.8)	24 (2.7)	<0.001	284 (4.3)	11 (0.9)	<0.001
Cilostazole, n (%)	1146 (16.7)	139 (15.6)	0.406	1226 (18.7)	241 (19.6)	0.438
ACEIs, n (%)	3784 (55.3)	356 (40.0)	<0.001	3893 (59.4)	539 (43.9)	<0.001
ARBs, n (%)	2023 (29.5)	238 (26.8)	0.087	1665 (25.4)	280 (22.8)	0.057
BBs, n (%)	5984 (87.4)	605 (68.1)	<0.001	5666 (86.4)	839 (68.4)	<0.001
CCBs, n (%)	313 (4.6)	44 (4.9)	0.613	389 (5.9)	70 (5.7)	0.792
Statin, n (%)						
Atorvastatin, n (%)	3556 (51.9)			3552 (54.2)		
Rosuvastatin, n (%)	2254 (32.9)			2025 (30.9)		
Simvastatin, n (%)	378 (5.5)			412 (6.3)		
Pitavastatin, n (%)	559 (8.1)			478 (7.3)		
Pravastatin, n (%)	86 (1.3)			76 (1.2)		
Fluvastatin, n (%)	14 (0.2)			14 (0.2)		
Infarct-related artery						
Left main, n (%)	111 (1.6)	20 (2.2)	0.172	106 (1.6)	14 (1.1)	0.256
LAD, n (%)	3440 (50.2)	434 (48.8)	0.347	3126 (47.7)	593 (48.3)	0.747
LCx, n (%)	1232 (18.0)	163 (18.3)	0.803	1085 (16.5)	190 (15.5)	0.356
RCA, n (%)	2064 (30.1)	272 (30.6)	0.783	2240 (34.2)	430 (35.0)	0.550
Treated vessel						
Left main, n (%)	175 (2.6)	26 (2.9)	0.516	179 (2.7)	21 (1.7)	0.039
LAD, n (%)	4105 (60.0)	508 (57.1)	0.108	3770 (57.5)	676 (55.1)	0.119
LCx, n (%)	1875 (27.4)	228 (25.6)	0.273	1675 (25.5)	274 (22.3)	0.018
RCA, n (%)	2509 (36.6)	318 (35.8)	0.611	2672 (40.8)	492 (40.1)	0.669
ACC/AHA lesion type						
Type B1, n (%)	827 (12.1)	161 (18.1)	<0.001	978 (14.9)	223 (18.2)	0.004
Type B2, n (%)	2643 (38.6)	296 (33.3)	0.002	2140 (32.6)	371 (30.2)	0.103
Type C, n (%)	3026 (44.2)	340 (38.2)	0.001	3002 (45.8)	494 (40.3)	<0.001
Extent of CAD						
Single-vessel, n (%)	3827 (55.9)	481 (54.1)	0.313	3250 (49.6)	614 (50.0)	0.760
2-vessel, n (%)	1925 (28.1)	242 (27.2)	0.606	1968 (30.0)	352 (28.7)	0.351
≥3-vessel, n (%)	1095 (16.0)	166 (18.7)	0.042	1339 (20.4)	261 (21.3)	0.499
Pre-PCI TIMI 0/1, n (%)	3857 (56.3)	544 (61.2)	0.006	3966 (60.5)	788 (64.2)	0.014
Type of stent						
ZES, n (%)	2219 (32.4)	347 (39.0)	<0.001	2404 (36.7)	526 (42.9)	<0.001
EES, n (%)	3335 (48.7)	389 (43.8)	0.005	3187 (48.6)	556 (45.3)	0.034
BES, n (%)	1161 (17.0)	123 (13.8)	0.019	944 (14.4)	122 (9.9)	<0.001
Others, n (%)	264 (3.9)	34 (3.8)	0.964	160 (2.4)	31 (2.5)	0.841
IVUS, n (%)	1358 (19.8)	169 (19.0)	0.591	1321 (20.1)	218 (17.8)	0.056
OCT, n (%)	61 (0.9)	7 (0.8)	0.756	47 (0.7)	7 (0.6)	0.709
FFR, n (%)	135 (2.0)	3 (0.3)	0.001	69 (1.0)	0	<0.001
Stent diameter (mm)	3.16 ± 0.42	3.18 ± 0.43	0.344	3.16 ± 0.43	3.17 ± 0.43	0.274
Stent length (mm)	26.9 ± 11.6	24.1 ± 8.1	<0.001	26.9 ± 11.5	24.7 ± 8.5	<0.001
Number of stents	1.45 ± 0.77	1.40 ± 0.72	0.039	1.48 ± 0.79	1.40 ± 0.75	0.002

Values are means ± SDs or numbers and percentages. The p values for continuous data were obtained from the unpaired t-test. The p values for categorical data were obtained from the chi-square or Fisher's exact test. eGFR, estimated glomerular filtration rate; LVEF, left ventricular ejection fraction; BMI, body mass index; SBP, systolic blood pressure; DBP, diastolic blood pressure; CPR, cardiopulmonary resuscitation; STEMI, ST-segment elevation myocardial infarction; PCI, percutaneous coronary intervention; NSTEMI, non-STEMI; MI, myocardial infarction; CABG, coronary artery bypass graft; HF, heart failure; CVA, cerebrovascular accidents; CK-MB, creatine kinase myocardial band; NT-ProBNP, N-terminal pro-brain natriuretic peptide; CRP, C-reactive protein; HDL, high-density lipoprotein; LDL, low-density lipoprotein; ACEIs, angiotensin-converting enzyme inhibitors; ARBs, angiotensin receptor blockers; BBs, beta blockers; CCBs, calcium channel blockers; LAD, left anterior descending coronary artery; LCx, left circumflex coronary artery; RCA, right coronary artery; ACC/AHA, American College of Cardiology/American Heart Association; CAD, coronary artery disease; TIMI, thrombolysis in myocardial infarction; ZES, zotarolimus-eluting stent; EES, everolimus-eluting stent; BES, biolimus-eluting stent; IVUS, intravascular ultrasound; OCT, optical coherence tomography; FFR, fractional flow reserve.

Table 4. Baseline characteristics between statin users and nonusers 2.

Variables	Group A3 eGFR 30–59 mL/min/1.73 m^2 (n = 2144)	Group B3 eGFR 30–59 mL/min/1.73 m^2 (n = 537)	p Value	Group A4 eGFR < 30 mL/min/1.73 m^2 (n = 507)	Group B4 eGFR < 30 mL/min/1.73 m^2 (n = 167)	p Value
Male, n (%)	1225 (57.1)	317 (59.0)	0.427	304 (60.0)	99 (59.3)	0.877
Age (years)	70.8 ± 10.4	70.8 ± 10.5	0.884	68.9 ± 10.9	69.8 ± 10.4	0.376
LVEF (%)	50.0 ± 12.3	48.4 ± 13.1	0.020	48.1 ± 11.9	44.2 ± 12.8	0.001
BMI (kg/m^2)	23.9 ± 3.2	23.7 ± 3.5	0.414	23.5 ±3.4	23.1 ±3.4	0.276
SBP (mmHg)	126.6 ± 30.2	120.0 ± 32.1	<0.001	132.2 ± 33.3	128.0 ± 25.8	0.183
DBP (mmHg)	75.7 ± 17.1	72.0 ± 17.5	<0.001	77.4 ± 18.0	73.7 ± 19.6	0.035
Cardiogenic shock, n (%)	160 (7.5)	58 (10.8)	0.011	44 (8.7)	25 (15.0)	0.020
CPR on admission, n (%)	129 (6.0)	51 (9.5)	0.004	24 (4.7)	11 (6.6)	0.349
Killip class III/IV, n (%)	416 (19.4)	146 (27.2)	<0.001	138 (27.2)	54 (32.3)	0.204
STEMI, n (%)	1160 (54.1)	309 (57.5)	0.152	173 (34.1)	65 (38.9)	0.260
Primary PCI, n (%)	1115 (96.1)	297 (96.1)	0.997	165 (95.4)	64 (98.5)	0.266
NSTEMI, n (%)	984 (45.9)	228 (42.5)	0.152	334 (65.9)	102 (61.1)	0.260
PCI within 24 h	791 (80.4)	170 (74.6)	0.051	263 (78.7)	77 (75.5)	0.488
Hypertension, n (%)	1489 (69.4)	340 (63.3)	0.006	412 (81.3)	135 (80.8)	0.903
Diabetes mellitus, n (%)	903 (42.1)	216 (40.2)	0.434	318 (62.7)	109 (65.3)	0.553
Dyslipidemia, n (%)	271 (12.6)	48 (8.9)	0.017	58 (11.4)	18 (10.8)	0.815
Previous MI, n (%)	140 (6.5)	27 (5.0)	0.231	46 (9.1)	15 (9.0)	0.972
Previous PCI, n (%)	215 (10.0)	52 (9.7)	0.872	72 (14.2)	17 (10.2)	0.235
Previous CABG, n (%)	23 (1.1)	6 (1.0)	0.929	8 (1.6)	1 (0.6)	0.464
Previous HF, n (%)	54 (2.5)	19 (3.5)	0.194	20 (3.9)	11 (6.6)	0.157
Previous CVA, n (%)	241 (11.2)	57 (10.6)	0.759	64 (12.6)	25 (15.0)	0.437
Current smokers, n (%)	566 (26.4)	158 (29.4)	0.159	110 (21.7)	30 (18.0)	0.302
Peak CK-MB (mg/dL)	103.5 ± 151.0	133.8 ± 201.7	<0.001	70.8 ± 127.9	91.7 ± 144.5	0.076
Peak troponin-I (ng/mL)	46.4 ± 94.5	48.2 ± 92.3	0.700	97.1 ± 204.6	55.3 ± 145.3	0.445
NT-ProBNP (pg/mL)	3188.7 ± 5091.2	3802.2 ± 5998.2	0.016	9248.5 ± 8231.4	9948.8 ± 9432.6	0.589
High-sensitivity CRP (mg/dL)	8.9 ± 38.6	12.7 ± 47.9	0.093	10.1 ± 32.4	15.2 ± 48.2	0.209
Serum creatinine (mg/L)	1.4 ± 0.3	1.4 ± 0.3	0.074	5.1 ± 4.6	5.1 ± 3.7	0.965
eGFR (mL/min/1.73 m^2)	49.2 ± 8.0	48.6 ± 8.2	0.130	16.5 ± 8.5	15.8 ± 8.2	0.305
Blood glucose (mg/L)	197.3 ± 101.1	207.9 ± 108.3	0.044	209.0 ± 129.7	217.0 ± 124.4	0.479
Total cholesterol (mg/dL)	177.1 ± 47.9	163.9 ± 41.6	<0.001	162.4 ± 52.3	148.2 ± 45.6	0.001
Triglyceride (mg/L)	128.3 ± 96.9	113.2 ± 73.0	<0.001	125.7 ± 111.3	117.5 ± 68.7	0.282
HDL cholesterol (mg/L)	42.7 ± 16.5	42.5 ± 17.6	0.828	39.3 ± 12.7	37.9 ± 14.8	0.302
LDL cholesterol (mg/L)	109.5 ± 46.5	100.7 ± 41.8	<0.001	95.9 ± 38.8	83.9 ± 36.4	0.001
Discharge medications, n (%)						
Aspirin, n (%)	2127 (99.2)	518 (96.5)	<0.001	498 (98.2)	156 (93.4)	0.001
Clopidogrel, n (%)	1941 (90.5)	523 (91.1)	0.798	457 (90.1)	160 (95.8)	0.606
Ticagrelor, n (%)	145 (6.8)	10 (1.9)	<0.001	35 (6.9)	5 (3.0)	0.087
Prasugrel, n (%)	58 (2.7)	4 (0.7)	0.006	15 (3.0)	2 (1.2)	0.266
Cilostazole, n (%)	434 (20.2)	82 (15.3)	0.008	97 (19.1)	21 (12.6)	0.060
ACEIs, n (%)	1122 (52.3)	189 (35.2)	<0.001	178 (35.1)	43 (25.7)	0.029
ARBs, n (%)	677 (31.6)	124 (23.1)	<0.001	215 (42.4)	35 (21.0)	<0.001
BBs, n (%)	1775 (82.8)	315 (58.7)	<0.001	431 (85.0)	79 (47.3)	<0.001
CCBs, n (%)	177 (8.3)	41 (7.6)	0.724	81 (16.0)	21 (12.6)	0.321
Statin, n (%)						
Atorvastatin, n (%)	1202 (56.1)			326 (64.3)		
Rosuvastatin, n (%)	608 (28.4)			116 (22.9)		
Simvastatin, n (%)	133 (6.2)			26 (5.1)		
Pitavastatin, n (%)	154 (7.2)			20 (3.9)		
Pravastatin, n (%)	40 (1.9)			12 (2.4)		
Fluvastatin, n (%)	7 (0.3)			7 (1.4)		
Infarct-related artery						
Left main, n (%)	51 (2.4)	16 (3.0)	0.425	26 (5.1)	8 (4.8)	0.863
LAD, n (%)	917 (42.8)	228 (42.4)	0.963	221 (43.6)	69 (41.3)	0.472
LCx, n (%)	324 (15.1)	69 (12.8)	0.195	72 (14.2)	29 (17.4)	0.320
RCA, n (%)	852 (39.7)	224 (41.7)	0.404	188 (37.1)	61 (36.5)	0.927
Treated vessel						
Left main, n (%)	82 (3.8)	17 (3.2)	0.524	32 (6.3)	13 (7.8)	0.508
LAD, n (%)	1175 (54.8)	278 (51.8)	0.207	298 (58.8)	90 (53.9)	0.268
LCx, n (%)	568 (26.5)	127 (23.6)	0.179	121 (23.9)	41 (24.6)	0.857
RCA, n (%)	997 (46.5)	253 (47.1)	0.799	223 (44.0)	99 (41.3)	0.589
ACC/AHA lesion type						
Type B1, n (%)	303 (14.1)	109 (20.3)	<0.001	72 (14.2)	16 (9.6)	0.145
Type B2, n (%)	720 (33.6)	133 (24.8)	<0.001	174 (34.3)	57 (34.1)	0.965
Type C, n (%)	983 (45.8)	224 (41.7)	0.090	238 (46.9)	83 (49.7)	0.536
Extent of CAD						
Single-vessel, n (%)	875 (40.8)	211 (39.3)	0.521	198 (39.1)	63 (37.7)	0.760
2-vessel, n (%)	671 (31.3)	172 (32.0)	0.743	148 (29.2)	52 (31.1)	0.633
≥3-vessel, n (%)	598 (27.9)	154 (28.7)	0.717	161 (31.8)	52 (31.1)	0.924
Pre-PCI TIMI 0/1, n (%)	1258 (58.7)	330 (61.5)	0.242	227 (44.8)	83 (49.7)	0.268
Type of stent						
ZES, n (%)	801 (37.4)	233 (43.4)	0.010	167 (32.9)	65 (38.9)	0.158
EES, n (%)	1092 (50.9)	245 (45.9)	0.030	274 (54.0)	79 (47.3)	0.153
BES, n (%)	249 (11.6)	52 (9.7)	0.222	64 (12.6)	18 (10.8)	0.587

Table 4. *Cont.*

Variables	Group A3 eGFR 30–59 mL/min/1.73 m² (*n* = 2144)	Group B3 eGFR 30–59 mL/min/1.73 m² (*n* = 537)	*p* Value	Group A4 eGFR < 30 mL/min/1.73 m² (*n* = 507)	Group B4 eGFR < 30 mL/min/1.73 m² (*n* = 167)	*p* Value
Others, *n* (%)	43 (2.0)	12 (2.2)	0.738	8 (1.6)	7 (4.2)	0.065
IVUS, *n* (%)	401 (18.7)	85 (15.8)	0.133	89 (17.6)	30 (18.0)	0.907
OCT, *n* (%)	4 (0.2)	3 (0.6)	0.131	1 (0.2)	0	0.566
FFR, *n* (%)	5 (0.2)	3 (0.6)	0.216	2 (0.4)	1 (0.6)	0.575
Stent diameter (mm)	3.11 ± 0.42	3.11 ± 0.44	0.887	3.09 ± 0.43	3.11 ± 0.44	0.555
Stent length (mm)	27.8 ± 12.3	26.0 ± 11.1	0.002	29.0 ± 13.7	28.1 ± 14.4	0.497
Number of stents	1.54 ± 0.82	1.53 ± 0.82	0.648	1.60 ± 0.87	1.51 ± 0.76	0.196

Values are means ± SDs or numbers and percentages. The *p* values for continuous data were obtained from the unpaired *t*-test. The *p* values for categorical data were obtained from the chi-square or Fisher's exact test. eGFR, estimated glomerular filtration rate; LVEF, left ventricular ejection fraction; BMI, body mass index; SBP, systolic blood pressure; DBP, diastolic blood pressure; CPR, cardiopulmonary resuscitation; STEMI, ST-segment elevation myocardial infarction; PCI, percutaneous coronary intervention; NSTEMI, non-STEMI; MI, myocardial infarction; CABG, coronary artery bypass graft; HF, heart failure; CVA, cerebrovascular accidents; CK-MB, creatine kinase myocardial band; NT-ProBNP, N-terminal pro-brain natriuretic peptide; CRP, C-reactive protein; HDL, high-density lipoprotein; LDL, low-density lipoprotein; ACEIs, angiotensin-converting enzyme inhibitors; ARBs, angiotensin receptor blockers; BBs, beta blockers; CCBs, calcium channel blockers; LAD, left anterior descending coronary artery; LCx, left circumflex coronary artery; RCA, right coronary artery; ACC/AHA, American College of Cardiology/American Heart Association; CAD, coronary artery disease; TIMI, thrombolysis in myocardial infarction; ZES, zotarolimus-eluting stent; EES, everolimus-eluting stent; BES, biolimus-eluting stent; IVUS, intravascular ultrasound; OCT, optical coherence tomography; FFR, fractional flow reserve.

3.1.1. Group A (Statin Users)

Group A1 (eGFR $\geq$ 90 mL/min/1.73 m^2) included the highest number of male patients; patients who received PCI within 24 h; current smokers; those with left anterior descending coronary artery (LAD) and left circumflex coronary artery (LCx) as the IRA and treated vessels, American College of Cardiology/American Heart Association (ACC/AHA) type B2 lesion, single-vessel disease and biolimus-eluting stent (BES) as the deployed stent; those who used optical coherence tomography and fraction flow reserve; and those prescribed with aspirin, ticagrelor, prasugrel, ACEI, BB and rosuvastatin as the discharge medications. The mean levels of LVEF, BMI, SBP, DBP, total cholesterol, triglyceride and LDL cholesterol and the mean diameter of deployed stents were highest in group A1. In group A2 (eGFR 60–89 mL/min/1.73 m^2), the number of patients with STEMI and pre-PCI TIMI 0/1 and the mean levels of peak creatine kinase myocardial band (CK-MB) and HDL cholesterol were highest. In group A3 (eGFR 30–59 mL/min/1.73 m^2), including patients who required CPR on admission, who received clopidogrel and cilostazol as the discharge medications, with the right coronary artery (RCA) as the IRA and treated vessel, with 2-vessel disease and with zotarolimus-eluting stent as a deployed stent, the mean age of the enrolled patients was highest. In group A4 (eGFR < 30 mL/min/1.73 m^2), including patients with cardiogenic shock, Killip class III/IV, non-STEMI (NSTEMI), hypertension, DM, previous MI, previous PCI, previous coronary artery bypass graft (CABG), previous HF, previous CVA, LM IRA and treated vessel, ACC/AHA type C lesion, $\geq$3-vessel disease, everolimus-eluting stent as a deployed stent and atorvastatin as a discharge medication, the mean values of peak troponin-I, NT-ProBNP, high-sensitivity C-reactive protein (hs-CRP), blood glucose and stent length and mean number of deployed stents were highest.

3.1.2. Group B (Statin Nonusers)

Group B1 (eGFR $\geq$ 90 mL/min/1.73 m^2) included the highest number of male patients, patients who received PCI within 24 h, current smokers and patients with LAD and LCx as the IRA and treated vessels, single-vessel disease, BES as a deployed stent and aspirin, prasugrel and ACEI as the discharge medications. The mean levels of LVEF, BMI, SBP, DBP, total cholesterol, triglyceride and LDL cholesterol and the mean diameter of deployed stents were highest in group B1. In group B2 (eGFR 60–89 mL/min/1.73 m^2), including patients with STEMI, ACC/AHA type B1 lesion and pre-PCI TIMI 0/1, the mean levels of peak CK-MB and HDL cholesterol and the prescription rates of clopidogrel and BB as the discharge medications were highest. In group B3 (eGFR 30–59 mL/min/1.73 m^2), including patients who needed CPR on admission and those with previous CABG, RCA as the IRA and treated vessel and 2-vessel disease, the mean age of enrolled patients and mean number of deployed stents were highest. In group B4 (eGFR < 30 mL/min/1.73 m^2), including patients with cardiogenic shock, Killip class III/IV, NSTEMI, hypertension, DM, previous MI, previous PCI, previous CABG, previous HF, previous CVA, LM IRA and treated vessel, ACC/AHA type C lesion, ≥3-vessel disease, everolimus-eluting stent as a deployed stent and atorvastatin as a discharge medication, the mean values of peak troponin-I, NT-ProBNP, hs-CRP, blood glucose, stent length and mean number of deployed stents were highest.

3.2. Clinical Outcomes

The 2-year major clinical outcomes are summarized in Table 5 and Table S2 and Figure 2.

Table 5. Hazard ratios for the 2-year major clinical outcomes in statin users.

	Hazard Ratio (95% CI) Unadjusted	p Value	Event Rates at 2 Years [a]	Hazard Ratio (95% CI) Adjusted [b]	p Value
MACE					
Group A1 vs.	-		5.2 %	-	-
Group A2	1.228 (1.059–1.425)	0.017	6.4 %	1.139 (0.969–1.339)	0.114
Group A3	2.015 (1.689–2.404)	<0.001	10.1 %	1.465 (1.183–1.813)	<0.001
Group A4	3.804 (2.991–4.837)	<0.001	18.5 %	2.082 (1.514–2.863)	<0.001
Group A2 vs. Group A3	1.641 (1.383–1.946)	<0.001		1.249 (1.027–1.520)	0.026
Group A2 vs. Group A4	3.096 (2.445–3.922)	<0.001		1.701 (1.263–2.290)	<0.001
Group A3 vs. Group A4	1.881 (1.458–2.427)	<0.001		1.439 (1.059–1.954)	0.020
All-cause death					
Group A1 vs.			0.9 %		-
Group A2	2.076 (1.494–2.886)	<0.001	1.8 %	1.937 (1.348–2.784)	<0.001
Group A3	5.454 (3.887–7.652)	<0.001	4.6 %	3.691 (2.452–5.554)	<0.001
Group A4	15.55 (10.71–22.56)	<0.001	12.9 %	5.068 (3.037–8.459)	<0.001
Group A2 vs. Group A3	2.625 (1.985–3.471)	<0.001		1.843 (1.342–2.531)	<0.001
Group A2 vs. Group A4	7.512 (5.457–10.34)	<0.001		3.160 (2.104–4.745)	<0.001
Group A3 vs. Group A4	2.853 (2.052–3.966)	<0.001		2.060 (1.396–3.039)	<0.001
Cardiac death					
Group A1 vs.			0.4 %		-
Group A2	2.364 (1.504–3.714)	<0.001	1.0 %	1.964 (1.215–3.177)	0.006
Group A3	6.001 (3.764–9.568)	<0.001	2.6 %	3.429 (1.993–5.898)	<0.001
Group A4	15.28 (9.047–25.81)	<0.001	6.8 %	4.512 (2.318–8.783)	<0.001
Group A2 vs. Group A3	2.537 (1.752–3.675)	<0.001		1.647 (1.087–2.495)	0.019
Group A2 vs. Group A4	6.476 (4.166–10.07)	<0.001		2.829 (1.674–4.781)	<0.001
Group A3 vs. Group A4	2.540 (1.610–4.008)	<0.001		2.040 (1.218–3.418)	0.007
Recurrent MI					
Group A1 vs.			1.6 %		-
Group A2	1.040 (0.785–1.377)	0.786	1.6 %	1.060 (0.778–1.444)	0.712
Group A3	1.738 (1.244–2.429)	0.001	2.8 %	1.070 (0.708–1.616)	0.750
Group A4	2.658 (1.607–4.395)	<0.001	4.3 %	1.486 (0.786–2.806)	0.223
Group A2 vs. Group A3	1.675 (1.675–2.340)	0.002		1.218 (0.821–1.807)	0.327
Group A2 vs. Group A4	2.556 (1.546–4.225)	<0.001		1.430 (0.762–2.682)	0.265
Group A3 vs. Group A4	1.531 (0.897–2.614)	0.118		1.192 (0.627–2.265)	0.593
Any repeat revascularization					
Group A1 vs.			3.4 %		
Group A2	1.092 (0.902–1.323)	0.367	3.6 %	1.036 (0.843–1.274)	0.735
Group A3	1.308 (1.013–1.689)	0.039	4.3 %	1.010 (0.743–1.372)	0.950
Group A4	1.582 (1.019–2.456)	0.041	5.2 %	1.161 (0.680–1.981)	0.585
Group A2 vs. Group A3	1.197 (0.929–1.542)	0.164		1.057 (0.791–1.413)	0.706
Group A2 vs. Group A4	1.442 (0.930–2.236)	0.102		1.053 (0.629–1.762)	0.845
Group A3 vs. Group A4	1.202 (0.751–1.924)	0.442		1.019 (0.587–1.771)	0.945

[a] Event rates at 2 years were calculated by Kaplan–Meyer analysis. [b] Adjusted model included male, age, LVEF, BMI, cardiogenic shock, CPR on admission, Killip class III/IV, STEMI hypertension, diabetes mellitus, previous MI, PCI and CVA, current smoker, NT-ProBNP, blood glucose, total cholesterol, HDL cholesterol, ACEI, ARB, BB, LM (IRA and treated vessel), ACC/AHA type B2 lesion, single-vessel disease, ≥3-vessel disease, stent diameter, stent length and number of stents. Group A1, statin users and eGFR ≥ 90 mL/min/1.73 m^2; Group A2, statin users and eGFR 60–89 mL/min/1.73 m^2; Group A3, statin users and eGFR 30–59 mL/min/1.73 m^2; Group A4, statin users and eGFR < 30 mL/min/1.73 m^2; Group B1, statin nonusers and eGFR ≥ 90 mL/min/1.73 m^2; Group B2, statin nonusers and eGFR 60–89 mL/min/1.73 m^2; Group B3, statin nonusers and eGFR 30–59 mL/min/1.73 m^2; Group B4, statin nonusers and eGFR < 30 mL/min/1.73 m^2; eGFR, estimated glomerular filtration rate; CI, confidence interval; LVEF, left ventricular ejection fraction; BMI, body mass index; CPR, cardiopulmonary resuscitation; STEMI, ST-segment elevation myocardial infarction; MI, myocardial infarction; PCI, percutaneous coronary intervention; CVA, cerebrovascular accident; HDL, high-density lipoprotein; ACEI, angiotensin-converting enzyme inhibitor; ARB, angiotensin receptor blocker; BB, beta blocker; ACC/AHA, American College of Cardiology/American Heart Association.

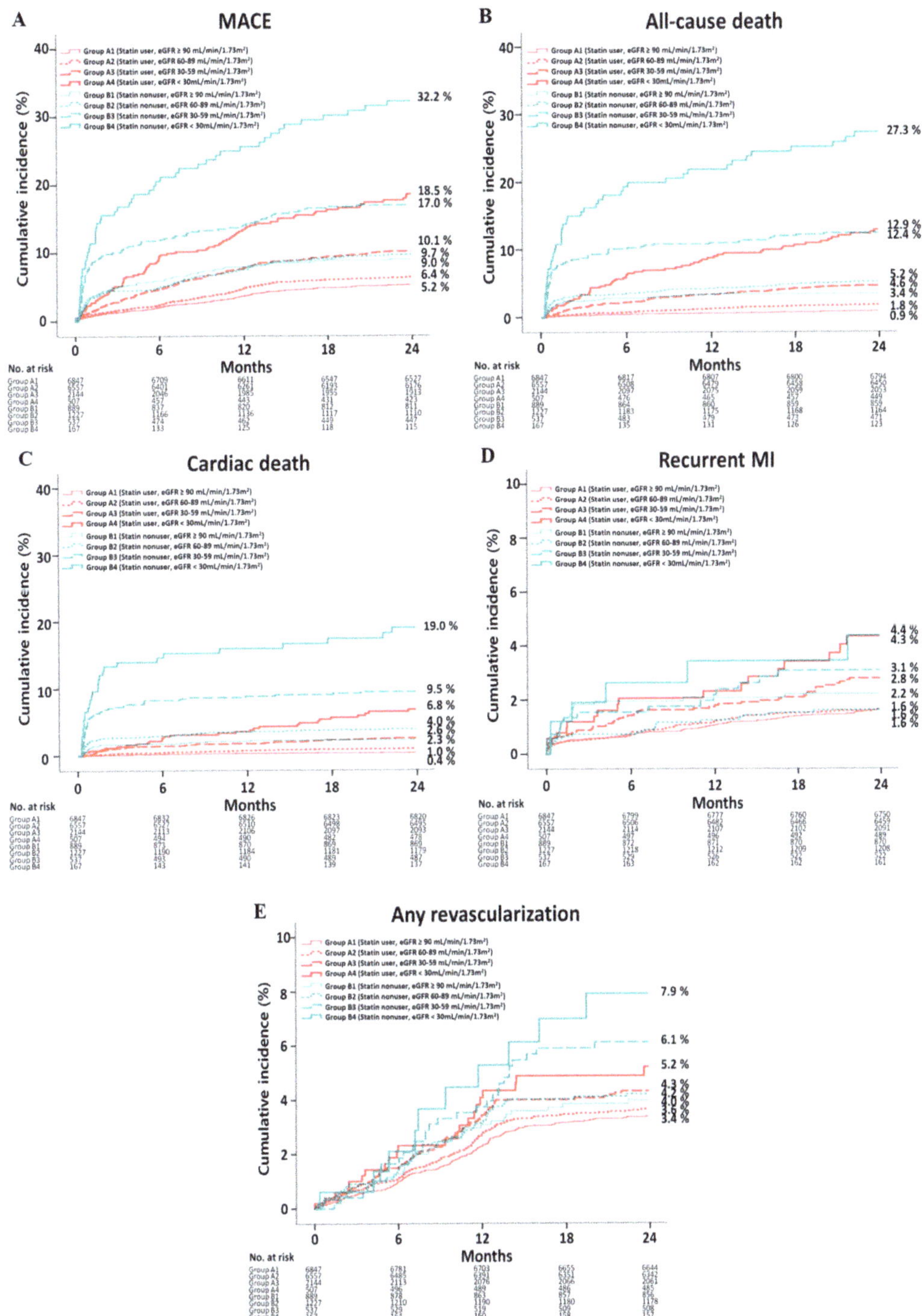

Figure 2. Kaplan–Meier analysis for the MACE (**A**), all-cause death (**B**), cardiac death (**C**), recurrent MI (**D**) and any repeat revascularization (**E**) during a 2-year follow-up period.

3.2.1. Group A

After adjustment, although the MACE (Table 5 and Figure 2A) rate was not significantly different between groups A1 and A2, it was significantly higher in groups A3 (adjusted hazard ratio (aHR), 1.465; 95% CI, 1.183–1.813; $p < 0.001$) and A4 (aHR, 2.082; 95% CI, 1.514–2.863; $p < 0.001$) than that in group A1, higher in groups A3 (aHR, 1.249; 95% CI, 1.027–1.520; $p = 0.026$) and A4 (aHR, 1.701; 95% CI, 1.263–2.290; $p < 0.001$) than that in group A2 and higher in group A4 than that in group A3 (aHR, 1.439; 95% CI, 1.059–1.954; $p = 0.020$). The all-cause death (Figure 2B) rates were significantly higher in groups A2 (aHR, 1.937; 95% CI, 1.348–2.784; $p < 0.001$), A3 (aHR, 3.691; 95% CI, 2.452–5.554; $p < 0.001$) and A4 (aHR, 5.068; 95% CI, 3.037–8.459; $p < 0.001$) than that in group A1, higher in groups A3 (aHR, 1.843; 95% CI, 1.342–2.531; $p < 0.001$) and A4 (aHR, 3.160; 95% CI, 2.104–4.745; $p < 0.001$) than that in group A2 and higher in group A4 than that in group A3 (aHR, 2.060; 95% CI, 1.396–3.039; $p < 0.001$). The CD (Figure 2C) rates were significantly higher in groups A2 (aHR, 1.964; 95% CI, 1.215–3.177; $p = 0.006$), A3 (aHR, 3.429; 95% CI, 1.993–5.898; $p < 0.001$) and A4 (aHR, 4.512; 95% CI, 2.318–8.783; $p < 0.001$) than that in group A1, higher in groups A3 (aHR, 1.647; 95% CI, 1.087–2.495; $p = 0.019$) and A4 (aHR, 2.829; 95% CI, 1.674–4.781; $p < 0.001$) than that in group A2 and higher in group A4 than that in group A3 (aHR, 2.040; 95% CI, 1.218–3.418; $p = 0.007$). However, the re-MI (Figure 2D) and any repeat revascularization (Figure 2E) rates were not significantly different among the four groups after adjustment (Table 5).

3.2.2. Group B

Table S2 shows the HRs for the 2-year major clinical outcomes in statin nonusers. After adjustment, the rate of MACE (Figure 2A) was not significantly different between groups B1 and B2, B1 and B3 and B2 and B3. However, it was significantly higher in group B4 than those in groups B1 (aHR, 2.648; 95% CI, 1.526–4.596; $p = 0.001$), B2 (aHR, 2.055; 95% CI, 1.297–3.254; $p = 0.002$) and B3 (aHR, 1.676; 95% CI, 1.056–2.661; $p = 0.029$). The all-cause death (Figure 2B) rates were not significantly different between groups B1 and B2 and groups B2 and B3. However, they were higher in group B3 than that in group B1 (aHR, 2.014; 95% CI, 1.076–3.769; $p = 0.029$) and higher in group B4 than that in group B1 (aHR, 6.891; 95% CI, 3.114–12.25; $p < 0.001$). Moreover, the all-cause death rate was higher in group B4 than that in groups B2 (aHR, 2.914; 95% CI, 1.681–5.050; $p < 0.001$) and B3 (aHR, 2.091; 95% CI, 1.238–3.233; $p = 0.006$). Similarly, the CD (Figure 2C) rate was higher in group B3 than that in group B1 (aHR, 2.201; 95% CI, 1.054–4.596; $p = 0.036$) and higher in group B4 than that in group B1 (aHR, 8.727; 95% CI, 3.295–14.11; $p < 0.001$). Moreover, the CD rates were higher in group B4 than that in groups B2 (aHR, 2.681; 95% CI, 1.400–5.135; $p = 0.003$) and B3 (aHR, 2.022; 95% CI, 1.166–3.184; $p = 0.014$). The re-MI (Figure 2D) and any repeat revascularization (Figure 2E) rates were not significantly different among the four groups after adjustment (Table S2).

3.2.3. Group A vs. B

Table 6 shows clinical outcomes between the statin user and nonuser groups at 2 years. In the four baseline renal function groups, the rates of MACE (group A1 vs. B1, aHR, 1.573; 95% CI, 1.181–2.096; $p = 0.002$; group A2 vs. B2, aHR, 1.381; 95% CI, 1.092–1.747; $p = 0.007$; group A3 vs. B3, aHR, 1.732; 95% CI, 1.329–2.266; $p < 0.001$; and group A4 vs. B4, aHR, 1.949; 95% CI, 1.347–2.822; $p < 0.001$), all-cause death (aHR, 2.242; 95% CI, 1.261–3.984; $p = 0.006$; aHR, 2.139; 95% CI, 1.471–3.110; $p < 0.001$; aHR, 2.510; 95% CI, 1.780–3.541; $p < 0.001$; and aHR, 2.476; 95% CI, 1.629–3.755; $p < 0.001$, respectively) and CD (aHR, 2.956; 95% CI, 1.412–6.189; $p = 0.004$; aHR, 2.422; 95% CI, 1.536–3.819; $p < 0.001$; aHR, 3.150; 95% CI, 2.069–4.795; $p < 0.001$; aHR, 3.341; 95% CI, 1.975–5.706; $p < 0.001$, respectively) were higher in statin nonusers than in statin users. However, the re-MI and any repeat revascularization rates were not significantly different between the statin user and nonuser groups.

Table 6. Clinical outcomes between statin users and nonusers at 2 years.

	Statin Users	Statin Nonusers					
Outcomes	**Group A1 (n = 6847)**	**Group B1 (n = 889)**	**Log-Rank**	**Unadjusted**		**Adjusted [a]**	
				HR (95% CI)	**p Value**	**HR (95% CI)**	**p Value**
MACE	320 (5.2)	78 (9.0)	<0.001	1.821 (1.421–2.332)	<0.001	1.573 (1.181–2.096)	0.002
All-cause death	53 (0.9)	30 (3.4)	<0.001	4.235 (2.705–6.629)	<0.001	2.242 (1.261–3.984)	0.006
Cardiac death	27 (0.4)	20 (2.3)	<0.001	5.567 (3.121–9.929)	<0.001	2.956 (1.412–6.189)	0.004
Re-MI	97 (1.6)	19 (2.2)	0.138	1.448 (0.886–2.369)	0.140	1.578 (0.918–2.711)	0.099
Any revascularization	203 (3.4)	33 (4.0)	0.353	1.190 (0.824–1.720)	0.354	1.191 (0.796–1.783)	0.395
Outcomes	**Group A2 (n = 6557)**	**Group B2 (n = 1227)**	**Log-Rank**	**Unadjusted**		**Adjusted [b]**	
				HR (95% CI)	**p Value**	**HR (95% CI)**	**p Value**
MACE	381 (6.4)	117 (9.7)	<0.001	1.573 (1.279–1.935)	<0.001	1.381 (1.092–1.747)	0.007
All-cause death	107 (1.8)	63 (5.2)	<0.001	3.031 (2.220–4.138)	<0.001	2.139 (1.471–3.110)	<0.001
Cardiac death	62 (1.0)	48 (4.0)	<0.001	4.023 (2.759–5.864)	<0.001	2.422 (1.536–3.819)	<0.001
Re-MI	98 (1.6)	19 (1.6)	0.980	1.006 (0.616–1.645)	0.980	1.199 (0.719–2.001)	0.487
Any revascularization	215 (3.6)	49 (4.2)	0.345	1.161 (0.851–1.584)	0.345	1.196 (0.856–1.671)	0.294
Outcomes	**Group A3 (n = 2144)**	**Group B3 (n = 537)**	**Log-Rank**	**Unadjusted**		**Adjusted [c]**	
				HR (95% CI)	**p Value**	**HR (95% CI)**	**p Value**
MACE	201 (10.1)	90 (17.0)	<0.001	1.817 (1.417–2.330)	<0.001	1.732 (1.329–2.266)	<0.001
All-cause death	91 (4.6)	66 (12.4)	<0.001	2.978 (2.169–4.088)	<0.001	2.510 (1.780–3.541)	<0.001
Cardiac death	51 (2.6)	50 (9.5)	<0.001	4.034 (2.731–5.958)	<0.001	3.150 (2.069–4.795)	<0.001
Re-MI	53(2.8)	15 (3.1)	0.661	1.137 (0.641–2.017)	0.661	1.311 (0.735–2.409)	0.346
Any revascularization	83 (4.3)	29 (6.1)	0.111	1.407 (0.922–2.148)	0.113	1.532 (1.018–2.428)	0.086
Outcomes	**Group A4 (n = 507)**	**Group B4 (n = 167)**	**Log-Rank**	**Unadjusted**		**Adjusted [d]**	
				HR (95% CI)	**p Value**	**HR (95% CI)**	**p Value**
MACE	84 (18.5)	52 (32.2)	<0.001	2.009 (1.422–2.840)	<0.001	1.949 (1.347–2.822)	<0.001
All-cause death	58 (12.9)	44 (27.3)	<0.001	2.493 (1.685–3.690)	<0.001	2.476 (1.629–3.755)	<0.001
Cardiac death	29 (6.8)	30 (19.0)	<0.001	3.378 (2.027–5.628)	<0.001	3.341 (1.975–5.706)	<0.001
Re-MI	18 (4.3)	6 (4.4)	0.901	1.060 (0.421–2.672)	0.901	1.065 (0.410–2.764)	0.898
Any revascularization	22 (5.2)	10 (7.9)	0.293	1.490 (0.705–3.146)	0.296	1.412 (0.639–3.118)	0.394

[a] Adjusted by male, age, BMI, LVEF, cardiogenic shock, CPR on admission, STEMI, PCI within 24 h, hypertension, DM, NT-ProBNP, total cholesterol, LDL cholesterol, aspirin, clopidogrel, ticagrelor, prasugrel, ACEI, ARB, BB, ACC/AHA type B1 lesion, ≥3-vessel disease, ZES and stent length (Tables S1 and S3). [b] Adjusted by male, age, BMI, LVEF, cardiogenic shock, CPR on admission, STEMI, PCI within 24 h, hypertension, DM, dyslipidemia, NT-ProBNP, total cholesterol, LDL cholesterol, aspirin, clopidogrel, ticagrelor, prasugrel, ACEI, ARB, BB, ACC/AHA type C lesion, ≥3-vessel disease, ZES, BES, FFR and stent length (Tables S1 and S3). [c] Adjusted by male, age, BMI, SBP, DBP, LVEF, cardiogenic shock, CPR on admission, Killip class III/IV, STEMI, hypertension, DM, peak CK-MB, NT-ProBNP, total cholesterol, triglyceride, LDL cholesterol, aspirin, ticagrelor, ACEI, ARB, BB, ACC/AHA type B1/B2 lesions and ≥3-vessel disease (Tables S1 and S4). [d] Adjusted by male, age, BMI, LVEF, cardiogenic shock, CPR on admission, STEMI, hypertension, DM, NT-ProBNP, LDL cholesterol, ACE, ARB, BB and ≥3-vessel disease (Tables S1 and S4). Group A1, eGFR ≥ 90 mL/min/1.73 m^2; Group A2, eGFR 60–89 mL/min/1.73 m^2; Group A3, eGFR 30–59 mL/min/1.73 m^2; Group A4, GFR < 30 mL/min/1.73 m^2; Group B1, eGFR ≥ 90 mL/min/1.73 m^2; Group B2, eGFR 60–89 mL/min/1.73 m^2; Group B3, eGFR 30–59 mL/min/1.73 m^2; Group B4, eGFR < 30 mL/min/1.73 m^2; eGFR, estimated glomerular filtration rate; HR, hazard ratio; CI, confidence interval; MACE, major adverse cardiac events; Re-MI, recurrent myocardial infarction; BMI, body mass index; LVEF, left ventricular ejection fraction; CPR, cardiopulmonary resuscitation; STEMI, ST-segment elevation myocardial infarction; PCI, percutaneous coronary intervention; DM, diabetes mellitus; NT-ProBNP, N-terminal pro-brain natriuretic peptide; LDL, low-density lipoprotein; ACEI, angiotensin-converting enzyme inhibitors; ARB, angiotensin receptor blockers; BB, beta blocker; ACC/AHA, American College of Cardiology/American Heart Association; ZES, zotarolimus-eluting stent; BES, biolimus-eluting stent; FFR, fractional flow reserve; SBP, systolic blood pressure; DBP, diastolic blood pressure; CK-MB, creatine kinase myocardial band.

3.2.4. Independent Predictors

Table 7 and Table S3 show the independent predictors for MACE and all-cause death in statin users and nonusers. Older age (≥65 years), STEMI, reduced LVEF (<40%), cardiogenic shock, CPR on admission, NT-ProBNP, LDL cholesterol, ACEI levels, ≥3-vessel disease and LM (IRA) were common independent predictors for both MACE and all-cause mortality in the statin user group (Table 7). Reduced LVEF, cardiogenic shock, CPR on admission, NT-ProBNP and LDL cholesterol levels and BB were common independent predictors for both MACE and all-cause death in the statin nonuser group (Table S3).

Table 7. Independent predictors for MACE and all-cause death in statin users.

Variables	MACE				All-Cause Death			
	Unadjusted		Adjusted		Unadjusted		Adjusted	
	HR (95% CI)	p Value	HR (95% CI)	p Value	HR (95% CI)	p Value	HR (95% CI)	p Value
Group A1 vs. Group A2	1.228 (1.059–1.425)	0.017	1.106 (0.940–1.301)	0.226	2.076 (1.494–2.886)	<0.001	1.146 (1.007–1.345)	0.040
Group A1 vs. Group A3	2.015 (1.689–2.404)	<0.001	1.314 (1.066–1.687)	0.012	5.454 (3.887–7.652)	<0.001	2.365 (1.544–3.625)	<0.001
Group A1 vs. Group A4	3.804 (2.991–4.837)	<0.001	1.779 (1.239–2.554)	0.002	15.55 (10.71–22.56)	<0.001	3.807 (2.151–6.736)	<0.001
Group A2 vs. Group A3	1.641 (1.383–1.946)	<0.001	1.342 (1.028–1.483)	0.040	2.625 (1.985–3.471)	<0.001	1.510 (1.085–2.100)	0.015
Group A2 vs. Group A4	3.096 (2.445–3.922)	<0.001	1.946 (1.522–2.415)	0.017	7.512 (5.457–10.34)	<0.001	2.175 (1.345–3.518)	0.002
Group A3 vs. Group A4	1.881 (1.458–2.427)	<0.001	1.521 (1.189–2.027)	0.034	2.853 (2.052–3.966)	<0.001	1.797 (1.162–2.779)	0.008
Male	1.325 (1.157–1.518)	<0.001	1.047 (0.888–1.235)	0.584	1.587 (1.255–2.006)	<0.001	1.146 (1.007–1.345)	0.040
Age, ≥65 years	1.577 (1.391–1.788)	<0.001	1.276 (1.094–1.488)	0.002	4.502 (3.430–5.910)	<0.001	3.985 (2.860–5.534)	<0.001
STEMI	1.300 (1.148–1.473)	<0.001	1.180 (1.028–1.355)	0.019	1.727 (1.377–2.166)	<0.001	1.425 (1.102–1.842)	0.007
LVEF, <40%	2.031 (1.724–2.393)	<0.001	1.491 (1.236–1.797)	<0.001	3.671 (2.865–4.703)	<0.001	2.088 (1.557–2.800)	<0.001
Cardiogenic shock	1.431 (1.074–1.907)	<0.001	1.369 (1.037–1.897)	0.005	2.304 (1.519–3.495)	<0.001	1.987 (1.269–3.231)	0.024
CPR on admission	2.680 (2.132–3.368)	<0.001	2.308 (1.787–2.982)	<0.001	3.979 (2.822–5.610)	<0.001	2.842 (1.900–4.252)	<0.001
Hypertension	1.498 (1.320–1.700)	<0.001	1.164 (1.007–1.345)	0.040	2.123 (1.676–2.678)	<0.001	1.390 (1.056–1.829)	0.019
Diabetes mellitus	1.791 (1.575–2.036)	<0.001	1.428 (1.234–1.653)	<0.001	2.391 (1.911–2.991)	<0.001	1.524 (1.172–1.980)	0.002
Previous heart failure	1.250 (0.690–2.266)	<0.001	1.613 (0.799–3.253)	0.182	2.590 (1.224–5.479)	0.013	1.058 (0.466–2.405)	0.892
Current smoker	1.309 (1.150–1.489)	<0.001	1.022 (0.873–1.197)	0.786	1.731 (1.360–2.202)	<0.001	1.214 (0.904–1.629)	0.197
NT-ProBNP	1.002 (0.999–1.004)	<0.001	1.003 (1.000–1.005)	<0.001	1.001 (0.998–1.002)	<0.001	1.002 (0.999–1.003)	<0.001
Total cholesterol	0.997 (0.995–0.998)	<0.001	1.001 (0.998–1.003)	0.637	0.994 (0.991–0.997)	<0.001	1.002 (0.998–1.007)	0.372
Triglyceride	0.999 (0.998–1.000)	<0.001	0.998 (0.997–0.999)	0.121	0.998 (0.996–0.999)	0.003	0.999 (0.997–1.001)	0.370
HDL cholesterol	0.990 (0.984–0.995)	<0.001	0.993 (0.988–1.001)	0.245	0.981 (0.976–0.997)	0.011	0.987 (0.975–0.999)	0.425
LDL cholesterol	0.998 (0.996–0.999)	<0.001	0.999 (0.997–1.000)	0.009	0.995 (0.992–0.999)	0.005	0.997 (0.992–1.001)	0.029
Aspirin	2.527 (1.491–4.283)	0.001	1.083 (0.553–2.121)	0.817	1.784 (1.356–2.351)	0.010	1.481 (0.661–3.318)	0.340
Ticagrelor	1.134 (0.874–1.471)	0.344	1.297 (0.972–1.730)	0.077	1.477 (0.877–2.486)	0.143	1.826 (0.993–3.360)	0.053
Prasugrel	1.344 (0.972–1.859)	0.074	1.256 (0.890–1.771)	0.194	3.224 (1.332–7.803)	0.009	2.356 (0.953–5.826)	0.063
ACEI	1.542 (1.360–1.747)	<0.001	1.369 (1.194–1.570)	<0.001	1.922 (1.532–2.411)	<0.001	1.613 (1.245–2.089)	<0.001
BB	1.360 (1.153–1.560)	<0.001	1.033 (0.856–1.245)	0.738	1.547 (1.167–2.051)	0.002	1.230 (0.902–1.679)	0.191
≥3-vessel disease	1.893 (1.656–2.164)	<0.001	1.572 (1.355–1.823)	<0.001	2.112 (1.671–2.668)	<0.001	1.374 (1.052–1.794)	0.020
Stent diameter <3.0 mm	1.189 (1.039–1.361)	0.012	1.038 (0.897–1.202)	0.614	1.075 (0.834–1.386)	0.575	1.333 (1.011–1.758)	0.041
Stent length ≥30 mm	1.250 (1.095–1.427)	0.001	1.096 (0.951–1.264)	0.206	1.499 (1.190–1.889)	0.001	1.263 (0.981–1.625)	0.070

MACE, major adverse cardiac events; HR, hazard ratio; CI, confidence interval; Group A1, statin users and eGFR ≥ 90 mL/min/1.73 m^2; Group A2, statin users and eGFR 60–89 mL/min/1.73 m^2; Group A3, statin users and eGFR 30–59 mL/min/1.73 m^2; Group A4, statin users and eGFR < 30 mL/min/1.73 m^2, eGFR, estimated glomerular filtration rate; STEMI, ST-elevation myocardial infarction; LVEF, left ventricular ejection fraction, CPR, cardiopulmonary resuscitation; NT-ProBNP, N-terminal pro-brain natriuretic peptide; HDL, high-density lipoprotein; LDL, low-density lipoprotein; ACEI, angiotensin-converting enzyme inhibitor; BB, beta blocker.

4. Discussion

The main findings of this retrospective observational study including patients with AMI who underwent successful PCI with newer-generation DES implantation were as follows: (1) regardless of the baseline renal function, individuals who underwent statin treatment had reduced rates of MACE, all-cause mortality and CD than those in statin nonusers; (2) despite these beneficial effects of statin therapy, the MACE, all-cause death and CD rates were significantly increased as the baseline eGFR decreased; (3) older age, STEMI, reduced LVEF, cardiogenic shock, CPR on admission, NT-ProBNP, LDL cholesterol, ACEI levels, ≥3-vessel disease and LM (IRA) were common independent predictors for both MACE and all-cause mortality in the statin user group.

To date, in the current guidelines [7,8], despite an MVE reducing the benefit of statin therapy in predialysis patients, this beneficial effect of statin therapy was not distinguished according to renal function (e.g., CKD grade 3, 4, or 5), and there is no convincing evidence among patients on dialysis [10]. In our study, we only included patients with AMI who did not require dialysis. Additionally, we directly compared major clinical outcomes between the statin user and nonuser groups according to baseline renal function to evaluate the presence or absence of benefit of statin treatment in these different renal function groups. In Table 6, in all four groups (eGFR ≥ 90, 60–89, 30–59 and <30 mL/min/1.73 m^2), statin therapy significantly reduced the rates of MACE, all-cause mortality and CD compared with those in statin nonusers. Moreover, the rates of MACE, all-cause mortality and CD significantly increased as the baseline eGFR decreased in group A (Table 5). These findings could be related to the poorer baseline characteristics of the statin nonuser group (e.g., reduced LVEF, high numbers of patients with cardiogenic shock or CPR on admission and high mean level of NT-ProBNP; Tables 3 and 4) compared with statin users. However, our results were consistent with those of previous reports [15,27,28]. Palmer et al. [15] showed that statins reduced the all-cause mortality (relative risk (RR), 0.81; 95% CI, 0.74–1.88) and

CD (RR, 0.78; 95% CI, 0.68–0.89) rates compared with placebo or no treatment in individuals not receiving dialysis. Sarnak et al. [10] also mentioned that the benefit of reducing MVE with statin-based therapy decreases as eGFR declines. Similarly, Herrington et al. [14] demonstrated that smaller relative effects of MVE were observed as eGFR declined (RR, 0.78; 99% CI, 0.75–0.82 for eGFR $\geq$ 60 mL/min/1.73 m^2; RR, 0.76; 99% CI, 0.70–0.81 for eGFR 45–60 mL/min/1.73 m^2; RR, 0.85; 99% CI, 0.75–0.96 for eGFR 30 to <45 mL/min/1.73 m^2; RR, 0.85; 95% CI, 0.71–1.02 for eGFR <30 mL/min/1.73 m^2). In group B, the MACE rates between groups B1 and B3 and between groups B2 and B3 and all-cause mortality and CD rates between groups B1 and B2 and between groups B2 and B3 were not significantly different (Table S2). However, after statin treatment (group A), the rates of MACE between groups A1 and A3 (aHR, 1.465; $p < 0.001$) and groups A2 and A3 (aHR, 1.249; $p = 0.026$) and all-cause mortality and CD rates between groups A1 and A3 (aHR, 3.691; $p < 0.001$, aHR, 3.429; $p < 0.001$, respectively) and between groups A2 and A3 (aHR, 1.843; $p < 0.001$, aHR, 1.647; $p = 0.019$, respectively) were significantly different. These results could reflect the trend that if GFR is reduced, the relative beneficial effects of statins might be smaller, in accordance with previous reports. [10,14]. Although the precise mechanisms responsible for the pattern of diminished benefit of statin with lower renal function are not well-known, the peculiar characteristics of the patients with CKD could be related to this pattern [14]. Patients with CKD are often excluded from randomized trials that evaluate cardioprotective drugs, and the quality and coverage of evidence on which to guide decision making in this population is suboptimal [29]. This lack of evidence on optimal treatment strategies for such patients may result in worse outcomes [30]. Additionally, the cause of CD is influenced by misclassification of their atypical clinical presentation [31]. The difficulty of interpreting elevated levels of biomarkers of cardiac damage in CKD is a possible contributing factor [32]. As the GFR declines, vascular calcification increases, and the calcification of the intima and media of large vessels in CKD is associated with all-cause death and cardiovascular mortality [10,33,34]. These cardiovascular changes in CKD are related to traditional (e.g., diabetes and hypertension) and nontraditional CKD-related cardiovascular disease risk factors (e.g., mineral and bone disease abnormalities, inflammation and oxidative stress) [10]. Because there is geographical variation in the prevalence of DM, the absolute magnitude of beneficial effects of statin therapy can vary regionally [35].

In our study, the re-MI and any repeat revascularization rates were not significantly different between the statin user and nonuser groups. Similar results were reported by Natsuaki et al. [36]. Among 14,706 patients who underwent PCI [36], the number of patients with AMI was approximately 30%. During a median follow-up of 956 days, the re-MI and any repeat revascularization rates were not significantly different between the statin user and nonuser groups according to the three different renal function groups (eGFR $\geq$ 60, $\leq$30 to <60 and <30 mL/min/1.73 m^2). They [36] suggested that patients with advanced CKD (eGFR < 30 mL/min/1.73 m^2) generally have advanced atherosclerosis, typically characterized by heavy calcification, and statins may no longer provide significant benefits in patients with end-stage vascular pathology. Another randomized study [37] failed to show the effects of statin therapy in decreasing restenosis. Although the study population was not confined to individuals with AMI or CKD, according to the Cholesterol Treatment Trialists' (CTT) Collaboration report, intensive statin therapy reduced the coronary revascularization rate by about 19% (95% CI, 11–18; $p < 0.0001$) [38]. Walter et al. [39] found that patients receiving prolonged statin treatment developed lower in-stent restenosis rates in comparison with nonreceivers (25% vs. 38%). Therefore, our results showing similar re-MI and any repeat revascularization rates between statin users and nonusers could be related to low number of enrolled patients in groups A4, B1, B3 and B4 and relatively low incidences of these events compared with previous studies [17,30]. According to recent meta-analysis data that evaluated CKD patients [40], in which CKD was defined as eGFR < 60 mL/min/1.73 m^2, results showed that the TLR/TVR (RR, 0.69; 95% CI, 0.57–0.84) was significantly reduced with DESs compared with bare-metal stents (BMS). Additionally, the use of second-generation DESs were associated with relative

27% reduction in TLR/TVR compared with first-generation DESs. Another study's meta-analysis data [41] showed that DESs were associated with lower TVR (RR, 0.61; 95% CI, 0.47–0.80) when compared with BMSs in patients with CKD. However, we think that future studies specifically focused on advanced CKD may help to clarify the benefit of statin treatment after PCI in this group. Interestingly, the number of patients with NSTEI was increased as their renal function deteriorated (Tables 1 and 2). Although, the precise underlying mechanisms of this phenomenon are not well known, some suggest that plaque erosion may be more predominant in the CKD group, in those patients who tend to be older and in those who have more established atherosclerosis, whereas the incidence of plaque rupture may be more common in younger non-CKD patients in whom less mature plaques are more vulnerable to rupture [42,43]. In both the statin user and nonuser groups, reduced LVEF, cardiogenic shock, CPR on admission and NT-ProBNP and LDL cholesterol levels were common independent predictors for both MACE and all-cause mortality. These variables are well-known unfavorable risk factors for mortality in patients with AMI [7,8].

Because the study populations of previous studies [14–17,27,28,36] regarding the long-term effects of statin treatment on major adverse events in patients with CKD were not confined to individuals with AMI and who received newer-generation DESs, we investigated the long-term major clinical outcomes of statin therapy confined to those patients to reflect current real-world practice. Moreover, as mentioned [29], evidence on optimal treatment strategies in patients with CKD is not abundant. More than 50 high-volume universities or community hospitals in South Korea participated in this study, but the study population was insufficient to provide meaningful results. Despite this weak point, we believe that our results could provide helpful information to interventional cardiologists in terms of current real-world information showing long-term effects of statin treatment according to the different renal function groups.

This study had other limitations. First, there may have been some underreporting and/or missing data and selection bias because this was a nonrandomized study. Second, although microalbuminuria is an early marker of chronic renal damage and a risk factor of cardiovascular disease [44], there was likely some misclassification of study groups due to the lack of information concerning the total amount of proteinuria and the presence or absence of microalbuminuria. Third, the estimation of renal function was based on a single measurement of eGFR at the time of presentation to the hospital. However, there is a possibility that eGFR may have worsened during the follow-up period. Unfortunately, we could not provide follow-up eGFR values because of a limitation of these registry data. Fourth, according to the current guidelines [7], the treatment goal is an LDL cholesterol level <1.8 mmol/L (<70 mg/dL) or at least 50% reduction in LDL cholesterol if the baseline LDL cholesterol level is 1.8–3.5 mmol/L. However, information regarding the follow-up levels of blood LDL cholesterol was incomplete in our registry data. This is a major shortcoming of this study and may be an important bias. Fifth, because the registry data did not include detailed or complete data on prescription doses, long-term adherence, discontinuation and drug-related adverse events, we could not provide this information during the follow-up period, which could have caused bias. Sixth, despite multivariable analyses, the variables that were not included in the data registry might have affected the study outcome. Seventh, because statins have a longer duration of use, the 2-year follow-up period in this study was relatively short for estimating long-term clinical outcomes. Eighth, because this retrospective study enrolled patients who underwent PCI between January 2006 and June 2015, this broad timeframe could have affected the clinical outcomes. Finally, during a 2-year follow-period, patients experienced definite or probable stent thrombosis (ST). Both in group A (group A1 vs. A2 vs. A3 vs. A4 = 37/6847 (0.5%) vs. 46/6557 (0.7%) vs. 22/2144 (1.0%) vs. 5/507 (1.0%), $p = 0.091$) and B (9/889 (1.0%) vs. 7/1227 (0.6%) vs. 4/537 (0.7%) vs. 4/537 (0.7%) vs. 1/167 (0.6%), $p = 0.702$, respectively), the cumulative incidences of ST were very low. Therefore, although ST is an important major determinant variable in patients with AMI [18], we inevitably could not include this variable as an endpoint in our study.

5. Conclusions

In the era of newer-generation DESs, although statin treatment was effective in reducing mortality, this beneficial effect was diminished in accordance with the deterioration of baseline renal function in patients with AMI who underwent successful PCI. These results could be helpful in understanding the current real-world effects of statins on patients with AMI with different renal functions. However, more large-scale, long-term follow-up studies are warranted to confirm these results.

Supplementary Materials: The following are available online at https://www.mdpi.com/article/10.3390/jcm10163504/s1, Table S1: Univariate analysis for MACE, Table S2: Hazard ratios for the 2-year major clinical outcomes in statin nonusers, Table S3: Independent predictors for MACE and all-cause death in statin nonusers.

Author Contributions: Conceptualization, Y.H.K., A.-Y.H., M.-K.H. and Y.J.; data curation, Y.H.K., A.-Y.H., S.-J.H. and S.K.; formal analysis, Y.H.K., A.-Y.H., S.-J.H. and S.K.; funding acquisition, M.H.J.; project administration, Y.H.K., A.-Y.H., M.H.J., B.-K.K., S.-J.H., S.K., C.-M.A., J.-S.K., Y.-G.K., D.C., M.-K.H. and Y.J.; resources, M.H.J., B.-K.K., S.-J.H., S.K., C.-M.A., J.-S.K., Y.-G.K., D.C., M.-K.H. and Y.J.; supervision, Y.H.K., M.H.J., D.C., M.-K.H. and Y.J.; validation, Y.H.K., A.-Y.H., M.H.J., B.-K.K., S.-J.H., S.K., C.-M.A., J.-S.K., Y.-G.K., D.C., M.-K.H. and Y.J.; visualization, Y.H.K., A.-Y.H., M.H.J., B.-K.K., S.-J.H., S.K., C.-M.A., J.-S.K., Y.-G.K., D.C., M.-K.H. and Y.J.; writing—original draft, Y.H.K. and A.-Y.H.; writing—review and editing, Y.H.K., A.-Y.H., M.H.J., B.-K.K., S.-J.H., S.K., C.-M.A., J.-S.K., Y.-G.K., D.C., M.-K.H. and Y.J. All authors have read and agreed to the published version of the manuscript.

Funding: This research was supported by a fund (2016-ER6304-02) by Research of Korea Centers for Disease Control and Prevention.

Institutional Review Board Statement: The study was conducted according to the guidelines of the Declaration of Helsinki and approved by the Chonnam National University Hospital Institutional Review Board (IRB) ethics committee (protocol code CNUH-2011-172 and 1 March 2011).

Informed Consent Statement: Informed written consent was obtained from all subjects involved in this study.

Data Availability Statement: Data are contained within the article or Supplementary Materials.

Acknowledgments: Korea Acute Myocardial infarction Registry (KAMIR) investigators: Myung Ho Jeong, Youngkeun Ahn, Sung Chul Chae, Jong Hyun Kim, Seung-Ho Hur, Young Jo Kim, In Whan Seong, Donghoon Choi, Jei Keon Chae, Taek Jong Hong, Jae Young Rhew, Doo-Il Kim, In-Ho Chae, Junghan Yoon, Bon-Kwon Koo, Byung-Ok Kim, Myoung Yong Lee, Kee-Sik Kim, Jin-Yong Hwang, Myeong Chan Cho, Seok Kyu Oh, Nae-Hee Lee, Kyoung Tae Jeong, Seung-Jea Tahk, Jang-Ho Bae, Seung-Woon Rha, Keum-Soo Park, Chong Jin Kim, Kyoo-Rok Han, Tae Hoon Ahn, Moo-Hyun Kim, Ki Bae Seung, Wook Sung Chung, Ju-Young Yang, Chong Yun Rhim, Hyeon-Cheol Gwon, Seong-Wook Park, Young-Youp Koh, Seung Jae Joo, Soo-Joong Kim, Dong Kyu Jin, Jin Man Cho, Sang-Wook Kim, Jeong Kyung Kim, Tae Ik Kim, Deug Young Nah, Si Hoon Park, Sang Hyun Lee, Seung Uk Lee, Hang-Jae Chung, Jang-Hyun Cho, Seung Won Jin, Myeong-Ki Hong, Yangsoo Jang, Jeong Gwan Cho, Hyo-Soo Kim, and Seung-Jung Park.

Conflicts of Interest: The authors declare that they do not have anything to disclose regarding conflict of interest with respect to this manuscript.

References

1. Szummer, K.; Wallentin, L.; Lindhagen, L.; Alfredsson, J.; Erlinge, D.; Held, C.; James, S.; Kellerth, T.; Lindahl, B.; Ravn-Fischer, A.; et al. Relations between implementation of new treatments and improved outcomes in patients with non-ST-elevation myocardial infarction during the last 20 years: Experiences from SWEDEHEART registry 1995 to 2014. *Eur. Heart J.* **2018**, *39*, 3766–3776. [CrossRef]
2. Puymirat, E.; Simon, T.; Cayla, G.; Cottin, Y.; Elbaz, M.; Coste, P.; Lemesle, G.; Motreff, P.; Popovic, B.; Khalife, K.; et al. Acute Myocardial Infarction: Changes in Patient Characteristics, Management, and 6-Month Outcomes Over a Period of 20 Years in the FAST-MI Program (French Registry of Acute ST-Elevation or Non-ST-Elevation Myocardial Infarction) 1995 to 2015. *Circulation* **2017**, *136*, 1908–1919. [CrossRef] [PubMed]

3. Townsend, N.; Wilson, L.; Bhatnagar, P.; Wickramasinghe, K.; Rayner, M.; Nichols, M. Cardiovascular disease in Europe: Epidemiological update 2016. *Eur. Heart J.* **2016**, *37*, 3232–3245. [CrossRef]
4. Kim, Y.; Ahn, Y.; Cho, M.C.; Kim, C.J.; Kim, Y.J.; Jeong, M.H. Current status of acute myocardial infarction in Korea. *Korean J. Intern. Med.* **2019**, *34*, 1–10. [CrossRef]
5. Larsen, A.I.; Tomey, M.I.; Mehran, R.; Nilsen, D.W.; Kirtane, A.J.; Witzenbichler, B.; Guagliumi, G.; Brener, S.J.; Généreux, P.; Kornowski, R.; et al. Comparison of outcomes in patients with ST-segment elevation myocardial infarction discharged on versus not on statin therapy (from the Harmonizing Outcomes with Revascularization and Stents in Acute Myocardial Infarction Trial). *Am. J. Cardiol.* **2014**, *113*, 1273–1279. [CrossRef]
6. Baigent, C.; Keech, A.; Kearney, P.M.; Blackwell, L.; Buck, G.; Pollicino, C.; Kirby, A.; Sourjina, T.; Peto, R.; Collins, R.; et al. Efficacy and safety of cholesterol-lowering treatment: Prospective meta-analysis of data from 90,056 participants in 14 randomised trials of statins. *Lancet* **2005**, *366*, 1267–1278.
7. Ibanez, B.; James, S.; Agewall, S.; Antunes, M.J.; Bucciarelli-Ducci, C.; Bueno, H.; Caforio, A.L.P.; Crea, F.; Goudevenos, J.A.; Halvorsen, S.; et al. 2017 ESC Guidelines for the management of acute myocardial infarction in patients presenting with ST-segment elevation: The Task Force for the management of acute myocardial infarction in patients presenting with ST-segment elevation of the European Society of Cardiology (ESC). *Eur. Heart J.* **2018**, *39*, 119–177.
8. Roffi, M.; Patrono, C.; Collet, J.P.; Mueller, C.; Valgimigli, M.; Andreotti, F.; Bax, J.J.; Borger, M.A.; Brotons, C.; Chew, D.P.; et al. 2015 ESC Guidelines for the management of acute coronary syndromes in patients presenting without persistent ST-segment elevation: Task Force for the Management of Acute Coronary Syndromes in Patients Presenting without Persistent ST-Segment Elevation of the European Society of Cardiology (ESC). *Eur. Heart J.* **2016**, *37*, 267–315. [PubMed]
9. Mafham, M.; Emberson, J.; Landray, M.J.; Wen, C.P.; Baigent, C. Estimated glomerular filtration rate and the risk of major vascular events and all-cause mortality: A meta-analysis. *PLoS ONE* **2011**, *6*, e25920. [CrossRef]
10. Sarnak, M.J.; Amann, K.; Bangalore, S.; Cavalcante, J.L.; Charytan, D.M.; Craig, J.C.; Gill, J.S.; Hlatky, M.A.; Jardine, A.G.; Landmesser, U.; et al. Chronic Kidney Disease and Coronary Artery Disease: JACC State-of-the-Art Review. *J. Am. Coll. Cardiol.* **2019**, *74*, 1823–1838. [CrossRef] [PubMed]
11. Sharma, K.; Ramachandrarao, S.; Qiu, G.; Usui, H.K.; Zhu, Y.; Dunn, S.R.; Ouedraogo, R.; Hough, K.; McCue, P.; Chan, L.; et al. Adiponectin regulates albuminuria and podocyte function in mice. *J. Clin. Investig.* **2008**, *118*, 1645–1656. [CrossRef]
12. Mason, R.P.; Dawoud, H.; Jacob, R.F.; Sherratt, S.C.R.; Malinski, T. Eicosapentaenoic acid improves endothelial function and nitric oxide bioavailability in a manner that is enhanced in combination with a statin. *Biomed. Pharmacother.* **2018**, *103*, 1231–1237. [CrossRef]
13. Ghayda, R.A.; Lee, J.Y.; Yang, J.W.; Han, C.H.; Jeong, G.H.; Yoon, S.; Hong, S.H.; Lee, K.H.; Gauckler, P.; Kronbichler, A.; et al. The effect of statins on all-cause and cardiovascular mortality in patients with non-dialysis chronic kidney disease, patients on dialysis, and kidney transplanted recipients: An umbrella review of meta-analyses. *Eur. Rev. Med. Pharmacol. Sci.* **2021**, *25*, 2696–2710.
14. Herrington, W.G.; Emberson, J.; Mihaylova, B.; Blackwell, L.; Reith, C.; Solbu, M.D.; Mark, P.B.; Fellström, B.; Jardine, A.G.; Wanner, C.; et al. Impact of renal function on the effects of LDL cholesterol lowering with statin-based regimens: A meta-analysis of individual participant data from 28 randomised trials. *Lancet Diabetes Endocrinol.* **2016**, *4*, 829–839. [PubMed]
15. Palmer, S.C.; Craig, J.C.; Navaneethan, S.D.; Tonelli, M.; Pellegrini, F.; Strippoli, G.F. Benefits and harms of statin therapy for persons with chronic kidney disease: A systematic review and meta-analysis. *Ann. Intern. Med.* **2012**, *157*, 263–275. [CrossRef] [PubMed]
16. Major, R.W.; Cheung, C.K.; Gray, L.J.; Brunskill, N.J. Statins and Cardiovascular Primary Prevention in CKD: A Meta-Analysis. *Clin. J. Am. Soc. Nephrol.* **2015**, *10*, 732–739. [CrossRef]
17. Baigent, C.; Landray, M.J.; Reith, C.; Emberson, J.; Wheeler, D.C.; Tomson, C.; Wanner, C.; Krane, V.; Cass, A.; Craig, J.; et al. The effects of lowering LDL cholesterol with simvastatin plus ezetimibe in patients with chronic kidney disease (Study of Heart and Renal Protection): A randomised placebo-controlled trial. *Lancet* **2011**, *377*, 2181–2192. [CrossRef]
18. Kim, Y.H.; Her, A.Y.; Jeong, M.H.; Kim, B.K.; Hong, S.J.; Kim, J.S.; Ko, Y.G.; Choi, D.; Hong, M.K.; Jang, Y. Impact of stent generation on 2-year clinical outcomes in ST-segment elevation myocardial infarction patients with multivessel disease who underwent culprit-only or multivessel percutaneous coronary intervention. *Catheter. Cardiovasc. Interv.* **2020**, *95*, E40–E55. [CrossRef]
19. Kim, Y.H.; Her, A.Y.; Jeong, M.H.; Kim, B.K.; Hong, S.J.; Kim, S.; Ahn, C.M.; Kim, J.S.; Ko, Y.G.; Choi, D.; et al. Effects of stent generation on clinical outcomes after acute myocardial infarction compared between prediabetes and diabetes patients. *Sci. Rep.* **2021**, *11*, 9364. [CrossRef]
20. National Kidney Foundation. K/DOQI clinical practice guidelines for chronic kidney disease: Evaluation, classification, and stratification. *Am. J. Kidney Dis.* **2002**, *39*, S1–S266.
21. Kim, J.H.; Chae, S.C.; Oh, D.J.; Kim, H.S.; Kim, Y.J.; Ahn, Y.; Cho, M.C.; Kim, C.J.; Yoon, J.H.; Park, H.Y.; et al. Multicenter Cohort Study of Acute Myocardial Infarction in Korea-Interim Analysis of the Korea Acute Myocardial Infarction Registry-National Institutes of Health Registry. *Circ. J.* **2016**, *80*, 1427–1436. [CrossRef] [PubMed]
22. Grech, E.D. ABC of interventional cardiology: Percutaneous coronary intervention. II: The procedure. *BMJ* **2003**, *326*, 1137–1140. [CrossRef] [PubMed]

23. Chen, K.Y.; Rha, S.W.; Li, Y.J.; Poddar, K.L.; Jin, Z.; Minami, Y.; Wang, L.; Kim, E.J.; Park, C.G.; Seo, H.S.; et al. Triple versus dual antiplatelet therapy in patients with acute ST-segment elevation myocardial infarction undergoing primary percutaneous coronary intervention. *Circulation* **2009**, *119*, 3207–3214. [CrossRef]
24. Lee, S.W.; Park, S.W.; Hong, M.K.; Kim, Y.H.; Lee, B.K.; Song, J.M.; Han, K.H.; Lee, C.W.; Kang, D.H.; Song, J.K.; et al. Triple versus dual antiplatelet therapy after coronary stenting: Impact on stent thrombosis. *J. Am. Coll. Cardiol.* **2005**, *46*, 1833–1837. [CrossRef] [PubMed]
25. Levey, A.S.; Stevens, L.A.; Schmid, C.H.; Zhang, Y.L.; Castro, A.F., 3rd; Feldman, H.I.; Kusek, J.W.; Eggers, P.; Van Lente, F.; Greene, T.; et al. A new equation to estimate glomerular filtration rate. *Ann. Intern. Med.* **2009**, *150*, 604–612. [CrossRef] [PubMed]
26. Lee, J.M.; Rhee, T.M.; Hahn, J.Y.; Kim, H.K.; Park, J.; Hwang, D.; Choi, K.H.; Kim, J.; Park, T.K.; Yang, J.H.; et al. Multivessel Percutaneous Coronary Intervention in Patients With ST-Segment Elevation Myocardial Infarction With Cardiogenic Shock. *J. Am. Coll. Cardiol.* **2018**, *71*, 844–856. [CrossRef]
27. Zhang, X.; Xiang, C.; Zhou, Y.H.; Jiang, A.; Qin, Y.Y.; He, J. Effect of statins on cardiovascular events in patients with mild to moderate chronic kidney disease: A systematic review and meta-analysis of randomized clinical trials. *BMC Cardiovas. Disord.* **2014**, *14*, 19. [CrossRef]
28. Palmer, S.C.; Navaneethan, S.D.; Craig, J.C.; Johnson, D.W.; Perkovic, V.; Hegbrant, J.; Strippoli, G.F. HMG CoA reductase inhibitors (statins) for people with chronic kidney disease not requiring dialysis. *Cochrane Database Syst. Rev.* **2014**, *31*, Cd007784.
29. Strippoli, G.F.; Craig, J.C.; Schena, F.P. The number, quality, and coverage of randomized controlled trials in nephrology. *J. Am. Soc. Nephrpol.* **2004**, *15*, 411–419. [CrossRef]
30. Hashimoto, Y.; Ozaki, Y.; Kan, S.; Nakao, K.; Kimura, K.; Ako, J.; Noguchi, T.; Suwa, S.; Fujimoto, K.; Dai, K.; et al. Impact of Chronic Kidney Disease on In-Hospital and 3-Year Clinical Outcomes in Patients With Acute Myocardial Infarction Treated by Contemporary Percutaneous Coronary Intervention and Optimal Medical Therapy-Insights From the J-MINUET Study. *Circ. J.* **2021**, CJ-20. [CrossRef]
31. Herzog, C.A.; Littrell, K.; Arko, C.; Frederick, P.D.; Blaney, M. Clinical characteristics of dialysis patients with acute myocardial infarction in the United States: A collaborative project of the United States Renal Data System and the National Registry of Myocardial Infarction. *Circulation* **2007**, *116*, 1465–1472. [CrossRef]
32. Tsutamoto, T.; Kawahara, C.; Yamaji, M.; Nishiyama, K.; Fujii, M.; Yamamoto, T.; Horie, M. Relationship between renal function and serum cardiac troponin T in patients with chronic heart failure. *Eur. J. Heart Fail.* **2009**, *11*, 653–658. [CrossRef] [PubMed]
33. Manjunath, G.; Tighiouart, H.; Ibrahim, H.; MacLeod, B.; Salem, D.N.; Griffith, J.L.; Coresh, J.; Levey, A.S.; Sarnak, M.J. Level of kidney function as a risk factor for atherosclerotic cardiovascular outcomes in the community. *J. Am. Coll. Cardiol.* **2003**, *41*, 47–55. [CrossRef]
34. London, G.M.; Guérin, A.P.; Marchais, S.J.; Métivier, F.; Pannier, B.; Adda, H. Arterial media calcification in end-stage renal disease: Impact on all-cause and cardiovascular mortality. *Nephrol. Dial. Transplant.* **2003**, *18*, 1731–1740. [CrossRef] [PubMed]
35. Fox, C.S.; Matsushita, K.; Woodward, M.; Bilo, H.J.; Chalmers, J.; Heerspink, H.J.; Lee, B.J.; Perkins, R.M.; Rossing, P.; Sairenchi, T.; et al. Associations of kidney disease measures with mortality and end-stage renal disease in individuals with and without diabetes: A meta-analysis. *Lancet* **2012**, *380*, 1662–1673. [CrossRef]
36. Natsuaki, M.; Furukawa, Y.; Morimoto, T.; Sakata, R.; Kimura, T. Renal function and effect of statin therapy on cardiovascular outcomes in patients undergoing coronary revascularization (from the CREDO-Kyoto PCI/CABG Registry Cohort-2). *Am. J. Cardiol.* **2012**, *110*, 1568–1577. [CrossRef]
37. Petronio, A.S.; Amoroso, G.; Limbruno, U.; Papini, B.; De Carlo, M.; Micheli, A.; Ciabatti, N.; Mariani, M. Simvastatin does not inhibit intimal hyperplasia and restenosis but promotes plaque regression in normocholesterolemic patients undergoing coronary stenting: A randomized study with intravascular ultrasound. *Am. Heart J.* **2005**, *149*, 520–526. [CrossRef]
38. Baigent, C.; Blackwell, L.; Emberson, J.; Holland, L.E.; Reith, C.; Bhala, N.; Peto, R.; Barnes, E.H.; Keech, A.; Simes, J.; et al. Efficacy and safety of more intensive lowering of LDL cholesterol: A meta-analysis of data from 170,000 participants in 26 randomised trials. *Lancet* **2010**, *376*, 1670–1681.
39. Walter, D.H.; Schächinger, V.; Elsner, M.; Mach, S.; Auch-Schwelk, W.; Zeiher, A.M. Effect of statin therapy on restenosis after coronary stent implantation. *Am. J. Cardiol.* **2000**, *85*, 962–968. [CrossRef]
40. Crimi, G.; Gritti, V.; Galiffa, V.A.; Scotti, V.; Leonardi, S.; Ferrario, M.; Ferlini, M.; De Ferrari, G.M.; Oltrona Visconti, L.; Klersy, C. Drug eluting stents are superior to bare metal stents to reduce clinical outcome and stent-related complications in CKD patients, a systematic review, meta-analysis and network meta-analysis. *J. Interv. Cardiol.* **2018**, *31*, 319–329. [CrossRef]
41. Volodarskiy, A.; Kumar, S.; Pracon, R.; Sidhu, M.; Kretov, E.; Mazurek, T.; Bockeria, O.; Kaul, U.; Bangalore, S. Drug-Eluting vs. Bare-Metal Stents in Patients with Chronic Kidney Disease and Coronary Artery Disease: Insights From a Systematic Review and Meta-Analysis. *J. Invasive Cardiol.* **2018**, *30*, 10–17. [PubMed]
42. Arbustini, E.; Dal Bello, B.; Morbini, P.; Burke, A.P.; Bocciarelli, M.; Specchia, G.; Virmani, R. Plaque erosion is a major substrate for coronary thrombosis in acute myocardial infarction. *Heart* **1999**, *82*, 269–272. [CrossRef]
43. Ozaki, Y.; Okumura, M.; Ismail, T.F.; Motoyama, S.; Naruse, H.; Hattori, K.; Kawai, H.; Sarai, M.; Takagi, Y.; Ishii, J.; et al. Coronary CT angiographic characteristics of culprit lesions in acute coronary syndromes not related to plaque rupture as defined by optical coherence tomography and angioscopy. *Eur. Heart J.* **2011**, *32*, 2814–2823. [CrossRef] [PubMed]
44. Özyilmaz, A.; Bakker, S.J.; de Zeeuw, D.; de Jong, P.E.; Gansevoort, R.T. Selection on albuminuria enhances the efficacy of screening for cardiovascular risk factors. *Nephrol. Dial. Transplant.* **2010**, *25*, 3560–3568. [CrossRef] [PubMed]

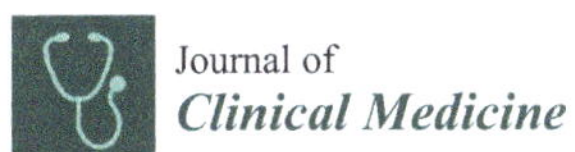
Journal of
Clinical Medicine

MDPI

Article

Incremental Diagnostic Value of CT Fractional Flow Reserve Using Subtraction Method in Patients with Severe Calcification: A Pilot Study

Yuki Kamo [1], Shinichiro Fujimoto [1,*], Yui O. Nozaki [1], Chihiro Aoshima [1], Yuko O. Kawaguchi [1], Tomotaka Dohi [1], Ayako Kudo [1], Daigo Takahashi [1], Kazuhisa Takamura [1], Makoto Hiki [1], Iwao Okai [1], Shinya Okazaki [1], Nobuo Tomizawa [2], Kanako K. Kumamaru [2], Shigeki Aoki [2] and Tohru Minamino [1,3]

1 Department of Cardiovascular Biology and Medicine, Juntendo University Graduate School of Medicine, Tokyo 113-8421, Japan; y-kawai@juntendo.ac.jp (Y.K.); y-nozaki@juntendo.ac.jp (Y.O.N.); caoshima@juntendo.ac.jp (C.A.); yukawagu@juntendo.ac.jp (Y.O.K.); tdohi@juntendo.ac.jp (T.D.); a.kudo.gt@juntendo.ac.jp (A.K.); d-takahashi@juntendo.ac.jp (D.T.); k-takamu@juntendo.ac.jp (K.T.); m-hiki@juntendo.ac.jp (M.H.); okaiwao@juntendo.ac.jp (I.O.); shinya@juntendo.ac.jp (S.O.); t.minamino@juntendo.ac.jp (T.M.)

2 Department of Radiology, Juntendo University Graduate School of Medicine, Tokyo 113-8421, Japan; n-tomizawa@juntendo.ac.jp (N.T.); k-kumamaru@juntendo.ac.jp (K.K.K.); s-aoki@juntendo.ac.jp (S.A.)

3 Japan Agency for Medical Research and Development-Core Research for Evolutionary Medical Science and Technology (AMED-CREST), Japan Agency for Medical Research and Development, Tokyo 100-0004, Japan

* Correspondence: s-fujimo@tj8.so-net.ne.jp; Tel.: +81-3-5802-1056

Citation: Kamo, Y.; Fujimoto, S.; Nozaki, Y.O.; Aoshima, C.; Kawaguchi, Y.O.; Dohi, T.; Kudo, A.; Takahashi, D.; Takamura, K.; Hiki, M.; et al. Incremental Diagnostic Value of CT Fractional Flow Reserve Using Subtraction Method in Patients with Severe Calcification: A Pilot Study. *J. Clin. Med.* **2021**, *10*, 4398. https://doi.org/10.3390/jcm10194398

Academic Editors: Koichi Node and Atsushi Tanaka

Received: 10 August 2021
Accepted: 22 September 2021
Published: 26 September 2021

Abstract: Although on-site workstation-based CT fractional flow reserve (CT-FFR) is an emerging method for assessing vessel-specific ischemia in coronary artery disease, severe calcification is a significant factor affecting CT-FFR's diagnostic performance. The subtraction method significantly improves the diagnostic value with respect to anatomic stenosis for patients with severe calcification in coronary CT angiography (CCTA). We evaluated the diagnostic capability of CT-FFR using the subtraction method (subtraction CT-FFR) in patients with severe calcification. This study included 32 patients with 45 lesions with severe calcification (Agatston score >400) who underwent both CCTA and subtraction CCTA using 320-row area detector CT and also received invasive FFR within 90 days. The diagnostic capabilities of CT-FFR and subtraction CT-FFR were compared. The sensitivities, specificities, positive predictive values (PPVs), and negative predictive values (NPVs) of CT-FFR vs. subtraction CT-FFR for detecting hemodynamically significant stenosis, defined as FFR ≤ 0.8, were 84.6% vs. 92.3%, 59.4% vs. 75.0%, 45.8% vs. 60.0%, and 90.5% vs. 96.0%, respectively. The area under the curve for subtraction CT-FFR was significantly higher than for CT-FFR (0.84 vs. 0.70) ($p = 0.04$). The inter-observer and intra-observer variabilities of subtraction CT-FFR were 0.76 and 0.75, respectively. In patients with severe calcification, subtraction CT-FFR had an incremental diagnostic value over CT-FFR, increasing the specificity and PPV while maintaining the sensitivity and NPV with high reproducibility.

Keywords: coronary CT angiography; subtraction; fractional flow reserve; coronary artery disease; Agatston score

1. Introduction

Multiple methods for non-invasively calculating fractional flow reserve (FFR) have been developed based on coronary computed tomography angiography (CCTA) images, and all have been reported to add an incremental diagnostic value to conventional CCTA using invasive FFR as a reference [1–6]. However, variations have been reported in specificity and the positive predictive value, compared to sensitivity and the negative predictive value [7–9].

A FFR calculation algorithm was developed from CCTA acquired via 320-row area detector CT (320-ADCT) using fluid–structure interaction as a method for CT-derived FFR (CT-FFR). This is considered to be capable of setting conditions unique to each patient in CT-FFR calculations, based on the shape, movement, cross-sectional area, and changes in the volume of the coronary artery, by acquiring multiple optimum cardiac phases from 70–99% of the cardiac phase data within one heartbeat and analyzing these data based on the hierarchical Bayes and Markov chain Monte Carlo method [10,11]. In addition, on-site analysis at a workstation is possible by calculating the 1D computational fluid dynamics. The diagnostic performance of CT-FFR with the positivity criterion defined as the invasive FFR $\leq$0.8 has previously been demonstrated, with the rate of accurate diagnosis being significantly higher than that of conventional CCTA; however, similarly to other methods, the specificity was lower than the sensitivity [12,13]. Contributing factors may be overestimation of the severity of stenosis or underestimation of the vascular diameter due to the spatial resolution and the influence of artifacts generated by calcification in the case of CCTA [14]. We previously reported that the specificity of CT-FFR markedly decreases in cases with severe calcification (Agatston score $\geq$400) and the presence of calcified plaques was identified as the strongest factor predicting false positivity in CT-FFR [12,15].

A method termed "subtraction" has recently been developed in which the influence of calcification is removed from the vascular lumen in order to observe the degree of stenosis of lesions by differentiating non-contrast-enhanced CT information from contrast-enhanced CT information [16]. Improvements have been achieved in the diagnostic performance of CCTA for invasive coronary angiography by using the subtraction method in severe calcification cases [17]; however, it has not yet been applied to CT-FFR.

The present study investigated the incremental diagnostic value of CT-FFR evaluated via CCTA where calcification was removed using the subtraction method in patients with severe calcification (Agatston score $\geq$ 400).

2. Materials and Methods

2.1. Study Population

Data accounting for 70–99% of the R-R interval within one heartbeat, from which CT-FFR may be calculated, were collected from 1594 out of 2742 patients who were examined for suspected coronary artery disease by CCTA using 320-ADCT between 1 January 2016 and 31 December 2019. The coronary artery calcification score (Agatston score) measured using a non-contrast CT scan was 400 or higher in 264 patients. Following the exclusion of patients judged as having difficulty in breath-holding for 25 s before imaging and those with large variations in heart rate during breath-holding (judged as inappropriate for the subtraction method), the final number of patients from whom images were acquired using the subtraction method was 195.

Invasive FFR was performed within 90 days of CCTA in 42 out of the 195 patients, consent to participation in the study was obtained from 37 patients (53 vessels), and the CT-FFR analysis was ultimately performed on 32 patients (45 vessels).

The present study was approved by the institutional Human Research Ethics Committee and all participants gave written informed consent. All procedures followed the principles of the Declaration of Helsinki.

2.2. Subtraction CCTA Acquisition

Patients with a pre-scan heart rate of $\geq$60 beats per minute were orally administered 20 to 40 mg of metoprolol. If their heart rate remained $\geq$60 beats per minute after 1 h, they were given an intravenous injection of landiolol (0.125 mg/kg) (Corebeta; Ono Pharmaceutical, Tokyo, Japan). Patients for whom beta-blockers were contraindicated (due to severe aortic stenosis, systolic blood pressure < 90 mmHg, bronchial asthma, symptomatic heart failure, or advanced atrioventricular block) did not receive these treatments. All patients received 0.6 mg of nitroglycerin sublingually (Myocor spray; Toa Eiyo, Tokyo, Japan).

CCTA was performed using 320-row CT equipment (Aquilion ONE Vision Edition, or GENESIS Edition; Canon Medical Systems Corporation, Otawara, Japan) with a collimation of 320 × 0.5 mm. All scans were performed at the fastest gantry rotation time of 275 ms using the prospective ECG-gated axial scan mode.

Each patient underwent an unenhanced scan at a tube voltage of 120 kVp and a tube current of 250 mA for calcium scoring. Images were reconstructed with a slice thickness of 3.0 mm and increments of 3.0 mm.

Patients received 18.0 mg of iodine/kg/s of iopamidol (Iopamiron 370 mg of iodine/kg; Bayer Holding Ltd., Osaka, Japan). A contrast medium was injected for 12 s, followed by 30 mL of a saline chaser. Two CCTA scans were performed during the subtraction CCTA examination [16,18–20]. Patients were asked to hold their breath immediately after the contrast medium injection started. The first scan was performed 5 s after the contrast medium injection started. The bolus tracking method was used to select the scan timing for the second scan. The second scan was performed 2 s after the CT number for the descending aorta reached 270 Hounsfield units (HU). Patients were asked to continue holding their breath throughout the scan (≈25 s). The scanning parameters for CCTA were as follows: tube voltage, 100 kVp (body mass index <30 kg/m^2) or 120 kVp (body mass index ≥ 30 kg/m^2); target SD, 22.0; scan coverage 100–160 mm; acquisition window, 70–99% of the R-R interval. Half-reconstruction was performed with a slice thickness of 0.5 mm and an increment of 0.25 mm, using a medium-soft tissue kernel (FC04) with adaptive iterative dose reductions using three-dimensional processing (AIDR3D; Canon Medical Systems). In each scan, four phases (70, 80, 90, and 99%) were reconstructed for the CT-FFR analysis. In addition, the phase with the minimum number of artifacts was selected at the CT console using cardiac-phase search software (PhaseNavi; Canon Medical Systems Corporation) for the visual CCTA analysis.

The subtraction CCTA images were derived using dedicated software (^{SURE}Subtraction; Canon Medical Systems). Specifically, volume datasets of all parts of the images obtained by pre-contrast CT and post-contrast CT were used to create the subtraction image by subtracting the CT value of each pixel in the pre-contrast CT image from the CT value of the corresponding pixel in the post-contrast CT image. Global non-rigid registration followed by local rigid registration was performed to obtain the subtraction image. As a result, the obtained subtraction images were images of the target segments with calcification only [19–21].

During processing, images were transferred to a workstation (Zio M900; Ziosoft Inc., Tokyo, Japan and Vitrea; Canon Medical Systems Corporation, Otawara, Japan). The mean effective dose was derived from the dose–length product multiplied by a conversion coefficient for the chest (κ = 0.014 mSv/mGy/cm) [22].

2.3. Calcium Scoring

A calcified lesion was defined as ≥3 contiguous pixels with a peak attenuation of at least 130 Hounsfield units (HU) [23]. Lesion scores from the left main, left anterior descending, left circumflex, and right coronary arteries were summed to obtain the total calcium score.

2.4. CCTA Interpretation

Cross-sectional and longitudinal curved multi-planar reformation images were both analyzed for plaque detection. Coronary artery segments with diameters of ≥2 mm were evaluated for the degree of stenosis. The percent degree of stenosis was assessed by obtaining the percent ratio of the stenotic lumen to the normal vessel diameter proximal or distal to the stenosis. Stenosis was measured at the angle showing the narrowest degree of stenosis. The degree of stenosis was evaluated by consensus by three experienced cardiologists who were unaware of the clinical data. Lesions with >50% stenosis were defined as significant. When a lesion stenosis was considered to be impossible to assess due to heavy calcification, it was classified as significant (>50% stenosis).

2.5. CT-FFR Analysis

CT-FFR was calculated using non-commercial software (CT-FFR; Canon Medical Systems). Using the phase with the minimum number of artifacts, the vascular central line and contours were automatically identified and manually corrected when necessary. Vessel segmentation was applied to the other three phases. The boundary condition was identified using variations in the vascular cross-sectional area in the images of the four different phases (70, 80, 90, and 99%). Pressure and flow values throughout the coronary artery were then calculated by performing a fluid analysis. CT-FFR was calculated for the original and the subtracted data. CT-FFR was calculated using a previously reported method [11,12,15,24].

The CT-FFR analyses were performed by observers who had more than 50 h of experience using this software. Observers were blinded to the invasive angiography and FFR findings.

2.6. Reproducibility Analysis

To evaluate inter- and intra-observer variabilities in the subtraction CT-FFR calculation, another operator who had more than 50 h of experience using this software performed post-processing for 30 consecutive vessels. The second operator also repeated post-processing for 30 consecutive vessels approximately 1 month after the first analysis, to evaluate intra-observer variability. In each case, for each vessel and for each operator, subtraction CT-FFR values were compared with those measured at the same position in invasive FFR. Anatomical landmarks, such as calcium deposits and/or side branches, were used to obtain subtraction CT-FFR at the same location for different operators.

2.7. Invasive FFR

Pressure measurements were performed using a 0.014-inch pressure guide wire (Verrata Pressure Guide Wire, Volcano Corp., San Diego, CA, USA) and suitable software (s5x™ Imaging System, Volcano Corp., San Diego, CA, USA). The pressure wire was calibrated and equalized with aortic pressure before being placed distal to the stenosis and in the distal third of the coronary artery being interrogated.

FFR was measured as the mean distal coronary pressure (Pd) divided by the mean aortic pressure (Pa) during maximal hyperemia. In brief, FFR was measured with a coronary pressure guide wire at maximal hyperemia induced by adenosine triphosphate (ATP) administered at 140 μg/kg/min for at least 2 min through a large forearm vein using an infusion pump until heart rate began to increase and the Pd/Pa ratio remained constant. Pressure wire pullback was performed to check for FFR at each lesion segment and pressure drift. If a Pd/Pa ratio <0.98 or >1.02 at the catheter tip was documented, the protocol mandated a repeat assessment. An FFR value of ≤ 0.8 was selected to define hemodynamically significant stenosis [25,26].

2.8. Definition of Risk Factors

Hypertension was defined as either systolic or diastolic blood pressure $\geq$ 140/90 mmHg or the use of antihypertensive medications. Diabetes mellitus was defined as fasting blood sugar $\geq$ 7.0 mmol/L (126 mg/dL), postprandial blood sugar $\geq$ 11.0 mmol/L (200 mg/dL), hemoglobin A1c $\geq$ 6.5% (47.5 mmol/mol), or the use of antidiabetic medications. Dyslipidemia was defined as total cholesterol $\geq$ 5.7 mmol/L (220 mg/dL), low-density lipoprotein cholesterol > 3.6 mmol/L (140 mg/dL), fasting triglycerides $\geq$ 1.7 mmol/L (150 mg/dL), high density cholesterol < 1.0 mmol/L (40 mg/dL), or the use of lipid-lowering medications. Smokers were defined as patients who had smoked during the past 1 year from the time of CCTA acquisition.

2.9. Statistical Analysis

Continuous data were expressed as the mean ± standard deviation (SD). If the variables were non-normally distributed, the median and quartile values were used. When the median and quartile data were 0, the maximum and minimum results were added in the form of the median (quartile; range). Categorical data were expressed as frequencies (percentages). Intraclass correlation coefficients were used to evaluate inter- and intra-observer variabilities for the subtraction CT-FFR analysis. The sensitivities, specificities, positive predictive values, negative predictive values, and diagnostic accuracy values of CCTA > 50% vs. subtraction CCTA > 50% vs. CT-FFR vs. subtraction CT-FFR ≤ 0.8, with respect to detecting hemodynamically significant stenosis defined as invasive FFR ≤ 0.8, were calculated. Diagnostic accuracy values using the area under the curve (AUC) of the receiver operating characteristic (ROC) curve to detect invasive FFR ≤ 0.8 were compared for CCTA > 50% vs. subtraction CCTA > 50% vs. CT-FFR ≤ 0.8 vs. subtraction CT-FFR ≤ 0.8 using the DeLong test, and p-values of <0.05 were considered to be significant. The statistical analyses were performed using JMP software for Windows (SAS Institute Inc., Cary, CA, USA).

3. Results

3.1. Patient and Scan Characteristics

The patient and scan characteristics are shown in Table 1. The mean age of patients was 70.8 ± 7.8 years and the mean Agatston score was 1014.6 (523.9–1382.5). Twenty-two patients (68.8%) had taken β blockers before the acquisition of images and the mean heart rate at acquisition was 54.0 ± 4.6. None of the patients were administered intravenous iopamidol before imaging. All patients received nitroglycerin sublingually before imaging. The mean radiation exposure dose was 4.2 ± 1.1 mSv.

Table 1. Patient and scan characteristics.

32 Patients	
Age (years)	70.8 ± 7.8
Gender (M/F)	22/11
Body mass index (Kg/m^2)	24.3 ± 3.1
Diabetes mellitus (%)	16 (50.0)
Hypertension (%)	22 (68.8)
Dyslipidemia (%)	21 (65.6)
Smoking	
current/former/never	2/17/13
Heart rate (bpm)	54.0 ± 4.6
Total CACS [1] (Agatston score)	1014.6 (523.9–1382.5)
β blocker administered (%)	
None	10 (31.3)
Oral	22 (68.8)
Intravenous	0 (0)
Nitrates administered	32 (100)
Tube voltage (%)	
100 kVp	27 (84.4)
120 kVp	5 (15.6)
Tube current (mA)	559.6 ± 43.8
DLPe [2] (mGy.cm)	299.3 ± 80.3
Effective dose (mSV)	4.2 ± 1.1

[1] CACS: coronary artery calcium score; [2] DLPe: extended dose–length product.

3.2. Vessel Characteristics

Patient-based analysis gave the following results: CCTA > 50% (31 patients (96.9%)), subtraction CCTA > 50% (22 (68.8%)), CT-FFR ≤ 0.8 (19 (59.4%)), and subtraction CT-FFR ≤ 0.8 (12 (37.5%)). Eleven patients (34.4%) showed invasive FFR ≤ 0.8.

Vessel-based analysis gave the following results: CCTA > 50% (42 vessels (93.3%)), subtraction CCTA > 50% (32 (71.1%)), CT-FFR ≤ 0.8 (25 (55.6%)), and subtraction CT-FFR ≤ 0.8 (20 (44.4%)). Thirteen vessels (28.9%) showed invasive FFR ≤ 0.8 (Table 2).

Table 2. Vessel characteristics.

32 Patients, 45 Vessels		
	Patient	Vessel
CCTA [1] maximum stenosis > 50% (%)	31 (96.9)	42 (93.3)
Subtraction CCTA maximum stenosis > 50% (%)	22 (68.8)	32 (71.1)
CT-FFR [2] ≤ 0.8 (%)	19 (59.4)	25 (55.6)
Subtraction CT-FFR ≤ 0.8 (%)	12 (37.5)	20 (44.4)
Invasive FFR ≤ 0.8 (%)	11 (34.4)	13 (28.9)
RCA/LAD/LCX	13/20/12	
CACS [3]		
RCA [4]	343.7 (124.0–632.3)	
LAD [5]	348.4 (243.0–611.0)	
LCX [6]	116.5 (55.1–252.3)	

[1] CCTA: coronary computed tomography angiography; [2] FFR: fractional flow reserve; [3] CACS: coronary artery calcium score; [4] RCA: right coronary artery; [5] LAD: left anterior descending artery; [6] LCX: left circumflex artery.

3.3. Diagnostic Accuracy of CCTA Findings, CT-FFR, and Subtraction CT-FFR

Table 3 shows the measurements of the diagnostic performances of CCTA > 50%, subtraction CCTA > 50%, CT-FFR ≤ 0.8, and subtraction CT-FFR ≤ 0.8 in detecting hemodynamically significant stenosis defined as invasive FFR ≤ 0.80.

Table 3. Diagnostic accuracies of CCTA findings, CT-FFR, subtraction CCTA and subtraction CT-FFR on a per patient and per vessel basis.

	(a) Per Patient			
	CCTA [1] findings	Subtraction CTA	CT-FFR [2]	Subtraction CT-FFR
True positive (*n*)	12	10	10	10
True negative (*n*)	2	6	12	9
False positive (*n*)	18	14	9	2
False negative (*n*)	0	2	1	1
Sensitivity (%)	100	83.3	90.9	90.9
True negative (%)	10.0	30.0	57.1	90.5
False positive (%)	40.0	41.7	52.6	83.3
False negative (%)	100	75.0	92.3	95.0
Accuracy (%)	43.8	50.0	68.8	90.6
	(b) Per Vessel			
	CCTA findings	Subtraction CTA	CT-FFR	Subtraction CT-FFR
True positive (*n*)	13	11	11	12
True negative (*n*)	3	10	19	24
False positive (*n*)	29	22	13	8
False negative (*n*)	0	2	2	1
Sensitivity (%)	100	84.6	94.6	92.3
True negative (%)	9.4	31.3	59.4	75.0
False positive (%)	31.0	33.3	45.8	60.0
False negative (%)	100	83.3	90.5	96.0
Accuracy (%)	35.6	46.7	66.7	80.0

[1] CCTA: coronary computed tomography angiography; [2] FFR: fractional flow reserve.

In the patient-based analysis (Table 3a), the sensitivities, specificities, PPV, NPV, and accuracy values of CCTA > 50%, subtraction CCTA > 50%, CT-FFR ≤ 0.8, and subtraction CT-FFR ≤ 0.8 were 100% vs. 83.3% vs. 90.9% vs. 90.9%, 10.0% vs. 30.0% vs. 57.1% vs. 90.5%, 40.0% vs. 41.7% vs. 52.6% vs. 83.3%, 100% vs. 75.0% vs. 92.3% vs. 95.0%, and 43.8% vs. 50.0% vs. 68.8% vs. 90.6%, respectively.

In the vessel-based analysis (Table 3b), the sensitivities of CCTA > 50%, subtraction CCTA > 50%, CT-FFR ≤ 0.8, and subtraction CT-FFR ≤ 0.8 were 100% vs. 84.6% vs. 84.6% vs. 92.3%, the specificities were 9.4% vs. 31.3% vs. 59.4% vs. 75.0%, the PPV scores were 31.0% vs. 33.3% vs. 45.8% vs. 60.0%, the NPV scores were 100% vs. 83.3% vs. 90.5% vs. 96.0%, and the accuracy values were 35.6% vs. 46.7% vs. 66.7% vs. 80.0%, respectively.

Figure 1 shows that the vessel-based AUCs for CCTA > 50%, subtraction CCTA > 50%, CT-FFR ≤ 0.8, and subtraction CT-FFR ≤ 0.8 for invasive FFR ≤ 0.8 were 0.55 (95% confidence interval (CI): 0.50–0.60) vs. 0.60 (95% CI: 0.46–0.73) vs. 0.70 (95% CI: 0.57–0.84) vs. 0.84 (95% CI 0.73–0.94), respectively. Significant differences were noted between CCTA > 50% vs. CT-FFR ($p = 0.02$), CCTA > 50% vs. subtraction CT-FFR ≤ 0.8 ($p < 0.01$), CT-FFR ≤ 0.8 vs. subtraction CT-FFR ≤ 0.8 ($p = 0.04$), and subtraction CCTA > 50% vs. subtraction CT-FFR ≤ 0.8 ($p < 0.01$).

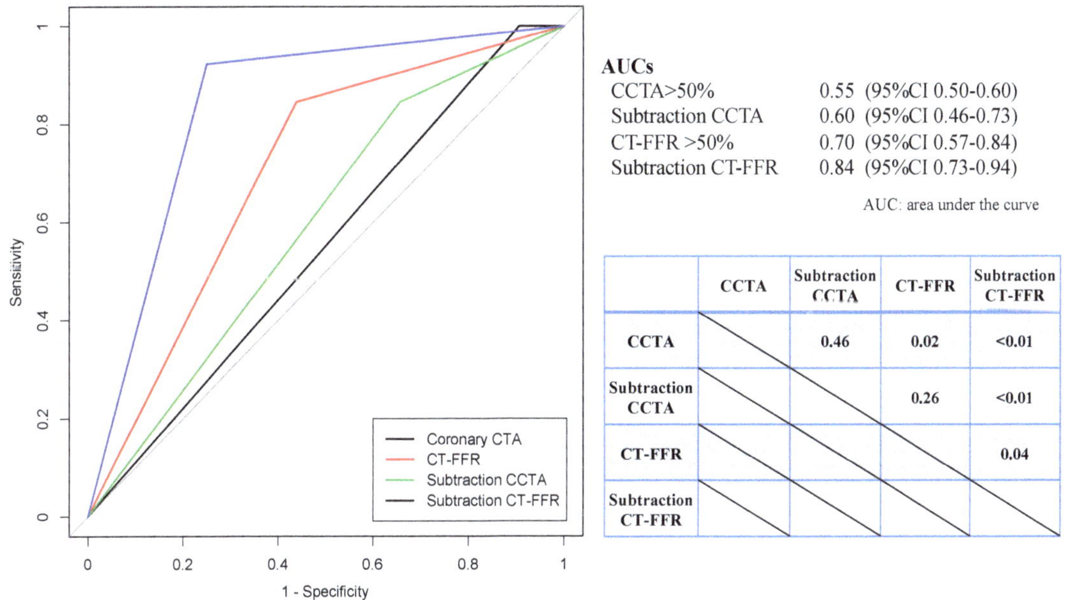

	CCTA	Subtraction CCTA	CT-FFR	Subtraction CT-FFR
CCTA		0.46	0.02	<0.01
Subtraction CCTA			0.26	<0.01
CT-FFR				0.04
Subtraction CT-FFR				

Figure 1. Comparison of areas under the curve (AUC) for the receiver operating characteristic curves of CCTA > 50%, subtraction CCTA > 50%, CT-FFR ≤ 0.8, subtraction CT-FFR ≤ 0.8.

A representative case is shown in Figure 2.

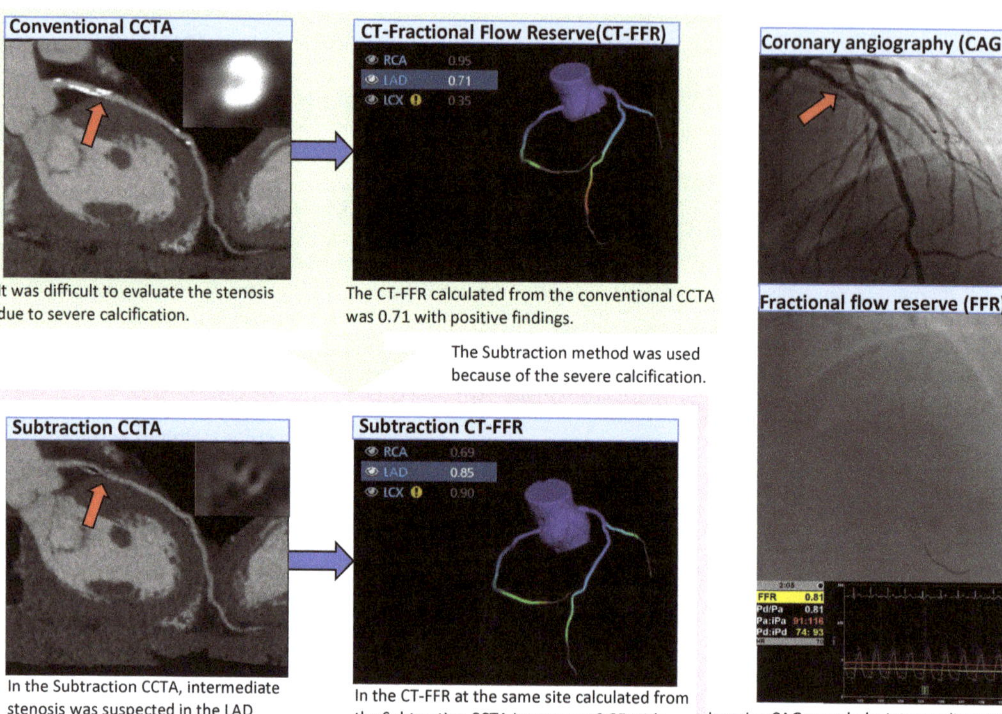

Figure 2. Representative case of subtraction CT-FFR. Since the Agatston score was 738.8, CCTA was performed using the subtraction method. In conventional CCTA, a calcified plaque was found in the LAD proximal.

3.4. Inter-Observer and Intra-Observer Reproducibility

In the analysis of 30 consecutive vessels, the correlation coefficient of inter-intra observer evaluation was 0.76 and the intra-observer–intraclass correlation coefficient was 0.75.

4. Discussion

To the best of our knowledge, this is the first study to apply the subtraction method to CT-FFR. Since the specificity of CT-FFR has previously been reported to be lower than the sensitivity using invasive FFR as a reference [12,13], unnecessary revascularization may result in an increase in false positive cases only, based on the results of CT-FFR. To overcome this problem, we reported the influence of pre-test probability on diagnostic performance as well as improvements in diagnostic performance using the correction formula for CT-FFR [24], and we also demonstrated that the strongest factor associated with false positivity was the presence of calcification [15]. Thus, we hypothesized that false positivity may be reduced by analyzing CT-FFR in images from which coronary arterial calcification had been removed using the subtraction method, particularly in cases with severe calcification. The subtraction CT-FFR method achieved a higher specificity and PPV than CT-FFR analyzed using conventional CCTA images, while maintaining the sensitivity and NPV, thereby reducing the false positive cases from nine to two patients in the patient-based analysis and from thirteen to eight lesions in the vessel-based analysis. Therefore, subtraction CT-FFR significantly increased the diagnostic accuracy, suggesting that overestimations of the degree of stenosis and underestimations of the vascular diameter due to the influence of spatial resolution and artifacts generated by calcification in the

CT-FFR analysis are the major factors leading to false positive cases, particularly in cases with severe calcification. However, in a previous study using FFR_{CT} (HeartFlow Inc., Redwood City, CA, USA), no significant difference in diagnostic performance due to the severity of calcification was noted, while the diagnostic performance of FFR_{CT} tended to be lower when limited to the subgroup with severe calcification similar to the calcification in this study [27]. The CT-FFR technique used in the present study is an on-site local computational analysis technique and the contours of the vascular wall and inner lumen are analyzed semi-automatically; therefore, manual correction may be necessary depending on individual cases. The images with severe calcification required more manual correction in the present study. The objectivity and accuracy of not only automatic extraction but also manual correction can be improved in subtraction images. We previously reported that analytical accuracy is stabilized by the training of analysts for CT-FFR [28,29] and that the inter-observer and intra-observer reproducibility of subtraction CT-FFR was also favorable.

However, among the 53 vessels remaining after participant consents were obtained, 3 vessels for both CT-FFR and subtraction CT-FFR, 1 vessel for CT-FFR alone, and 4 vessels for subtraction CT-FFR alone could not be analyzed. One of the reasons was that in conventional CT-FFR, the boundary between the inner lumen and wall became unclear due to calcification-induced artifacts and the inner lumen was visualized as narrower than it actually was. Moreover, in subtraction CT-FFR, calcified lesions were visualized as larger, due to the misregistration caused by the blurring of images in the differentiation of non-contrast-enhanced CT images from contrast-enhanced CT images in which the inner lumen is visualized as narrower. This may also be a factor contributing to false positivity in the 8 out of 45 vessels from which the analytical results of subtraction CT-FFR were acquired. Since non-contrast-enhanced and contrast-enhanced CT images cannot be simultaneously acquired, misregistration may be due to factors such as the heart rate [30], poor breath-holding [31], and body movement during imaging.

Misregistration is an important issue in the use of the subtraction method. In a previous study, misregistration was noted in approximately 50% of the segments of CCTA images acquired using the subtraction method and the frequency of misregistration increased as the lesion became a distal site [30]. However, in the present study, misregistration was found in only approximately 15% of vessels. To reduce the misregistration and increase the diagnostic accuracy of subtraction CT-FFR, appropriate cases should be selected.

Moreover, the radiation exposure dose was higher in the subtraction method than in conventional imaging because images were acquired twice for comparisons between contrast-enhanced and non-contrast-enhanced imaging. A previous study reported that the effective radiation dose in subtraction CCTA acquired using the single breath-holding method was 5.2–10 mSv [16]; however, the effective radiation dose was reduced to 4.2 ± 1.1 mSv in the present study by applying low-voltage imaging at 100 kVp in patients with a body mass index of 30 or lower [17], and this method was considered to be acceptable for clinical use.

Limitations

There are some limitations that need to be addressed. This was a single-center study with a small number of subjects. Among patients with severe calcification, CT-FFR analysis was only performed on the images with an R-R interval of 70–99% in the diastolic phase of one heartbeat. Furthermore, acquisition using the subtraction method was limited to those patients who were judged to be capable of holding their breath for at least 25 s. Accordingly, 195 out of 264 patients with severe calcification could actually be imaged using the subtraction method. In addition, although the radiation dose was relatively low because in most of the patients CCTA was performed with a tube voltage of 100 kVp as previously described, a higher radiation dose than that for ordinary CCTA is one of the weak points of this subtraction method. This method was only analyzed using 320-row CT equipment and the specific software mentioned, which is likely to represent limited versatility. Furthermore, the indication of invasive coronary angiography and invasive FFR within 90 days depended on the judgment of the attending physicians according to the results of CCTA, suggesting that case selection was biased.

5. Conclusions

By analyzing CT-FFR images of severely calcified lesions (Agatston score ≥400) acquired using the subtraction method, the number of false positive CT-FFR cases was reduced and the diagnostic performance was also significantly improved.

Author Contributions: Conceptualization, Y.K. and S.F.; methodology, Y.K. and S.F.; software, S.F.; formal analysis, Y.K.; investigation, Y.K., Y.O.N., C.A., Y.O.K., A.K., D.T., K.T., M.H., I.O., T.D., and S.O.; resources, S.F.; data curation, Y.K., Y.O.N., C.A., Y.O.K., A.K., D.T., and K.T.; writing—original draft preparation, Y.K.; writing—reviewing and editing, S.F., N.T., and K.K.K.; visualization, Y.K.; supervision, S.A. and T.M.; project administration, S.F.; funding acquisition, S.F. All authors have read and agreed to the published version of the manuscript.

Funding: This research was supported by Canon Medical Systems Corporation.

Institutional Review Board Statement: The study was conducted according to the guidelines of the Declaration of Helsinki and approved by the Ethics Committee of Juntendo University (protocol code 15-130, November 2015).

Informed Consent Statement: Informed consent was obtained from all subjects involved in the study. Written informed consent has been obtained from the patient(s) to the publication of this paper.

Acknowledgments: We are indebted to Yosuke Kogure, RT and Hidekazu Inage, RT for technical assistance in this study.

Conflicts of Interest: Shinichiro Fujimoto has a research agreement with Canon Medical Systems Corporation that is related to this study. All other authors declare no conflict of interest.

References

1. Koo, B.K.; Erglis, A.; Doh, J.H.; Daniels, D.V.; Jegere, S.; Kim, H.S.; Dunning, A.; DeFrance, T.; Lansky, A.; Leipsic, J.; et al. Diagnosis of ischemia-causing coronary stenoses by noninvasive fractional flow reserve computed from coronary computed tomographic angiograms. Results from the prospective multicenter DISCOVER-FLOW (Diagnosis of Ischemia-Causing Stenoses Obtained Via Noninvasive Fractional Flow Reserve) study. *J. Am. Coll. Cardiol.* **2011**, *58*, 1989–1997. [CrossRef]
2. Min, J.K.; Leipsic, J.; Pencina, M.J.; Berman, D.S.; Koo, B.K.; van Mieghem, C.; Erglis, A.; Lin, F.Y.; Dunning, A.M.; Apruzzese, P.; et al. Diagnostic accuracy of fractional flow reserve from anatomic CT angiography. *JAMA* **2012**, *308*, 1237–1245. [CrossRef]
3. Nørgaard, B.L.; Leipsic, J.; Gaur, S.; Seneviratne, S.; Ko, B.S.; Ito, H.; Jensen, J.M.; Mauri, L.; De Bruyne, B.; Bezerra, H.; et al. Diagnostic performance of noninvasive fractional flow reserve derived from coronary computed tomography angiography in suspected coronary artery disease: The NXT trial (Analysis of Coronary Blood Flow Using CT Angiography: Next Steps). *J. Am. Coll. Cardiol.* **2014**, *63*, 1145–1155. [CrossRef]
4. Coenen, A.; Lubbers, M.M.; Kurata, A.; Kono, A.; Dedic, A.; Chelu, R.G.; Dijkshoorn, M.L.; Gijsen, F.J.; Ouhlous, M.; van Geuns, R.-J.M.; et al. Fractional flow reserve computed from noninvasive CT angiography data: Diagnostic performance of an on-site clini-cian-operated computational fluid dynamics algorithm. *Radiology* **2015**, *274*, 674–683. [CrossRef]
5. De Geer, J.; Sandstedt, M.; Björkholm, A.; Alfredsson, J.; Janzon, M.; Engvall, J.; Persson, A. Software-based on-site estimation of fractional flow reserve using standard coronary CT angiography data. *Acta Radiol.* **2016**, *57*, 1186–1192. [CrossRef] [PubMed]
6. Tang, C.X.; Liu, C.Y.; Lu, M.J.; Schoepf, U.J.; Tesche, C.; Bayer, R.R.; Hudson, H.T.; Zhang, X.L.; Li, J.H.; Wang, Y.N.; et al. CT FFR for Ischemia-Specific CAD with a New Computational Fluid Dynamics Algorithm: A Chinese Multicenter Study. *JACC Cardiovasc. Imaging* **2020**, *13*, 980–990. [CrossRef]
7. Wu, W.; Pan, D.R.; Foin, N.; Pang, S.; Ye, P.; Holm, N.; Ren, X.-M.; Luo, J.; Nanjundappa, A.; Chen, S.-L. Noninvasive fractional flow reserve derived from coronary computed tomography angiography for identification of ischemic lesions: A systematic review and meta-analysis. *Sci. Rep.* **2016**, *6*, 29409. [CrossRef]
8. Baumann, S.; Renker, M.; Hetjens, S.; Fuller, S.R.; Becher, T.; Loßnitzer, D.; Lehmann, R.; Akin, I.; Borggrefe, M.; Lang, S.; et al. Comparison of Coronary Computed Tomography Angiography-Derived vs Invasive Fractional Flow Reserve Assessment: Meta-Analysis with Subgroup Evaluation of Intermediate Stenosis. *Acad. Radiol.* **2016**, *23*, 1402–1411. [CrossRef]
9. Cook, C.M.; Petraco, R.; Shun-Shin, M.J.; Ahmad, Y.; Nijjer, S.; Al-Lamee, R.; Kikuta, Y.; Shiono, Y.; Mayet, J.; Francis, D.P.; et al. Diagnostic Accuracy of Computed Tomography-Derived Fractional Flow Reserve: A Systematic Review. *JAMA Cardiol.* **2017**, *2*, 803–810. [CrossRef]

10. Hirohata, K.; Kano, A.; Goryu, A.; Ooga, J.; Hongo, T.; Higashi, S.; Fujisawa, Y.; Wakai, S.; Arakita, K.; Ikeda, Y.; et al. A novel CT-FFR method for the coronary artery based on 4D-CT image analysis and structural and fluid analysis. *Med. Imaging 2015 Phys. Med. Imaging* **2015**, *9412*, 94122O.
11. Kato, M.; Hirohata, K.; Kano, A.; Higashi, S.; Goryu, A.; Hongo, T.; Kaminaga, S.; Fujisama, Y. Fast CT-FFR Analysis Method for the Coronary Artery Based on 4D-CT Image Analysis and Structural and Fluid Analysis. In Proceedings of the ASME 2015 International Mechanical Engineering Congress and Exposition. Volume 3: Biomedical and Biotechnology Engineering, Houston, TX, USA, 13–19 November 2015; p. V003T03A023. [CrossRef]
12. Fujimoto, S.; Kawasaki, T.; Kumamaru, K.K.; Kawaguchi, Y.; Dohi, T.; Okonogi, T.; Ri, K.; Yamada, S.; Takamura, K.; Kato, E.; et al. Diagnostic performance of on-site computed CT-fractional flow reserve based on fluid structure interactions: Comparison with invasive fractional flow reserve and instantaneous wave-free ratio. *Eur. Hear. J. Cardiovasc. Imaging* **2019**, *20*, 343–352. [CrossRef]
13. Ko, B.S.; Cameron, J.D.; Munnur, R.K.; Wong, D.T.L.; Fujisawa, Y.; Sakaguchi, T.; Hirohata, K.; Hislop-Jambrich, J.; Fujimoto, S.; Takamura, K.; et al. Noninvasive CT-Derived FFR Based on Structural and Fluid Analysis: A Comparison With Invasive FFR for Detection of Functionally Significant Stenosis. *JACC Cardiovasc. Imaging* **2017**, *10*, 663–673. [CrossRef]
14. Kühl, J.T.; Hove, J.D.; Kristensen, T.S.; Norsk, J.B.; Engstrøm, T.; Køber, L.; Kelbæk, H.; Kofoed, K.F. Coronary CT angiography in clinical triage of patients at high risk of coronary artery disease. *Scand. Cardiovasc. J.* **2017**, *51*, 28–34. [CrossRef]
15. Kawaguchi, Y.O.; Fujimoto, S.; Kumamaru, K.K.; Kato, E.; Dohi, T.; Takamura, K.; Aoshima, C.; Kamo, Y.; Kato, Y.; Hiki, M.; et al. The predictive factors affecting false positive in on-site operated CT-fractional flow reserve based on fluid and structural interaction. *Int. J. Cardiol. Heart Vasc.* **2019**, *23*, 100372. [CrossRef]
16. Yoshioka, K.; Tanaka, R.; Muranaka, K. Subtraction coronary CT angiography for calcified lesions. *Cardiol. Clin.* **2012**, *30*, 93–102. [CrossRef]
17. Takamura, K.; Fujimoto, S.; Kawaguchi, Y.; Kato, E.; Aoshima, C.; Hiki, M.; Kumamaru, K.K.; Daida, H. The usefulness of low radiation dose subtraction coronary computed tomography angiography for patients with calcification using 320-row area detector CT. *J. Cardiol.* **2018**, *73*, 58–64. [CrossRef]
18. Tanaka, R.; Yoshioka, K.; Muranaka, K.; Chiba, T.; Ueda, T.; Sasaki, T.; Fusazaki, T.; Ehara, S. Improved evaluation of calcified segments on coronary CT angiography: A feasibility study of coronary calcium subtraction. *Int. J. Cardiovasc. Imaging* **2013**, *29*, 75–81. [CrossRef]
19. Yoshioka, K.; Tanaka, R.; Muranaka, K.; Sasaki, T.; Ueda, T.; Chiba, T.; Takeda, K.; Sugawara, T. Subtraction coronary CT angiography using second-generation 320-detector row CT. *Int. J. Cardiovasc. Imaging* **2015**, *31*, 51–58. [CrossRef]
20. Amanuma, M.; Kondo, T.; Sano, T.; Sekine, T.; Takayanagi, T.; Matsutani, H.; Arai, T.; Morita, H.; Ishizaka, K.; Arakita, K.; et al. Subtraction coronary computed tomography in patients with severe calcification. *Int. J. Cardiovasc. Imaging* **2015**, *31*, 1635–1642. [CrossRef]
21. Kawaguchi, Y.; Fujimoto, S.; Takamura, K.; Kato, E.; Suda, S.; Matsumori, R.; Hiki, M.; Daida, H.; Kumamaru, K.K. Submillisievert imaging protocol using full reconstruction and advanced patient motion correction in 320-row area detector coronary CT angiography. *Int. J. Cardiovasc. Imaging* **2018**, *34*, 465–474. [CrossRef]
22. Shrimpton, P.C.; Hillier, M.C.; Lewis, M.A.; Dunn, M. National survey of doses from CT in the UK: 2003. *Br. J. Radiol.* **2006**, *79*, 968–980. [CrossRef]
23. Agatston, A.S.; Janowitz, W.R.; Hildner, F.J.; Zusmer, N.R.; Viamonte, M., Jr.; Detrano, R. Quantification of coronary artery calcium using ultrafast computed tomography. *J. Am. Coll. Cardiol.* **1990**, *15*, 827–832. [CrossRef]
24. Kato, E.; Fujimoto, S.; Kumamaru, K.K.; Kawaguchi, Y.O.; Dohi, T.; Aoshima, C.; Kamo, Y.; Takamura, K.; Kato, Y.; Hiki, M.; et al. Adjustment of CT-fractional flow reserve based on fluid–structure interaction underestimation to minimize 1-year cardiac events. *Heart Vessel.* **2020**, *35*, 162–169. [CrossRef]
25. Götberg, M.; Christiansen, E.H.; Gudmundsdottir, I.J.; Sandhall, L.; Danielewicz, M.; Jakobsen, L.; Olsson, S.-E.; Öhagen, P.; Olsson, H.; Omerovic, E.; et al. Instantaneous Wave-free Ratio versus Fractional Flow Reserve to Guide PCI. *N. Engl. J. Med.* **2017**, *376*, 1813–1823. [CrossRef]
26. Cook, C.M.; Jeremias, A.; Petraco, R.; Sen, S.; Nijjer, S.; Shun-Shin, M.J.; Ahmad, Y.; de Waard, G.; van de Hoef, T.; Echavarria-Pinto, M.; et al. Fractional Flow Reserve/Instantaneous Wave-Free Ratio Discordance in Angiographically Intermediate Coronary Stenoses: An Analysis Using Doppler-Derived Coronary Flow Measurements. *JACC Cardiovasc. Interv.* **2017**, *10*, 2514–2524. [CrossRef]
27. Nørgaard, B.L.; Gaur, S.; Leipsic, J.; Ito, H.; Miyoshi, T.; Park, S.J.; Zvaigzne, L.; Tzemos, N.; Jensen, J.M.; Hansson, N.; et al. Influence of Coronary Calcification on the Diagnostic Performance of CT Angiography Derived FFR in Coronary Artery Disease: A Substudy of the NXT Trial. *JACC Cardiovasc. Imaging* **2015**, *8*, 1045–1055. [CrossRef]
28. Ri, K.; Kumamaru, K.K.; Fujimoto, S.; Kawaguchi, Y.; Dohi, T.; Yamada, S.; Takamura, K.; Kogure, Y.; Yamada, N.; Kato, E.; et al. Noninvasive Computed Tomography–Derived Fractional Flow Reserve Based on Structural and Fluid Analysis: Reproducibility of On-site Determination by Unexperienced Observers. *J. Comput. Assist. Tomogr.* **2018**, *42*, 256–262. [CrossRef]
29. Kumamaru, K.K.; Angel, E.; Sommer, K.N.; Iyer, V.; Wilson, M.F.; Agrawal, N.; Bhardwaj, A.; Kattel, S.B.; Kondziela, S.; Malhotra, S.; et al. Inter- and Intraoperator Variability in Measurement of On-Site CT-derived Fractional Flow Reserve Based on Structural and Fluid Analysis: A Comprehensive Analysis. *Radiol. Cardiothorac. Imaging* **2019**, *1*, e180012. [CrossRef]

30. Fuchs, A.; Kühl, J.T.; Chen, M.Y.; Medel, D.V.; Alomar, X.; Shanbhag, S.M.; Helqvist, S.; Kofoed, K. Subtraction CT angiography improves evaluation of significant coronary artery disease in patients with severe calcifications or stents—the C-Sub 320 multicenter trial. *Eur. Radiol.* **2018**, *28*, 4077–4085. [CrossRef]
31. Andrew, M.; John, H. The challenge of coronary calcium on coronary computed tomographic angiography (CCTA) scans: Effect on interpretation and possible solutions. *Int. J. Cardiovasc. Imaging* **2015**, *31*, 145–157. [CrossRef]

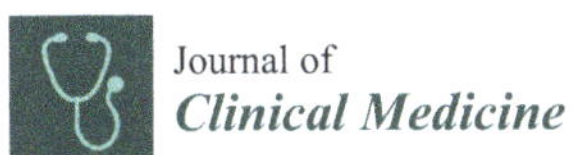
Journal of
Clinical Medicine
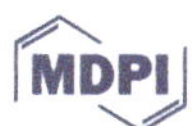

Article

Impact of Serum Uric Acid Level on Systemic Endothelial Dysfunction in Patients with a Broad Spectrum of Ischemic Heart Disease

Takashi Hiraga [1,†], Yuichi Saito [1,*,†], Naoto Mori [2], Kazuya Tateishi [1], Hideki Kitahara [1] and Yoshio Kobayashi [1]

1 Department of Cardiovascular Medicine, Chiba University Graduate School of Medicine, Chiba 260-0856, Japan; t_hiraga1990@yahoo.co.jp (T.H.); kazuyatateishi0926@gmail.com (K.T.); hidekita.0306@gmail.com (H.K.); yuiryosuke@msn.com (Y.K.)
2 Department of Internal Medicine, Chiba Aoba Municipal Hospital, Chiba 260-0852, Japan; polymol.3321@gmail.com
* Correspondence: saitoyuichi1984@gmail.com; Tel.: +81-42-222-7171
† Hiraga and Saito contributed equally.

Abstract: Previous studies indicated that serum uric acid (SUA) level is a marker of endothelial function in subsets of ischemic heart disease (IHD). In the present study, we aimed to evaluate the relation between the SUA level and endothelial function in patients with a broad spectrum of IHD, including obstructive coronary artery disease (CAD) and ischemia with no obstructive CAD (INOCA). Three prospective studies and one retrospective study were pooled, in which the SUA level was measured, and systemic endothelial function was assessed using the reactive hyperemia index (RHI). The primary endpoint of the present study was a correlation of the SUA level with RHI. A total of 181 patients with a broad spectrum of IHD were included, among whom, 46 (25%) had acute coronary syndrome presentation and 15 (8%) had INOCA. Overall, the SUA level was negatively correlated with the RHI ($r = -0.22$, $p = 0.003$). Multivariable analysis identified the SUA level and INOCA as significant factors associated with RHI values. In conclusion, in patients with a broad spectrum of IHD, including obstructive epicardial CAD (chronic and acute coronary syndromes) and INOCA, the SUA level was significantly and negatively correlated with systemic endothelial function assessed with the RHI. INOCA, rather than obstructive CAD, was more associated with endothelial dysfunction.

Keywords: uric acid; endothelial function; ischemic heart disease; ischemia with no obstructive coronary artery disease

Citation: Hiraga, T.; Saito, Y.; Mori, N.; Tateishi, K.; Kitahara, H.; Kobayashi, Y. Impact of Serum Uric Acid Level on Systemic Endothelial Dysfunction in Patients with a Broad Spectrum of Ischemic Heart Disease. *J. Clin. Med.* **2021**, *10*, 4530. https://doi.org/10.3390/jcm10194530

Academic Editors: Koichi Node and Carlos Gonzalez-Juanatey

Received: 4 September 2021
Accepted: 28 September 2021
Published: 30 September 2021

1. Introduction

Angina is a common clinical presentation of ischemic heart disease (IHD), which affects more than 100 million people worldwide [1]. The traditional understanding of IHD includes chronic coronary syndrome (CCS) and acute coronary syndrome (ACS) due to epicardial coronary artery narrowings and occlusions [2]. ACS is a part of the natural history of CCS, but from a clinical perspective, the two entities are different [3]. A large US registry showed that approximately one third of patients undergoing elective coronary angiography for the investigation of angina do not have obstructive epicardial coronary artery disease (CAD) [4], suggesting ischemia with no obstructive CAD (INOCA) accounts for a sizable proportion in IHD.

Uric acid, the end-product of purine metabolism in humans, is associated with inflammation, oxidative stress, and endothelial dysfunction, contributing to the development of atherosclerotic diseases including IHD [5]. Previous studies have indicated that urate lowering therapy had an effect on blood pressure and endothelial function [5], and we and others have reported that the serum uric acid (SUA) level was a marker or predictor of systemic endothelial dysfunction in patients with ACS and INOCA [6–8]. However, whether the SUA level is associated with impaired endothelial function in patients with a broad spectrum of IHD is unclear. Additionally, the impact of a subset of IHD on endothelial dysfunction remains unknown. The aim of the present study was to evaluate the relation between the SUA level and systemic endothelial function in patients with obstructive CAD (CCS and ACS) undergoing percutaneous coronary intervention (PCI) and coronary artery bypass grafting (CABG), and INOCA.

2. Methods

2.1. Study Population and Definitions

We have conducted three prospective studies and one retrospective study to evaluate systemic endothelial function at Chiba University Hospital, in which patients with various types of IHD were included. The present study was a post hoc analysis using pooled data of the four studies (Figure 1). All studies were approved by the institutional ethics committee and conducted in accordance with the Declaration of Helsinki. Each study included patients (1) undergoing elective CABG procedures, (2) undergoing elective PCI, (3) with ACS who underwent PCI, and (4) with INOCA including vasospastic angina (VSA) and/or microvascular dysfunction (MVD). In all studies, SUA levels were measured at baseline and systemic endothelial function was non-invasively assessed. Individual patient data were pooled to create the dataset and to evaluate the impact of SUA level on endothelial dysfunction in patients with a broad spectrum of IHD. Patients with antihyperuricemic agents were excluded.

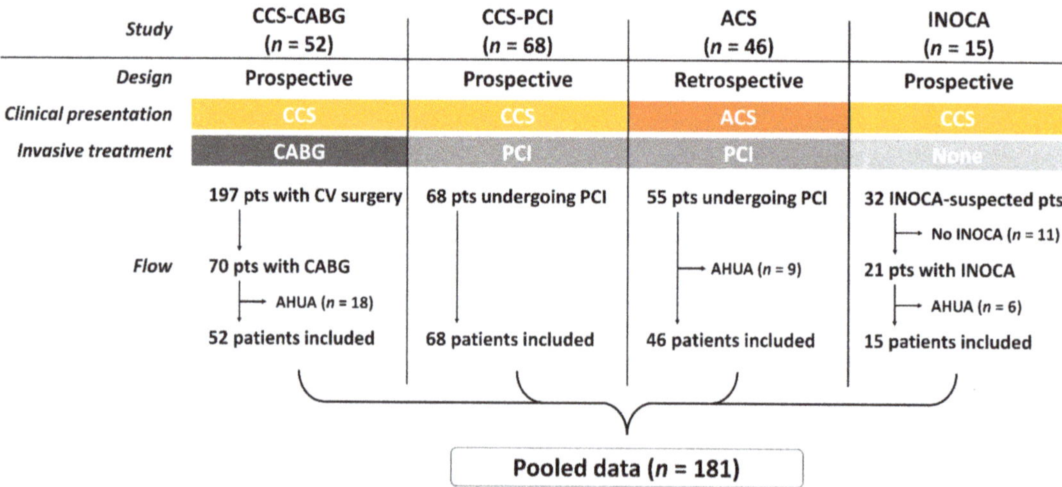

Figure 1. Study flow. ACS: acute coronary syndrome, AHUA: antihyperuricemic agent, CABG: coronary artery bypass grafting, CCS: chronic coronary syndrome, INOCA: ischemia with no obstructive coronary artery disease, PCI: percutaneous coronary intervention.

A study (n = 197) enrolled patients planned for elective cardiovascular surgery, among whom, 70 underwent isolated or concomitant CABG procedures (registered at the University Hospital Medical Information Network Clinical Trials Registry: UMIN000015135) [9,10]. After excluding 18 patients who received antihyperuricemic agents, 52 were included in the present analysis (CCS-CABG group). Another CCS cohort included 68 patients undergoing elective PCI procedures under intravascular ultrasound guidance (UMIN000027855) (CCS-PCI group) [11,12]. Patients with ACS (n = 46) were also included in the present pooled data from a retrospective study (ACS group) [6]. All patients in the CCS-PCI and ACS groups underwent PCI procedures per local standard practice. Patients received dual antiplatelet therapy before or at the time of PCI, and radial artery approach, intracoronary imaging, and contemporary drug-eluting stents were predominantly used [13–18]. The fourth study was a prospective investigation in which intracoronary acetylcholine (ACh) provocation tests and invasive wire-based physiological assessment were employed to diagnose vasospastic angina and/or coronary microvascular dysfunction in patients with suspected INOCA (UMIN000019863) [8,19]. INOCA was defined as having a positive ACh provocation test (angiographic coronary artery vasospasm accompanied by chest pain or ischemic electrocardiographic changes) and/or microvascular dysfunction (coronary flow reserve $\leq$ 2.5 or index of microcirculatory resistance $\geq$ 25) [8,19]. A total of 15 patients with INOCA (vasospastic angina and/or microvascular dysfunction) were included in the present pooled data (INOCA group).

Hypertension was defined as having a previous diagnosis of hypertension or previous antihypertensive medications. Diabetes mellitus was defined as a previous diagnosis of diabetes or previous glucose lowering medications, or hemoglobin A1c $\geq$ 6.5%. Dyslipidemia was defined as low-density lipoprotein cholesterol $\geq$ 140 mg/dL, high-density lipoprotein cholesterol < 40 mg/dL, or fasting triglycerides > 150 mg/dL, or a previous diagnosis of dyslipidemia. Current smoking was defined as a history of smoking within the past year [20]. In addition, hyperuricemia was defined as >7 mg/dL for men and >6 mg/dL for women. Estimated glomerular filtration rate was calculated with the modification of diet in renal disease equation using the Japanese coefficient according to the Kidney Disease Outcomes Quality Initiative clinical guidelines [21].

2.2. Endothelial Function Assessment

Systemic endothelial function was assessed with reactive hyperemic index (RHI) using the EndoPAT 2000 device (Itamar Medical Inc., Caesarea, Israel), which is validated to evaluate endothelial function non-invasively, operator-independently, and reproducibly [22]. RHI was measured as previously described [6,8–12,19]. Briefly, patients fasted and refrained from taking caffeine, tobacco, and all medications for at least eight hours. RHI was measured in a quiet and temperature-controlled room in the early morning. The dedicated probes to measure arterial pulse wave were placed on the index fingers and a blood pressure cuff was placed on either upper arm. The baseline pulse amplitude was evaluated for the first 5-min period. The cuff was subsequently inflated for five minutes, and then deflated to induce reactive hyperemia for the next five minutes. The EndoPAT 2000 device automatically calculated RHI, which is the ratio of amplitude of arterial pulse wave after deflation period divided by those before inflation period, indexed to the contralateral arm. RHI was measured before the invasive procedures (i.e., CABG, PCI, and intracoronary diagnostic investigations) in the CCS-CAGB, CCS-PCI, and INOCA groups, while in the ACS group, endothelial function was evaluated on the day of discharge or 1 day earlier [6]. Patients were divided into two groups according to a cut-off value of RHI of 1.67 [23].

2.3. Endpoint and Statistical Analysis

The primary endpoint of the present pooled study was a correlation of SUA level with endothelial function assessed with RHI. The impact of a subset in a broad spectrum of IHD on RHI was also evaluated. Exploratory analysis on clinical outcomes was performed to identify major adverse cardiovascular events (MACE), a composite of all-cause death, myocardial infarction, and stroke. Statistical analysis was performed with SAS software version 9.3 (SAS Institute, Cary, NC, USA). All data are expressed as mean $\pm$ standard deviation, median (interquartile range), or frequency (%), as appropriate. Continuous variables were compared with Student's *t*-test and analysis of variance, and categorical variables were assessed with Fisher's exact test. A normal distribution was visually assessed with P-P plots and was tested using Kolmogorov–Smirnov test. The correlation between variables were analyzed using Pearson's correlation coefficient. Kaplan–Meier analysis with the log-rank test was employed to assess MACE-free survival rates. Age, sex, and factors associated with variables on univariable analyses ($p < 0.10$) were included into multivariable analysis. Multiple linear regression analysis was performed to identify factors associated with RHI, and multivariable logistic regression analysis for RHI < 1.67

was also conducted as a sensitivity analysis, presented as odds ratio with 95% confidence intervals. A value of $p < 0.05$ was considered statistically significant.

3. Results

A total of 181 patients with a broad spectrum of IHD were included, of whom, 46 (25%) had ACS presentation and 15 (8%) had no obstructive epicardial CAD (i.e., INOCA) (Figure 1). Hyperuricemia was observed in 26 (19%) and 10 (22%) men and women ($p = 0.83$).

Table 1 and Table S1 list the overall baseline characteristics and those among the four groups. The mean SUA level was 5.7 ± 1.5 mg/dL, and RHI < 1.67 was observed in 75 (41%) patients.

Table 1. Baseline characteristics.

Variable	All
	(n = 181)
Age (years)	68.9 ± 10.9
Men	135 (75%)
Body mass index (kg/m^2)	24.0 ± 3.9
Hypertension	133 (73%)
Diabetes mellitus	73 (40%)
Dyslipidemia	129 (71%)
Current smoker	44 (24%)
Prior myocardial infarction	40 (22%)
eGFR (ml/min/1.73 m^2)	67.2 ± 19.9
Serum uric acid (mg/dL)	5.7 ± 1.5
LDL cholesterol (mg/dL)	107.5 ± 34.6
HDL cholesterol (mg/dL)	52.2 ± 16.0
Non-fasting triglyceride (mg/dL)	136.7 ± 80.7
Hemoglobin A1c (%)	6.4 ± 1.3
Clinical presentation	
Acute coronary syndrome	46 (25%)
Chronic coronary syndrome	135 (75%)
Medical treatment	
Aspirin	111 (61%)
P2Y12 inhibitor	56 (31%)
Oral hypoglycemic agent	48 (27%)
Metformin	20 (11%)
SGLT2 inhibitor	7 (4%)
ACE-I or ARB	90 (50%)
β-blocker	56 (31%)
Calcium channel blocker	86 (48%)
Diuretic	32 (18%)
Statin	108 (60%)
Fibrate	2 (1%)
Reactive hyperemia index	1.84 ± 0.53

ACE-I: angiotensin converting enzyme inhibitor, ARB: angiotensin II receptor blocker, eGFR: estimate glomerular filtration rate, HDL: high density lipoprotein, LDL: low density lipoprotein, SGLT: sodium-glucose cotransporter.

Overall, the SUA level was negatively correlated with the RHI ($r = -0.22$, $p = 0.003$). Multivariable analysis identified the SUA level and INOCA as significant factors associated with RHI values (Table 2). As a sensitivity analysis, logistic regression analysis confirmed the SUA level and INOCA as predictors of an RHI < 1.67 (Table S2). During the median follow-up period of 792 (362, 1540) days, 16 (8.8%) patients experienced MACE (Table S3). The patients with an RHI < 1.67 were non-significantly associated with an increased risk of MACE than those with an RHI ≥ 1.67 (Figure 2).

Table 2. Predictors of reactive hyperemia index.

Variable	Univariable		Multivariable	
	r	*p* Value	β	*p* Value
Age (years)	0.09	0.20	−0.01	0.94
Men	−0.03	0.65	0.004	0.95
Body mass index (kg/m^2)	−0.13	0.09	−0.07	0.37
Hypertension	−0.02	0.83		
Diabetes mellitus	−0.06	0.45		
Dyslipidemia	0.01	0.91		
Current smoker	−0.14	0.07	−0.09	0.25
Prior myocardial infarction	−0.02	0.82		
eGFR (ml/min/1.73 m^2)	0.12	0.11		
Serum uric acid (mg/dL)	−0.22	0.003	−0.22	0.004
LDL cholesterol (mg/dL)	0.003	0.97		
HDL cholesterol (mg/dL)	0.08	0.28		
Non-fasting triglyceride (mg/dL)	−0.07	0.33		
Hemoglobin A1c (%)	−0.04	0.63		
INOCA	−0.15	0.04	−0.16	0.03

eGFR: estimated glomerular filtration rate, HDL: high density lipoprotein, INOCA: ischemia with no obstructive coronary artery disease, LDL: low density lipoprotein.

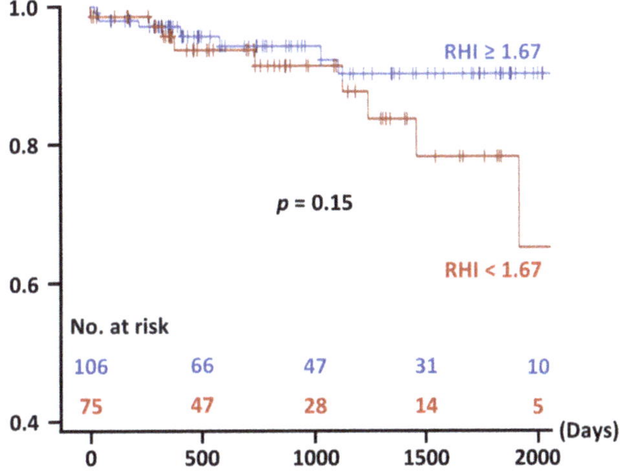

Figure 2. Probability free from major adverse cardiovascular events. MACE: major adverse cardiovascular events, RHI: reactive hyperemia index.

4. Discussion

The present study demonstrated that in patients with various types of IHD, including obstructive CAD (CCS and ACS) and INOCA, systemic endothelial dysfunction was found in 41%. The SUA level was significantly and negatively associated with the RHI. In addition to the SUA level, INOCA rather than other obstructive CAD was identified as a factor related to endothelial dysfunction in the present study population. To our knowledge, this is the first study investigating systemic endothelial function in a broad spectrum of IHD.

The current guidelines for the diagnosis and management of IHD are predominantly shaped by the burden of epicardial obstructive CAD, including CCS and ACS [3,24], while recent investigations have shown that a sizable proportion of patients with angina have no obstructive epicardial CAD but myocardial ischemia, namely INOCA [25]. Consequently, consensus documents have been published to provide definitions and guidance on the diagnostic approach and management of INOCA [26,27]. The European consensus document indicated that vasospastic angina and coronary microvascular dysfunction are the major endotypes of INOCA, and the present study determined both as the definition of the INOCA group. It is well known that endothelial dysfunction plays important roles in the development of obstructive CAD and INOCA [27,28]. However, few studies have investigated the relation of endothelial function to the entire spectrum of IHD. In this context, the present study confirmed that endothelial function is a key underlying mechanism in IHD. Interestingly, INOCA rather than obstructive CAD was identified as a factor strongly associated with systemic endothelial dysfunction in this study. Given that coronary vasospasm is not necessarily provoked in patients with established obstructive CAD when an ACh provocation test is performed, this finding may be reasonable and be translated into diagnostic and therapeutic approaches for INOCA. As indicated in the recent European guidelines (Class IIb) [3], an endothelium-dependent diagnostic procedure (i.e., an ACh provocation test) may be considered in suspected INOCA. Whether endothelium targeting therapy improves clinical outcomes and quality of life in INOCA remains largely unknown but deserves further investigation.

We and other groups have previously shown the SUA level as a marker or predictor of systemic endothelial dysfunction in patients with ACS and INOCA [6–8], and the present study supported the concept in the entire spectrum of IHD. While numerous epidemiological studies have reported the association of the SUA level with cardiovascular disease, including IHD [5], a therapeutic intervention targeting SUA in IHD has not been fully investigated. Noman et al. previously demonstrated that in CCS patients with angiographically confirmed obstructive CAD, allopurinol (600 mg/day) significantly improved exercise capacity in a randomized, placebo-controlled, cross-over setting [29]. Although it is unclear whether xanthin oxidase inhibition itself or the reduced SUA levels by allopurinol (or both) prolonged the exercise time, the improvement in peripheral and coronary endothelial function were suggested as the mechanism in their paper [29]. Despite the modest correlation ($r = -0.22$, $p = 0.003$), SUA lowering therapy might be beneficial in patients with IHD.

The present study has several limitations. The present pooled data consist of three prospective studies and one retrospective study and were assessed as a post hoc analysis. ACS presentation accounted for 28% among the patients with obstructive CAD, which is in line with current clinical practice in Japan, while only 8% of the patients had INOCA in the present study. Given that 30–50% of patients may reportedly have INOCA among those undergoing invasive coronary angiography [4,25], the impact of INOCA may have been underrepresented in the present pooled data. Nevertheless, multivariable analyses identified INOCA as a significant factor associated with a lower RHI, reinforcing a crucial role of systemic endothelial dysfunction in INOCA. Despite the multivariable analyses, there were several confounding factors and unmeasured variables including medications and detailed data on blood pressure and a smoking habit (e.g., 24-h ambulatory blood pressure monitoring, and number of cigarettes smoked per day). Although a meta-analysis reported the prognostic impact of the RHI [30], clinical outcomes were not significantly different between the patients with endothelial dysfunction (RHI < 1.67) and their counterpart in the present study, probably because of the small sample size.

5. Conclusions

In patients with a broad spectrum of IHD, including obstructive CAD (CCS and ACS) and INOCA, the SUA level was significantly and negatively correlated with systemic endothelial function assessed with the RHI. INOCA, rather than obstructive CAD, was more associated with endothelial dysfunction.

Supplementary Materials: The following are available online at https://www.mdpi.com/article/10.3390/jcm10194530/s1, Table S1: Baseline characteristics; Table S2: Predictors of reactive hyperemia index < 1.67; Table S3: Clinical outcomes.

Author Contributions: Conceptualization, Y.S.; methodology, T.H. and Y.S.; validation, T.H. and Y.S.; formal analysis, Y.S.; investigation, Y.S., N.M. and K.T.; data curation, T.H. and Y.S.; writing—original draft preparation, T.H.; writing—review and editing, Y.S. and H.K.; visualization, Y.S.; supervision, H.K. and Y.K.; project administration, Y.S. and Y.K. All authors have read and agreed to the published version of the manuscript.

Funding: This research received no external funding.

Institutional Review Board Statement: The study was conducted according to the guidelines of the Declaration of Helsinki, and approved by the Ethics Committee of Chiba University (protocol code 1645, 1908, 2677, and G27031; date of approval 11 October 2013, 22 October 2014, 5 June 2017, and 16 November 2015).

Informed Consent Statement: This study was approved by the institutional ethics committee and conducted in accordance with the Declaration of Helsinki. Informed consent was obtained or waived in the form of opt-out.

Data Availability Statement: Data sharing not applicable.

Conflicts of Interest: The authors declare no conflict of interest.

References

1. GBD 2015 Mortality and Causes of Death Collaborators. Global, regional, and national life expectancy, all-cause mortality, and cause-specific mortality for 249 causes of death, 1980-2015: A systematic analysis for the Global Burden of Disease Study 2015. *Lancet* **2016**, *388*, 1459–1544. [CrossRef]
2. Montalescot, G.; Sechtem, U.; Achenbach, S.; Andreotti, F.; Arden, C.; Budaj, A.; Bugiardini, R.; Crea, F.; Cuisset, T.; Di Mario, C.; et al. 2013 ESC guidelines on the management of stable coronary artery disease: The Task Force on the management of stable coronary artery disease of the European Society of Cardiology. *Eur. Heart J.* **2013**, *34*, 2949–3003.
3. Knuuti, J.; Wijns, W.; Saraste, A.; Capodanno, D.; Barbato, E.; Funck-Brentano, C.; Prescott, E.; Storey, R.F.; Deaton, C.; Cuisset, T.; et al. 2019 ESC Guidelines for the diagnosis and management of chronic coronary syndromes. *Eur. Heart J.* **2020**, *41*, 407–477. [CrossRef]
4. Patel, M.R.; Peterson, E.D.; Dai, D.; Brennan, J.M.; Redberg, R.F.; Anderson, H.V.; Brindis, R.G.; Douglas, P.S. Low diagnostic yield of elective coronary angiography. *N. Engl. J. Med.* **2010**, *362*, 886–895. [CrossRef]
5. Saito, Y.; Tanaka, A.; Node, K.; Kobayashi, Y. Uric acid and cardiovascular disease: A clinical review. *J. Cardiol.* **2021**, *78*, 51–57. [CrossRef]
6. Saito, Y.; Kitahara, H.; Nakayama, T.; Fujimoto, Y.; Kobayashi, Y. Relation of Elevated Serum Uric Acid Level to Endothelial Dysfunction in Patients with Acute Coronary Syndrome. *J. Atheroscler. Thromb.* **2019**, *26*, 362–367. [CrossRef] [PubMed]
7. Motoyama, T.; Kawano, H.; Kugiyama, K.; Hirashima, O.; Ohgushi, M.; Tsunoda, R.; Moriyama, Y.; Miyao, Y.; Yoshimura, M.; Ogawa, H.; et al. Vitamin E administration improves impairment of endothelium-dependent vasodilation in patients with coronary spastic angina. *J. Am. Coll. Cardiol.* **1998**, *32*, 1672–1679. [CrossRef]
8. Saito, Y.; Kitahara, H.; Nishi, T.; Fujimoto, Y.; Kobayashi, Y. Systemic endothelial dysfunction in patients with vasospastic and microvascular angina: Serum uric acid as a marker of reactive hyperemia index. *Coron. Artery Dis.* **2020**, *31*, 565–566. [CrossRef]
9. Saito, Y.; Kitahara, H.; Matsumiya, G.; Kobayashi, Y. Preoperative Assessment of Endothelial Function for Prediction of Adverse Events after Cardiovascular Surgery. *Circ. J.* **2017**, *82*, 118–122. [CrossRef]
10. Saito, Y.; Kitahara, H.; Matsumiya, G.; Kobayashi, Y. Preoperative endothelial function and long-term cardiovascular events in patients undergoing cardiovascular surgery. *Heart Vessels* **2019**, *34*, 318–323. [CrossRef] [PubMed]
11. Mori, N.; Saito, Y.; Saito, K.; Matsuoka, T.; Tateishi, K.; Kadohira, T.; Kitahara, H.; Fujimoto, Y.; Kobayashi, Y. Relation of Plasma Xanthine Oxidoreductase Activity to Coronary Lipid Core Plaques Assessed by Near-Infrared Spectroscopy Intravascular Ultrasound in Patients With Stable Coronary Artery Disease. *Am. J. Cardiol.* **2020**, *125*, 1006–1012. [CrossRef]
12. Saito, Y.; Mori, N.; Murase, T.; Nakamura, T.; Akari, S.; Saito, K.; Matsuoka, T.; Tateishi, K.; Kadohira, T.; Kitahara, H.; et al. Greater coronary lipid core plaque assessed by near-infrared spectroscopy intravascular ultrasound in patients with elevated xanthine oxidoreductase: A mechanistic insight. *Heart Vessels* **2021**, *36*, 597–604. [CrossRef] [PubMed]
13. Sakamoto, K.; Sato, R.; Tabata, N.; Ishii, M.; Yamashita, T.; Nagamatsu, S.; Motozato, K.; Yamanaga, K.; Hokimoto, S.; Sueta, D.; et al. Temporal trends in coronary intervention strategies and the impact on one-year clinical events: Data from a Japanese multi-center real-world cohort study. *Cardiovasc. Interv. Ther.* **2021**. [CrossRef]
14. Ozaki, Y.; Katagiri, Y.; Onuma, Y.; Amano, T.; Muramatsu, T.; Kozuma, K.; Otsuji, S.; Ueno, T.; Shiode, N.; Kawai, K.; et al. CVIT expert consensus document on primary percutaneous coronary intervention (PCI) for acute myocardial infarction (AMI) in 2018. *Cardiovasc. Interv. Ther.* **2018**, *33*, 178–203. [CrossRef] [PubMed]
15. Saito, Y.; Kobayashi, Y.; Fujii, K.; Sonoda, S.; Tsujita, K.; Hibi, K.; Morino, Y.; Okura, H.; Ikari, Y.; Honye, J. Clinical expert consensus document on standards for measurements and assessment of intravascular ultrasound from the Japanese Association of Cardiovascular Intervention and Therapeutics. *Cardiovasc. Interv. Ther.* **2020**, *35*, 1–12. [CrossRef]

16. Sonoda, S.; Hibi, K.; Okura, H.; Fujii, K.; Honda, Y.; Kobayashi, Y. Current clinical use of intravascular ultrasound imaging to guide percutaneous coronary interventions. *Cardiovasc. Interv. Ther.* **2020**, *35*, 30–36. [CrossRef] [PubMed]
17. Fujii, K.; Kubo, T.; Otake, H.; Nakazawa, G.; Sonoda, S.; Hibi, K.; Shinke, T.; Kobayashi, Y.; Ikari, Y.; Akasaka, T. Expert consensus statement for quantitative measurement and morphological assessment of optical coherence tomography. *Cardiovasc. Interv. Ther.* **2020**, *35*, 13–18. [CrossRef] [PubMed]
18. Saito, Y.; Kobayashi, Y. Contemporary coronary drug-eluting and coated stents: A mini-review. *Cardiovasc. Interv. Ther.* **2021**, *36*, 20–22. [CrossRef]
19. Saito, Y.; Kitahara, H.; Nishi, T.; Fujimoto, Y.; Kobayashi, Y. Decreased resting coronary flow and impaired endothelial function in patients with vasospastic angina. *Coron. Artery Dis.* **2019**, *30*, 291–296. [CrossRef]
20. Sawano, M.; Yamaji, K.; Kohsaka, S.; Inohara, T.; Numasawa, Y.; Ando, H.; Iida, O.; Shinke, T.; Ishii, H.; Amano, T. Contemporary use and trends in percutaneous coronary intervention in Japan: An outline of the J-PCI registry. *Cardiovasc. Interv. Ther.* **2020**, *35*, 218–226. [CrossRef]
21. Horio, M.; Imai, E.; Yasuda, Y.; Watanabe, T.; Matsuo, S. Modification of the CKD epidemiology collaboration (CKD-EPI) equation for Japanese: Accuracy and use for population estimates. *Am. J. Kidney Dis.* **2010**, *56*, 32–38. [CrossRef] [PubMed]
22. Sauder, K.A.; West, S.G.; McCrea, C.E.; Campbell, J.M.; Jenkins, A.L.; Jenkins, D.J.; Kendall, C.W. Test-retest reliability of peripheral arterial tonometry in the metabolic syndrome. *Diabetes Vasc. Dis. Res.* **2014**, *11*, 201–207. [CrossRef]
23. Saito, Y.; Kitahara, H.; Nakayama, T.; Fujimoto, Y.; Kobayashi, Y. Night-time blood pressure variability negatively correlated with reactive hyperemia index. *Int. J. Cardiol.* **2017**, *230*, 332–334. [CrossRef] [PubMed]
24. Kimura, K.; Kimura, T.; Ishihara, M.; Nakagawa, Y.; Nakao, K.; Miyauchi, K.; Sakamoto, T.; Tsujita, K.; Hagiwara, N.; Miyazaki, S.; et al. JCS 2018 Guideline on Diagnosis and Treatment of Acute Coronary Syndrome. *Circ. J.* **2019**, *83*, 1085–1196. [CrossRef] [PubMed]
25. Herscovici, R.; Sedlak, T.; Wei, J.; Pepine, C.J.; Handberg, E.; Bairey-Merz, C.N. Ischemia and No Obstructive Coronary Artery Disease (INOCA): What Is the Risk? *J. Am. Heart Assoc.* **2018**, *7*, e008868. [CrossRef] [PubMed]
26. Ong, P.; Camici, P.G.; Beltrame, J.F.; Crea, F.; Shimokawa, H.; Sechtem, U.; Kaski, J.C.; Bairey-Merz, C.N.; Coronary Vasomotion Disorders International Study Group (COVADIS). International standardization of diagnostic criteria for microvascular angina. *Int. J. Cardiol.* **2018**, *250*, 16–20. [CrossRef] [PubMed]
27. Kunadian, V.; Chieffo, A.; Camici, P.G.; Berry, C.; Escaned, J.; Maas, A.H.E.M.; Prescott, E.; Karam, N.; Appelman, Y.; Fraccaro, C.; et al. An EAPCI Expert Consensus Document on Ischaemia with Non-Obstructive Coronary Arteries in Collaboration with European Society of Cardiology Working Group on Coronary Pathophysiology & Microcirculation Endorsed by Coronary Vasomotor Disorders International Study Group. *Eur. Heart J.* **2020**, *41*, 3504–3520.
28. Förstermann, U.; Münzel, T. Endothelial nitric oxide synthase in vascular disease: From marvel to menace. *Circulation* **2006**, *113*, 1708–1714. [CrossRef] [PubMed]
29. Noman, A.; Ang, D.S.; Ogston, S.; Lang, C.C.; Struthers, A.D. Effect of high-dose allopurinol on exercise in patients with chronic stable angina: A randomised, placebo controlled crossover trial. *Lancet* **2010**, *375*, 2161–2167. [CrossRef]
30. Matsuzawa, Y.; Kwon, T.G.; Lennon, R.J.; Lerman, L.O.; Lerman, A. Prognostic Value of Flow-Mediated Vasodilation in Brachial Artery and Fingertip Artery for Cardiovascular Events: A Systematic Review and Meta-Analysis. *J. Am. Heart Assoc.* **2015**, *4*, e002270. [CrossRef]

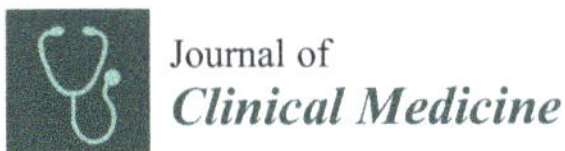
Journal of
Clinical Medicine

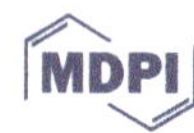

Article

Outcomes of Different Reperfusion Strategies of Multivessel Disease Undergoing Newer-Generation Drug-Eluting Stent Implantation in Patients with Non-ST-Elevation Myocardial Infarction and Chronic Kidney Disease

Yong Hoon Kim [1,*,†], Ae-Young Her [1,†], Myung Ho Jeong [2], Byeong-Keuk Kim [3], Sung-Jin Hong [3], Seung-Jun Lee [3], Chul-Min Ahn [3], Jung-Sun Kim [3], Young-Guk Ko [3], Donghoon Choi [3], Myeong-Ki Hong [3] and Yangsoo Jang [4]

1 Division of Cardiology, Department of Internal Medicine, Kangwon National University School of Medicine, Chuncheon 24289, Korea; hermartha1@gmail.com
2 Department of Cardiology, Cardiovascular Center, Chonnam National University Hospital, Gwangju 61469, Korea; myungho@chollian.net
3 Division of Cardiology, Severance Cardiovascular Hospital, Yonsei University College of Medicine, Seoul 03722, Korea; kimbk@yuhs.ac (B.-K.K.); HONGS@yuhs.ac (S.-J.H.); SJUNLEE@yuhs.ac (S.-J.L.); DRCELLO@yuhs.ac (C.-M.A.); kjs1218@yuhs.ac (J.-S.K.); ygko@yuhs.ac (Y.-G.K.); cdhlyj@yuhs.ac (D.C.); mkhong61@yuhs.ac (M.-K.H.)
4 Department of Cardiology, CHA Bundang Medical Center, CHA University School of Medicine, Seongnam 13496, Korea; jangys1212@cha.ac.kr
* Correspondence: yhkim02@kangwon.ac.kr
† Yong Hoon Kim and Ae-Young Her contributed equally to this work as the first authors.

Citation: Kim, Y.H.; Her, A.-Y.; Jeong, M.H.; Kim, B.-K.; Hong, S.-J.; Lee, S.-J.; Ahn, C.-M.; Kim, J.-S.; Ko, Y.-G.; Choi, D.; et al. Outcomes of Different Reperfusion Strategies of Multivessel Disease Undergoing Newer-Generation Drug-Eluting Stent Implantation in Patients with Non-ST-Elevation Myocardial Infarction and Chronic Kidney Disease. *J. Clin. Med.* **2021**, *10*, 4629. https://doi.org/10.3390/jcm10204629

Academic Editors: Koichi Node and Atsushi Tanaka

Received: 8 September 2021
Accepted: 5 October 2021
Published: 9 October 2021

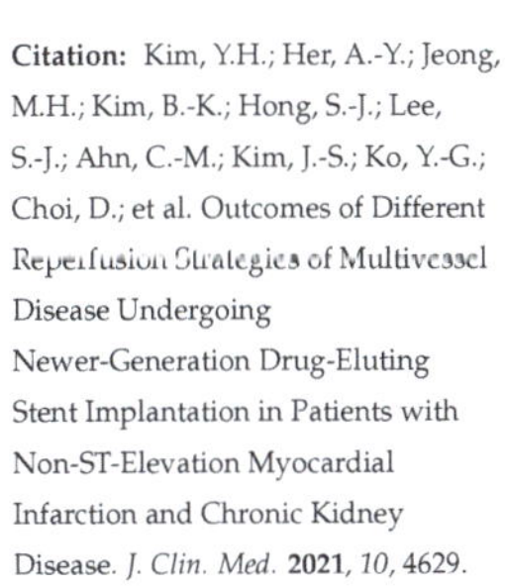

Abstract: Because available data are limited, we compared the 2-year clinical outcomes among different reperfusion strategies (culprit-only percutaneous coronary intervention (C-PCI), multivessel PCI (M-PCI), complete revascularization (CR) and incomplete revascularization (IR)) of multivessel disease (MVD) undergoing newer-generation drug-eluting stent implantation in patients with non-ST-elevation myocardial infarction (NSTEMI) and chronic kidney disease (CKD). In this nonrandomized, multicenter, retrospective cohort study, a total of 1042 patients (C-PCI, $n = 470$; M-PCI, $n = 572$; CR, $n = 432$; IR, $n = 140$) were recruited from the Korea Acute Myocardial Infarction Registry (KAMIR) and evaluated. The primary outcome was the occurrence of major adverse cardiac events, defined as all-cause death, recurrent myocardial infarction and any repeat coronary revascularization. The secondary outcome was probable or definite stent thrombosis. During the 2-year follow-up period, the cumulative incidences of the primary (C-PCI vs. M-PCI, adjusted hazard ratio (aHR), 1.020; $p = 0.924$; CR vs. IR, aHR, 1.012; $p = 0.967$; C-PCI vs. CR, aHR, 1.042; $p = 0.863$; or C-PCI vs. IR, aHR, 1.060; $p = 0.844$) and secondary outcomes were statistically insignificant in the four comparison groups. In the contemporary newer-generation DES era, C-PCI may be a better reperfusion option for patients with NSTEMI with MVD and CKD rather than M-PCI, including CR and IR, with regard to the procedure time and the risk of contrast-induced nephropathy. However, further well-designed, large-scale randomized studies are warranted to confirm these results.

Keywords: angioplasty; drug-eluting stents; non-ST-elevation myocardial infarction; multivessel disease

1. Introduction

The extent of coronary artery disease (CAD) is a marker of diffuse atherosclerosis and plaque burden and multivessel disease (MVD) is associated with worse outcomes in patients with infarction (AMI) [1]. The incidence of MVD in patients with non-ST-segment elevation myocardial infarction (NSTEMI) is more than 50% [2,3]. Even though percutaneous coronary intervention (PCI) for an infarct-related artery (IRA) is a well-established standard treatment [4,5], the treatment strategies for a non-IRA in the NSTEMI milieu are still debatable [6–9]. Revascularization of the non-IRA may reduce the incidence of recurrent ischemia, improve left ventricular function, reduce arrhythmias and potentially improve hemodynamics [10]. In contrast, procedural complexity might lead to overexposure to radiation and an increased risk of developing contrast-induced nephropathy and further ischemia [11–13] in patients with AMI and MVD. Approximately 25–30% of patients with NSTEMI have moderately reduced renal function [14]. A drop of 10 mL/min/1.73 m^2 in the glomerular filtration rate (GFR) leads to a 5% to 6% incremental increase in cardiovascular mortality rates [15]. Thus, patients with chronic kidney disease (CKD) and NSTEMI have worse prognosis than those with normal renal function [16]. Unfortunately, individuals with CKD are often excluded from or underrepresented in randomized trials and are less likely to receive guideline-recommended medical and revascularization therapy [17]. Yet, data on PCI patients with NSTEMI with MVD and CKD are limited. Additionally, according to a recent meta-analysis, the use of second-generation drug-eluting stent (2G-DES) resulted in an 18% reduction in all-cause death and a 27% reduction in target lesion revascularization/target vessel revascularization (TLR/TVR) compared to the use of first-generation DES (1G-DES) in patients with CKD [18]. Hence, after confining the study population who received newer-generation DES to reflect current real-world practice, we compared the 2-year clinical outcomes among different reperfusion strategies (culprit-only PCI (C-PCI), multivessel PCI (M-PCI), complete revascularization (CR) and incomplete revascularization (IR)) of MVD in patients with NSTEMI and CKD.

2. Methods

2.1. Study Population

In this nonrandomized, multicenter, retrospective cohort study, a total of 30,757 patients with AMI who underwent successful PCI during index hospitalization using DES and who were not receiving continuous renal replacement therapy, including hemodialysis or peritoneal dialysis, between May 2008 and June 2015 were recruited from the Korea AMI Registry (KAMIR) [19]. KAMIR is the first nationwide and multicenter registry that included >50 tertiary-care teaching hospitals in South Korea since November 2005. Detailed information on this registry can be found on the website (http://www.kamir.or.kr (accessed on 6 May 2021). Eligible patients were aged ≥18 years at the time of hospital admission. Patients with the following were also excluded: deployed 1G-DES (n = 4769, 15.5%), incomplete laboratory results (n = 6075, 19.8%), loss to follow-up (n = 1568, 5.1%) and in-hospital death (n = 307, 1.0%). A total of 18,038 patients with AMI who underwent successful PCI using newer-generation DES were enrolled. The types of newer-generation DESs used are listed in Table 1. After excluding those with estimated GFR (eGFR) ≥60 mL/min/1.73 m^2 (n = 14,697, 81.5%), 3341 patients (18.5%) with AMI with eGFR < 60 mL/min/1.73 m^2 remained. After excluding those with STEMI (n = 1704, 51%), 1637 patients (49%) with NSTEMI remained. Those with cardiogenic shock (n = 71, 4.3%), single-vessel disease (n = 481, 29.4%), and cardiopulmonary resuscitation (CPR) on admission (n = 43, 2.6%) were also excluded. Finally, 1042 patients with NSTEMI were included in the study. Patients were assigned to the C-PCI (n = 470, 45.1%) and M-PCI (n = 572, 54.9%) groups. In the case of M-PCI, 432 (75.5%) patients received CR and 140 (24.5%) patients received IR (Figure 1). All data were collected using a web-based case report form at each participating center. The study was conducted in accordance with the ethical guidelines of the 2004 Declaration of Helsinki and was approved by the ethics committee of each participating center and the Chonnam National University Hospital Institutional Review Board ethics committee (CNUH-2011-172). All 1042 patients included in the study provided written informed consent prior to enrollment. They also completed a 2-year clinical follow-up through face-to-face interviews, phone calls or chart reviews. The processes of event adjudication have been described in a previous publication by KAMIR investigators [20].

Table 1. Baseline clinical, laboratory, angiographic and procedural characteristics.

Variables	Culprit-Only PCI (n = 470)	Multivessel PCI (n = 572)	p Value	CR (n = 432)	IR (n = 140)	p Value
Age (years)	71.7 ± 9.7	71.3 ± 9.1	0.431	71.3 ± 9.2	71.2 ± 9.0	0.876
≥65 years, n (%)	364 (77.4)	434 (75.9)	0.551	328 (75.9)	106 (75.7)	0.959
Male, n (%)	278 (59.1)	298 (52.1)	0.023	217 (50.2)	81 (57.9)	0.117
LVEF (%)	48.3 ± 12.6	49.1 ± 12.8	0.283	49.9 ± 12.7	46.1 ± 12.5	0.010
<40%, n (%)	116 (24.7)	131 (22.9)	0.502	93 (21.5)	38 (27.1)	0.169
BMI (kg/m^2)	23.6 ± 3.3	23.8 ± 3.3	0.354	23.9 ± 3.3	23.54 ±3.3	0.081
SBP (mmHg)	133.9 ± 30.1	134.73 ± 29.7	0.664	134.5 ± 29.3	135.3 ± 31.0	0.774
DBP (mmHg)	78.3 ± 16.6	78.1 ± 15.5	0.884	78.1 ± 15.4	78.3 ± 15.6	0.864
Killip class III, n (%)	83 (17.7)	101 (17.7)	0.999	75 (17.4)	26 (18.6)	0.744
Hypertension, n (%)	363 (77.2)	439 (76.7)	0.853	323 (74.8)	116 (82.9)	0.049
Diabetes mellitus, n (%)	247 (52.6)	325 (56.8)	0.169	234 (54.2)	91 (65.0)	0.025
Dyslipidemia, n (%)	294 (62.6)	378 (66.1)	0.236	294 (68.1)	84 (60.0)	0.080
Previous MI, n (%)	37 (7.9)	48 (8.4)	0.761	33 (7.6)	15 (10.7)	0.254
Previous PCI, n (%)	71 (15.1)	68 (11.9)	0.128	42 (9.7)	26 (18.6)	0.007
Previous CABG, n (%)	11 (2.3)	8 (1.4)	0.352	3 (0.7)	5 (3.6)	0.024
Previous HF, n (%)	22 (4.7)	25 (4.4)	0.881	18 (4.2)	7 (5.0)	0.640
Previous CVA, n (%)	72 (15.3)	73 (12.8)	0.235	54 (12.5)	19 (13.6)	0.771
Current smokers, n (%)	98 (20.9)	103 (18.0)	0.247	80 (18.5)	23 (16.4)	0.615
Peak CK-MB (mg/dL)	61.1 ± 96.8	48.8 ± 80.8	0.049	47.6 ± 75.9	52.5 ± 94.5	0.578
Peak troponin-I (ng/mL)	35.6 ± 91.5	26.8 ± 97.2	0.216	24.4 ± 60.0	34.3 ± 88.7	0.491
NT-ProBNP (pg/mL)	7027.3 ± 9781.9	6152.7 ± 9097.5	0.166	5825.1 ± 8862.6	7015.4 ± 8725.4	0.151
Hs-CRP (mg/dL)	9.4 ± 32.9	9.5 ± 40.7	0.962	10.8 ± 45.8	5.5 ± 17.4	0.047
Serum creatinine (mg/L)	2.41 ± 2.45	2.36 ± 2.62	0.729	2.32 ± 2.64	2.45 ± 2.58	0.634
eGFR, mL/min/1.73 m^2	39.6 ± 16.7	40.2 ± 16.6	0.617	40.8 ± 16.5	38.3 ± 16.8	0.121
Blood glucose (mg/dL)	189.4 ± 100.3	198.5 ± 110.0	0.162	193.6 ± 108.1	213.6 ± 114.7	0.071
Total cholesterol (mg/dL)	169.7 ± 56.8	173.6 ± 46.3	0.224	174.1 ± 45.7	172.1 ± 48.1	0.666
Triglyceride (mg/L)	118.2 ± 71.0	128.6 ± 106.3	0.039	130.9 ± 116.3	121.8 ± 66.0	0.253
HDL cholesterol (mg/L)	42.5 ± 22.2	40.6 ± 10.9	0.088	40.2 ± 10.5	42.0 ± 12.0	0.097
LDL cholesterol (mg/L)	103.8 ± 41.9	107.2 ± 36.1	0.160	109.1 ± 35.4	101.5 ± 38.0	0.038
Discharge medications						
Aspirin, n (%)	451 (96.0)	554 (96.9)	0.437	418 (96.8)	136 (97.1)	0.821
Clopidogrel, n (%)	435 (92.6)	530 (92.5)	0.862	405 (93.8)	125 (89.3)	0.098
Ticagrelor, n (%)	23 (4.9)	31 (5.4)	0.779	19 (4.4)	12 (8.6)	0.083
Prasugrel, n (%)	12 (2.6)	11 (1.9)	0.530	8 (1.9)	3 (2.1)	0.735
Cilostazole, n (%)	77 (16.4)	138 (24.1)	0.002	121 (28.0)	17 (12.1)	<0.001
Beta-blocker, n (%)	368 (78.3)	449 (78.5)	0.938	339 (78.5)	110 (78.6)	0.980
ACEI, n (%)	202 (43.0)	233 (40.7)	0.465	180 (41.7)	53 (37.9)	0.489
ARB, n (%)	167 (35.5)	214 (37.4)	0.531	158 (36.6)	56 (40.0)	0.467
CCB, n (%)	81 (17.2)	88 (15.4)	0.420	64 (14.8)	24 (17.1)	0.507
Lipid lowering agent, n (%)	360 (76.6)	470 (82.2)	0.028	348 (80.6)	122 (87.1)	0.077
Angiographic & procedural characteristics						
IRA						
LM, n (%)	17 (3.6)	36 (6.3)	0.048	22 (5.1)	14 (10.0)	0.038
LAD, n (%)	190 (40.4)	202 (35.3)	0.104	151 (35.0)	51 (36.4)	0.751
LCx, n (%)	105 (22.3)	143 (25.0)	0.316	114 (26.4)	29 (20.7)	0.216
RCA, n (%)	158 (33.6)	191 (33.4)	0.939	145 (33.6)	46 (32.9)	0.918
Treated vessel						
LM, n (%)	21 (4.5)	56 (9.8)	0.001	38 (8.8)	18 (12.9)	0.160
LAD, n (%)	217 (46.2)	420 (73.4)	<0.001	321 (74.3)	99 (70.7)	0.403
LCx, n (%)	131 (27.9)	352 (61.5)	<0.001	284 (65.7)	68 (48.6)	<0.001
RCA, n (%)	180 (38.3)	317 (55.4)	<0.001	247 (57.2)	70 (50.0)	0.138
Extent of CAD						
2-vessel disease, n (%)	229 (48.7)	270 (47.2)	0.663	227 (52.5)	43 (30.7)	<0.001
≥3-vessel disease, n (%)	241 (51.3)	302 (52.8)	0.663	205 (47.5)	97 (69.3)	<0.001
ACC/AHA lesion type						
Type B1, n (%)	62 (13.2)	78 (13.6)	0.856	54 (12.5)	24 (17.1)	0.164
Type B2, n (%)	154 (32.8)	180 (31.5)	0.655	154 (35.6)	26 (18.6)	<0.001
Type C, n (%)	224 (47.7)	272 (47.6)	0.973	196 (45.4)	76 (54.3)	0.066
Pre-PCI TIMI flow grade 0/1, n (%)	185 (39.4)	228 (39.9)	0.870	179 (41.4)	49 (35.0)	0.197
In-hospital GP IIb/IIIa, n (%)	28 (6.0)	25 (4.4)	0.260	17 (3.9)	8 (5.7)	0.371
Drug-eluting stents [a]						
ZES, n (%)	168 (35.7)	203 (35.5)	0.932	164 (38.0)	39 (27.9)	0.033
EES, n (%)	248 (52.8)	321 (56.1)	0.279	233 (53.9)	88 (62.9)	0.064
BES, n (%)	54 (11.5)	66 (11.5)	0.980	47 (10.9)	19 (13.6)	0.386
Others, n (%)	6 (1.3)	7 (1.2)	0.939	6 (1.4)	1 (0.7)	0.528
IVUS, n (%)	68 (14.5)	138 (24.1)	<0.001	99 (22.9)	39 (27.9)	0.235
OCT, n (%)	1 (0.2)	2 (0.3)	0.682	1 (0.2)	1 (0.7)	0.430
FFR, n (%)	3 (0.6)	2 (0.3)	0.502	1 (0.2)	1 (0.7)	0.430

Table 1. *Cont.*

Variables	Culprit-Only PCI (*n* = 470)	Multivessel PCI (*n* = 572)	*p* Value	CR (*n* = 432)	IR (*n* = 140)	*p* Value
Completeness of multivessel PCI						
CR, *n* (%)	-	432 (75.5)	-	432 (100.0)	-	-
IR, *n* (%)		140 (24.5)	-	-	140 (100.0)	-
PCI for non-IRA	-					
During index PCI, *n* (%)	-	402 (70.3)	-	315 (72.9)	87 (62.1)	0.015
Staged PCI before discharge, *n* (%)	-	170 (29.7)	-	117 (27.1)	53 (37.9)	0.015
Time from admission to PCI (hours)	18.1 ± 54.6	22.6 ± 56.7	0.008	22.6 ± 57.3	22.9 ± 55.4	0.928
Stent diameter (mm)	3.03 ± 0.41	3.04 ± 0.40	0.689	3.02 ± 0.38	3.11 ± 0.45	0.028
Stent length (mm)	28.8 ± 13.4	29.1 ± 14.6	0.735	28.6 ± 14.6	30.5 ± 14.6	0.192
Number of stent	1.42 ± 0.70	2.31 ± 0.99	<0.001	2.40 ± 1.00	2.03 ± 0.92	<0.001
GRACE risk score	150.9 ± 27.3	150.1 ± 26.7.	0.640	149.7 ± 26.8	151.4 ± 26.7.	0.509
>140, *n* (%)	294 (62.6)	343 (60.0)	0.394	255 (59.0)	88 (62.9)	0.422

For continuous variables, intergroup differences were evaluated with the unpaired *t*-test and data are expressed as mean ± standard deviation. For categorical variables, intergroup differences were analyzed using the χ^2 test or, if not applicable, Fisher's exact test and the data are expressed as count and percentage. CR, complete revascularization; IR, incomplete revascularization; LVEF, left ventricular ejection fraction; BMI, body mass index; SBP, systolic blood pressure; DBP, diastolic blood pressure; MI, myocardial infarction; PCI, percutaneous coronary intervention; CABG, coronary artery bypass graft; HF, heart failure; CVA, cerebrovascular events; CK-MB, creatine kinase myocardial band; NT-ProBNP, N-terminal pro-brain natriuretic peptide; Hs-CRP, high-sensitivity C-reactive protein; eGFR, estimated glomerular filtration rate; HDL, high-density lipoprotein; LDL, low-density lipoprotein; ACEI, angiotensin converting enzyme inhibitors; ARB, angiotensin receptor blockers; CCB, calcium channel blockers; IRA, infarct-related artery; LM, left main coronary artery; LAD, left anterior descending coronary artery; LCx, left circumflex coronary artery; RCA, right coronary artery; CAD, coronary artery disease; ACC/AHA, American College of Cardiology/American Heart Association; TIMI, thrombolysis in myocardial infarction; GP, glycoprotein; ZES, zotarolimus-eluting stent; EES, everolimus-eluting stent; BES, biolimus-eluting stent; IVUS, intravascular ultrasound; OCT, optical coherence tomography; FFR, fractional flow reserve; GRACE, Global Registry of Acute Coronary Events; [a] Drug-eluting stents were composed of ZES (Resolute Integrity stent; Medtronic, Inc., Minneapolis, MN), EES (Xience Prime stent, Abbott Vascular, Santa Clara, CA; or Promus Element stent, Boston Scientific, Natick, MA) and BES (BioMatrix Flex stent, Biosensors International, Morges, Switzerland; or Nobori stent, Terumo Corporation, Tokyo, Japan).

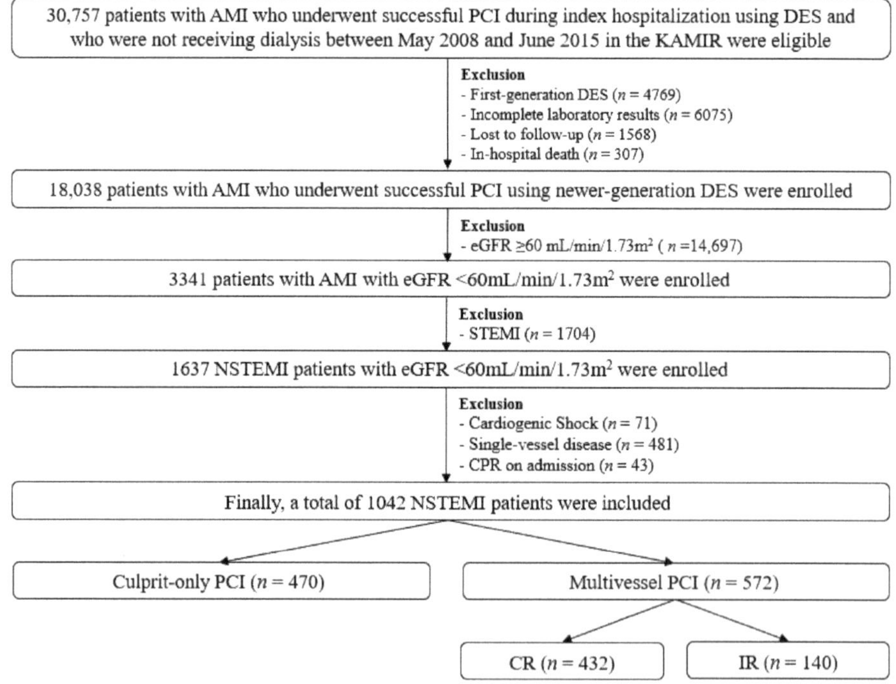

Figure 1. Flowchart. AMI, acute myocardial infarction; PCI, percutaneous coronary intervention; DES, drug-eluting stent; KAMIR, Korea AMI Registry; eGFR, estimated glomerular filtration rate; STEMI, ST-segment-elevation myocardial infarction; NSTEMI, non-STEMI; CPR, cardiopulmonary resuscitation; CR, complete revascularization; IR, incomplete revascularization.

2.2. Percutaneous Coronary Intervention and Medical Treatment

Following general guidelines [21], coronary angiography and PCI were performed via a transfemoral or transradial approach. Aspirin (200–300 mg) and clopidogrel (300–600 mg) when available, or ticagrelor (180 mg) or prasugrel (60 mg), were prescribed as loading doses to the individuals before PCI. After PCI, dual antiplatelet therapy (DAPT; a combination of aspirin (100 mg/day) with clopidogrel (75 mg/day) or ticagrelor (90 mg twice a day) or prasugrel (5–10 mg/day)) was recommended at least 12 months. Based on previous reports [22,23], triple antiplatelet therapy (TAPT; 100 mg of cilostazol was administered twice a day in addition, to DAPT) was administered at the discretion of the individual operator. Moreover, the access site, revascularization strategy and selection of DES were left to the discretion of the individual operators.

2.3. Study Definitions and Clinical Outcomes

Glomerular function was calculated using the Chronic Kidney Disease Epidemiology Collaboration equation for eGFR [24]. In this study, CKD was defined as eGFR <60 mL/min/1.73 m^2 [25,26]. If the patients showed the absence of persistent ST-segment elevation with increased cardiac biomarkers and if the clinical context was appropriate, these patients were considered to have NSTEMI [4,27]. MVD was defined as at least two major vessels ($\geq$2 mm diameter) with >70% stenosis of the vessel diameter [28]. Successful PCI was defined as residual stenosis <30% and thrombolysis in myocardial infarction grade III flow in the IRA after the procedure. The culprit vessel was evaluated by coronary angiographic findings, 12-lead electrocardiogram, two-dimensional echocardiogram and noninvasive stress test [29]. The M-PCI group comprised patients who underwent PCI of the non-IRA during index PCI of the IRA or who underwent staged PCI for the non-IRA within the index hospitalization. Hence, patients with NSTEMI and MVD who underwent staged PCI after discharge were excluded from this study (Figure 1). CR was defined as open IRA followed by dilatation of all other significantly narrowed arteries during the primary procedure or index hospitalization. IR was defined as successfully opened IRA followed by dilatation of only the significantly narrowed artery in $\geq$1 non-IRA vessel during the primary procedure or index hospitalization [30]. The Global Registry of Acute Coronary Events (GRACE) risk score [31] was calculated for all patients. The primary clinical outcome of this study was the occurrence of major adverse cardiac events (MACE), defined as all-cause death, recurrent myocardial infarction (re-MI), or any coronary repeat revascularization, including TLR, TVR and non-TVR. The secondary clinical outcome was definite or probable stent thrombosis (ST) during the 2-year follow-up period. All-cause death was considered cardiac death (CD) unless an undisputed noncardiac cause was present [32]. Any repeat revascularization was composed of TLR, TVR and non-TVR. The definitions of re-MI, TLR, TVR and non-TVR have been previously published [33,34]. The cumulative incidence of ST was defined according to the Academic Research Consortium [35]. However, the incidence of ST in this study, was low; hence, the total number of ST events was described instead of a separate cumulative incidence according to their time interval (acute, subacute, late and very late).

2.4. Statistical Analyses

For continuous variables, intergroup differences were evaluated using the unpaired *t*-test and data were expressed as mean ± standard deviation. For categorical variables, intergroup differences were analyzed using the χ^2 test or, if not applicable, Fisher's exact test and data were expressed as counts and percentages. Various clinical outcomes were estimated using the Kaplan–Meier method and intergroup differences were compared using the log-rank test. Significant confounding covariates ($p < 0.05$) were included in the multivariate Cox regression analysis. The variables included in the comparison between C-PCI and M-PCI were as follows: age; male sex; left ventricular ejection fraction (LVEF) <40%; blood levels of peak creatine kinase-myocardial band (CK-MB), peak troponin-I, N-terminal pro-brain natriuretic peptide (NT-proBNP) and triglyceride; discharge medications (cilostazol and lipid-lowering agent); IRA (left main coronary artery (LM)); treated vessels (LM, left anterior descending (LAD) artery, left circumflex artery (LCx) and right coronary artery (RCA)); use of intravascular ultrasound (IVUS); time from admission to PCI; number of deployed stents; and GRACE risk score. The variables included in the comparison between CR and IR, between C-PCI and CR and between C-PCI and IR are shown in Table 2. For all analyses, two-sided values of $p < 0.05$ were considered statistically significant. All statistical analyses were performed using the Statistical Package for the Social Sciences version 20 (IBM, Armonk, NY, USA).

Table 2. Clinical outcomes.

Outcomes	Cumulative Events (%)		Log-Rank	Unadjusted		Adjusted [a]	
	Culprit-Only (*n* = 470)	Multivessel (*n* = 572)		HR (95% CI)	*p* Value	HR (95% CI)	*p* Value
MACE	71 (16.0)	84 (15.7)	0.985	1.003 (0.731–1.376)	0.985	1.020 (0.675–1.542)	0.924
All-cause death	48 (10.8)	44 (8.2)	0.187	1.316 (0.874–1.981)	0.188	1.328 (0.774–2.278)	0.303
Cardiac death	24 (5.5)	25 (4.8)	0.606	1.159 (0.662–2.029)	0.606	1.280 (0.608–2.696)	0.516
Re-MI	14 (3.5)	22 (4.3)	0.410	0.755 (0.386–1.476)	0.412	1.178 (0.531–3.084)	0.582
Any revascularization	22 (5.3)	27 (5.3)	0.899	0.964 (0.549–1.693)	0.899	1.042 (0.496–2.188)	0.913
TVR	14 (3.4)	16 (3.1)	0.927	1.034 (0.505–2.119)	0.927	1.246 (0.490–3.167)	0.645
Non-TVR	9 (2.1)	11 (2.2)	0.968	0.982 (0.407–2.370)	0.968	1.628 (0.506–5.240)	0.414
ST (definite or probable)	4 (0.9)	9 (1.6)	0.295	0.538 (0.166–1.748)	0.303	1.367 (0.308–6.069)	0.681
Outcomes	Cumulative Events (%)		Log-Rank	Unadjusted		Adjusted [b]	
	CR (*n* = 432)	IR (*n* = 140)		HR (95% CI)	*p* Value	HR (95% CI)	*p* Value
MACE	63 (15.5)	21 (16.6)	0.871	0.960 (0.586–1.573)	0.871	1.012 (0.577–1.776)	0.967
All-cause death	35 (8.6)	9 (7.2)	0.543	1.254 (0.603–2.610)	0.544	1.271 (0.542–2.977)	0.581
Cardiac death	18 (4.5)	7 (5.7)	0.673	0.829 (0.346–1.985)	0.674	1.429 (0.517–3.947)	0.491
Re-MI	16 (4.2)	6 (5.0)	0.719	0.842 (0.329–2.153)	0.720	1.239 (0.414–3.709)	0.702
Any revascularization	19 (5.0)	8 (6.4)	0.538	0.772 (0.338–1.764)	0.539	1.385 (0.541–3.545)	0.497
TVR	11 (2.8)	5 (4.1)	0.550	0.726 (0.252–2.089)	0.552	1.750 (0.485–6.320)	0.393
Non-TVR	8 (2.1)	3 (2.3)	0.823	0.860 (0.228–3.240)	0.823	1.524 (0.272–8.544)	0.632
ST (definite or probable)	6 (1.4)	3 (2.7)	0.533	0.646 (0.162–2.584)	0.537	1.890 (0.357–10.00)	0.454
Outcomes	Cumulative Events (%)		Log-Rank	Unadjusted		Adjusted [c]	
	Culprit-Only (*n* = 470)	CR (*n* = 432)		HR (95% CI)	*p* Value	HR (95% CI)	*p* Value
MACE	71 (16.0)	63 (15.5)	0.956	1.010 (0.719–1.417)	0.956	1.042 (0.656–1.654)	0.863
All-cause death	48 (10.8)	35 (8.6)	0.308	1.254 (0.811–1.938)	0.309	1.223 (0.673–2.223)	0.509
Cardiac death	24 (5.5)	18 (4.5)	0.522	1.220 (0.662–2.248)	0.523	1.305 (0.569–2.993)	0.529
Re-MI	14 (3.5)	16 (4.2)	0.515	0.789 (0.385–1.616)	0.516	1.107 (0.434–2.823)	0.832
Any revascularization	22 (5.3)	19 (5.0)	0.907	1.037 (0.562–1.917)	0.907	1.096 (0.461–2.605)	0.836
TVR	14 (3.4)	11 (2.8)	0.750	1.137 (0.516–2.504)	0.751	1.906 (0.703–5.171)	0.205
Non-TVR	9 (2.1)	8 (2.1)	0.966	1.021 (0.394–2.646)	0.966	2.958 (0.683–12.81)	0.147
ST (definite or probable)	4 (0.9)	6 (1.4)	0.439	0.610 (0.172–2.161)	0.443	1.344 (0.276–6.654)	0.715
Outcomes	Cumulative Events (%)		Log-Rank	Unadjusted		Adjusted [d]	
	Culprit-Only (*n* = 470)	IR (*n* = 140)		HR (95% CI)	*p* Value	HR (95% CI)	*p* Value
MACE	71 (16.0)	21 (16.6)	0.853	0.955 (0.587–1.554)	0.853	1.060 (0.594–1.891)	0.844
All-cause death	48 (10.8)	9 (7.2)	0.222	1.553 (0.762–3.165)	0.226	2.007 (0.882–4.569)	0.097
Cardiac death	24 (5.5)	7 (5.7)	0.993	0.996 (0.429–2.313)	0.993	1.057 (0.381–2.929)	0.916
Re-MI	14 (3.5)	6 (5.0)	0.393	0.661 (0.254–1.721)	0.396	1.807 (0.517–6.312)	0.354
Any revascularization	22 (5.3)	8 (6.4)	0.562	0.788 (0.351–1.769)	0.563	1.524 (0.542–4.280)	0.424
TVR	14 (3.4)	5 (4.1)	0.672	0.802 (0.289–2.228)	0.672	1.592 (0.405–6.264)	0.506
Non-TVR	9 (2.1)	3 (2.3)	0.850	0.882 (0.239–3.257)	0.850	1.043 (0.183–5.931)	0.962
ST (definite or probable)	4 (0.9)	3 (2.7)	0.207	0.394 (0.088–1.762)	0.223	1.446 (0.172–12.16)	0.735

HR, hazard ratio; CI, confidence interval; MACE, major adverse cardiac events; Re-MI, recurrent myocardial infarction; TVR, target vessel revascularization; ST, stent thrombosis; CR, complete revascularization; IR, incomplete revascularization; LVEF, left ventricular ejection fraction; MI, myocardial infarction; PCI, percutaneous coronary intervention; CABG, coronary artery bypass graft; CK-MB, creatine kinase myocardial band; NT-ProBNP, N-terminal pro-brain natriuretic peptide; Hs-CRP, high-sensitivity C-reactive protein; HDL, high-density lipoprotein; LDL, low-density lipoprotein; IRA, infarct-related artery; LM, left main coronary artery; LAD, left anterior descending coronary artery; LCx, left circumflex coronary artery; RCA, right coronary artery; CAD, coronary artery disease; ACC/AHA, American College of Cardiology/American Heart Association; EES, everolimus-eluting stent; IVUS, intravascular ultrasound; GRACE, Global Registry of Acute Coronary Events. [a] Adjusted by age, male sex, LVEF <40%, peak CK-MB, peak troponin-I, NT-ProBNP, triglyceride, cilostazole, lipid lowering agents, IRA (LM), treated vessel (LM, LAD, LCx and RCA), IVUS, time from admission to PCI, number of stent and GRACE risk score. [b] Adjusted by age, male sex, LVEF, hypertension, DM, previous PCI, previous CABG, peak troponin-I, NT-ProBNP, Hs-CRP, LDL-cholesterol, cilostazole, IRA (LM), treated vessel (LCx), 2-vessel disease, 3-vessel disease, ACC/AHA type B2 lesion, ZES, PCI for non-IRA, stent diameter, number of stent and GRACE risk score. [c] Adjusted by age, male sex, LVEF <40%, previous PCI, peak CK-MB, peak troponin-I, NT-ProBNP, HDL-cholesterol, LDL-cholesterol, cilostazole, treated vessel (LM, LAD, LCx and RCA), IVUS, time from admission to PCI and number of stent and GRACE risk score. [d] Adjusted by age, male sex, LVEF, DM, peak troponin-I, NT-ProBNP, blood glucose, lipid lowering agent, IRA (LM), treated vessel (LM, LAD, LCx and RCA), 2-vessel disease, 3-vessel disease, ACC/AHA type B2 lesion, EES, IVUS, stent diameter, number of stent and GRACE risk score.

3. Results

3.1. Baseline Characteristics

The baseline clinical, laboratory and procedural characteristics of the study population are summarized in Table 1 and Table S1. In the comparison between C-PCI and M-PCI, the number of male patients and the mean value of peak CK-MB were higher in the C-PCI group and the mean time interval from admission to PCI, the prescription rate of lipid-lowering agent as a discharge medication, IRA (LM) and use of IVUS were significantly higher in the M-PCI group. In the comparison between CR and IR, the mean value of LVEF, the number of 2-vessel disease and American College of Cardiology/American Heart Association (ACC/AHA) type B2 lesion were higher in the CR group. In contrast, the number of patients with hypertension, diabetes mellitus (DM), previous history of PCI and coronary artery bypass graft (CABG), IRA (LM), ≥3-vessel disease and ACC/AHA type B2 lesion were higher in the IR group. In the comparison between C-PCI and CR, the number of male patients, those with a previous history of PCI and the mean value of peak CK-MB were higher in the C-PCI group. However, the mean time from admission to PCI, number of all treated vessels (LM, LAD, LCx and RCA), use of IVUS and mean diameter of deployed stent were higher in the CR group. In the comparison between C-PCI and IR, the mean value of LVEF and the number of ACC/AHA type B2 lesion were higher in the C-PCI group. The number of DM, lipid-lowering agents as a discharge medication, IRA (LM), all treated vessels, ≥3-vessel disease, use of IVUS and mean number of deployed stents were higher in the IR group. The mean value of the GRACE risk score and the number of patients with GRACE risk score >140 were similar between the C-PCI and M-PCI groups, between the CR and IR groups, between the C-PCI and CR groups and between the C-PCI and IR groups (Table 1 and Table S1).

3.2. Clinical Outcomes

The cumulative incidences of major clinical outcomes at 2 years are listed in Table 2, Figure 2 and Figure S1. In the comparison between C-PCI and M-PCI, after adjustment, the cumulative incidences of MACE (Figure 2A), all-cause death (Figure 2B), CD (Figure 2C), re-MI (Figure 2D), any repeat revascularization (Figure 2E), TVR (Figure 2F), non-TVR (Figure 2G) and ST (Figure 2H) were similar between the C-PCI and M-PCI groups. In the comparison between CR and IR, after adjustment, the cumulative incidences of all major clinical outcomes were similar between the CR and IR groups. Similarly, the primary and secondary clinical outcomes were similar between the C-PCI and CR groups and between the C-PCI and IR groups (Table 2 and Figure S1). Table 3 shows the independent predictors of MACE at 2 years. Reduced LVEF (<40%), peak troponin-I and NT-proBNP levels were significant independent predictors of MACE.

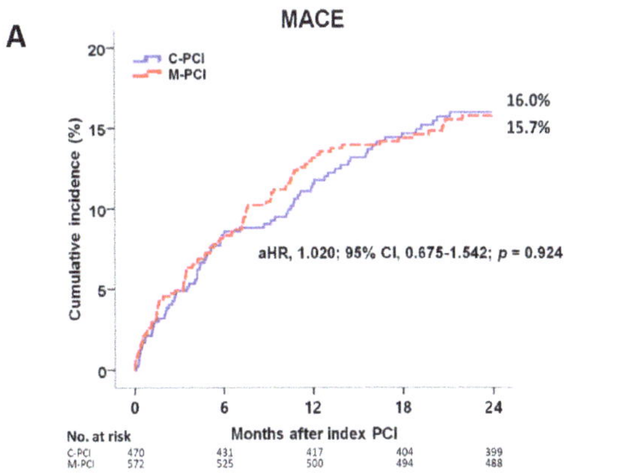

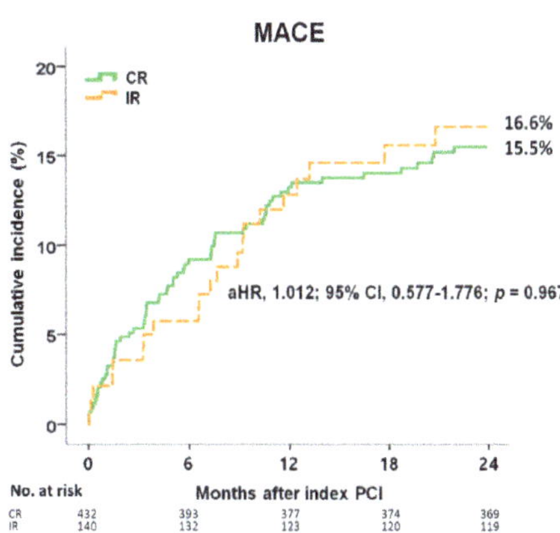

Figure 2. *Cont.*

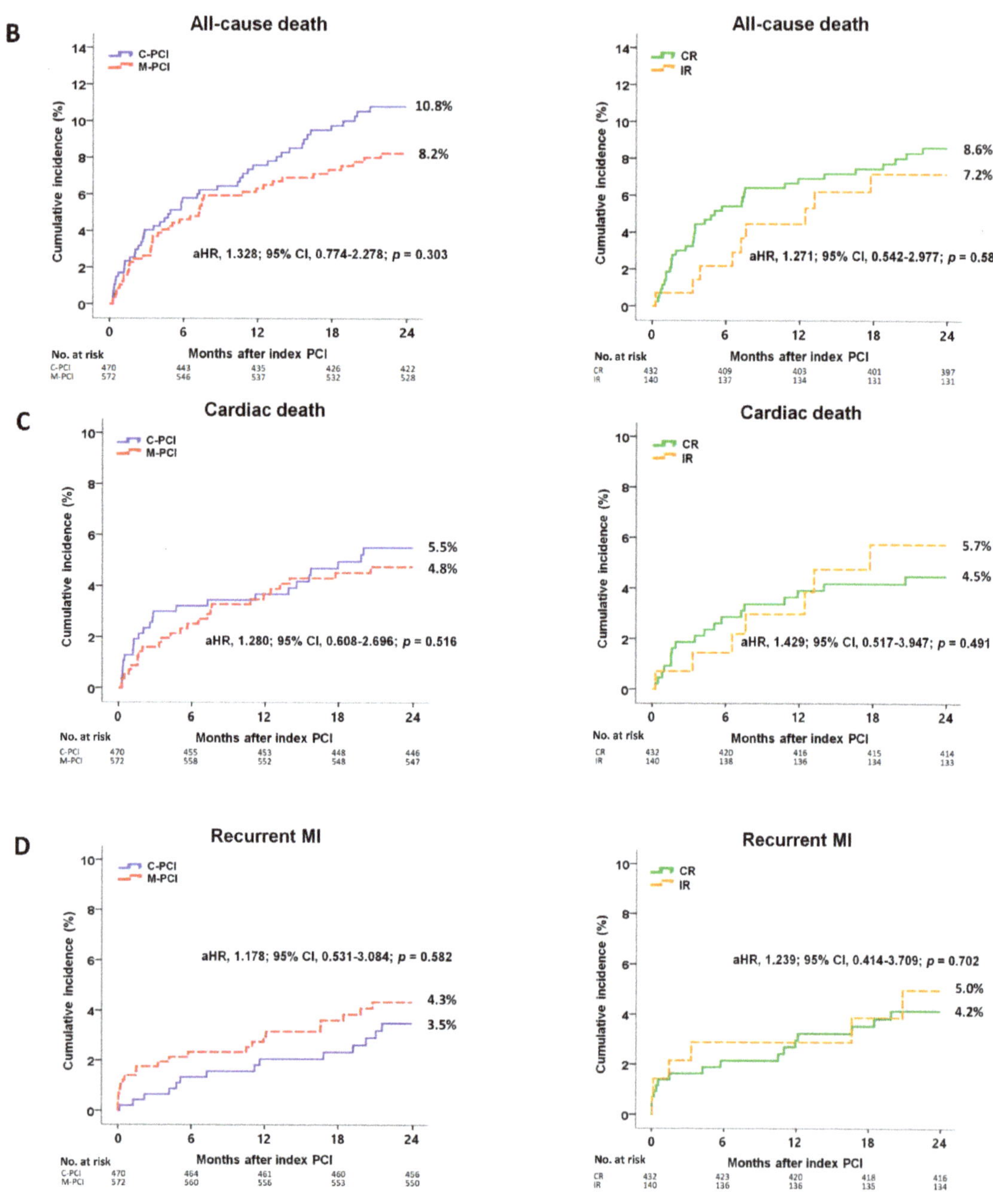

Figure 2. *Cont.*

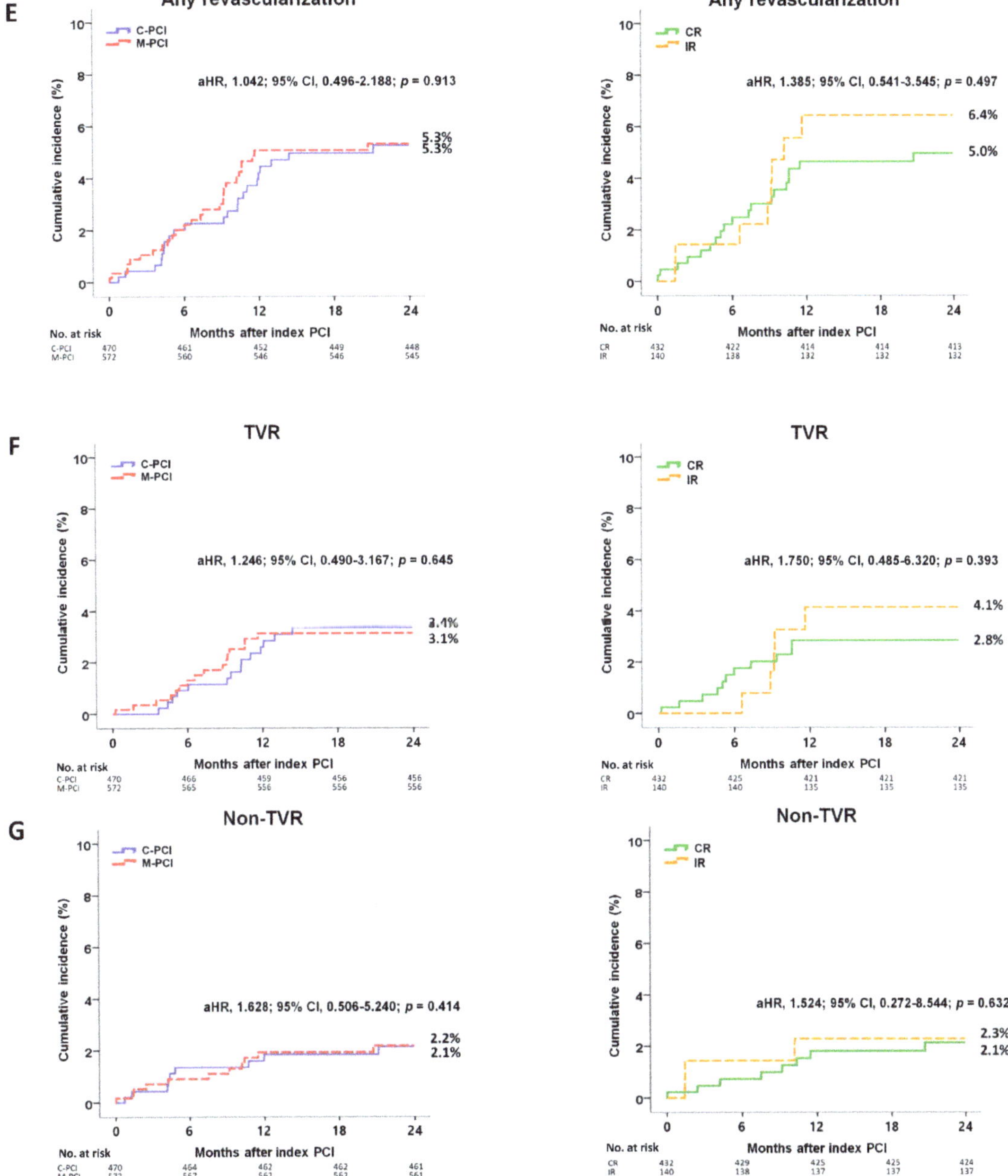

Figure 2. *Cont.*

H

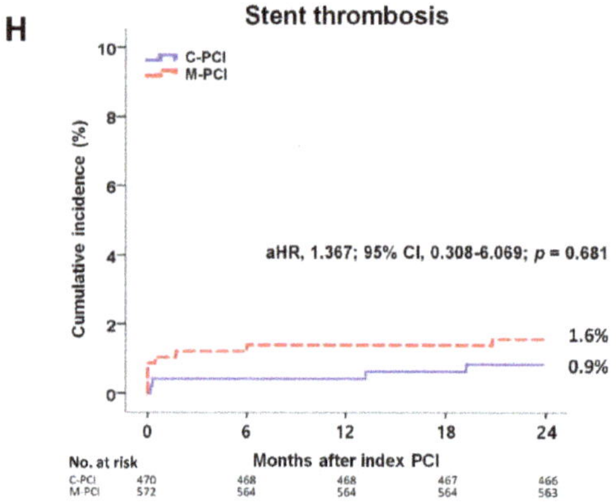

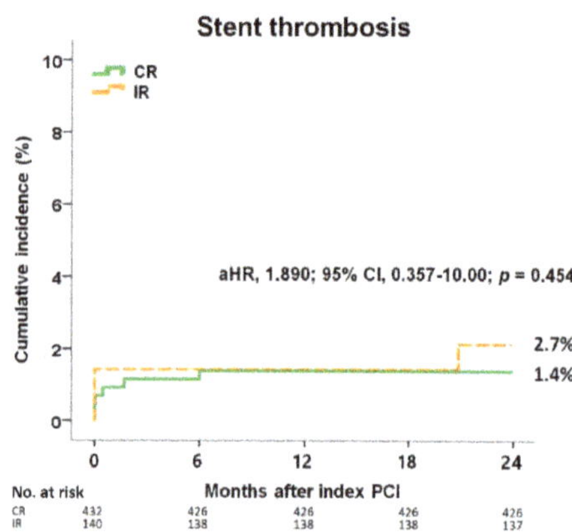

Figure 2. Kaplan-Meier analyses for the MACE (**A**), all-cause death (**B**), cardiac death (**C**), recurrent MI (**D**), any repeat revascularization (**E**), TVR (**F**), non-TVR (**G**) and ST (**H**) between the C-PCI group and the M-PCI group and the CR group and the IR group at 2 years. aHR, adjusted hazard ratio; CI, confidence interval; MACE, major adverse cardiac events; MI, myocardial infarction; TVR, target vessel revascularization; C-PCI, culprit-only PCI; M-PCI, multivessel PCI; CR, complete revascularization; IR, incomplete revascularization.

Table 3. Independent predictors for MACE.

Variables	Unadjusted		Adjusted	
	HR (95% CI)	*p*	HR (95% CI)	*p*
C-PCI vs. M-PCI	1.003 (0.731–1.376)	0.985	1.090 (0.706–1.684)	0.696
CR vs. IR	0.960 (0.586–1.573)	0.871	1.021 (0.552–1.888)	0.947
C-PCI vs. CR	1.010 (0.719–1.417)	0.956	1.192 (0.741–1.920)	0.469
C-PCI vs. IR	0.955 (0.587–1.554)	0.853	1.143 (0.592–2.206)	0.691
Age, ≥65 years	1.438 (1.019–2.030)	0.039	1.422 (0.951–2.010)	0.083
Male	1.317 (0.954–1.820)	0.095	1.282 (0.894–1.838)	0.177
LVEF, <40%	1.993 (1.438–2.763)	<0.001	1.482 (1.026–2.235)	0.029
Killip class III	1.691 (1.180–2.423)	0.004	1.349 (0.836–2.177)	0.220
Hypertension	1.169 (0.792–1.724)	0.432	1.146 (0.756–1.737)	0.520
Diabetes mellitus	1.471 (1.060–2.041)	0.021	1.387 (0.948–2.028)	0.092
Previous PCI	1.105 (0.704–1.735)	0.665	1.080 (0.667–1.748)	0.756
Previous CABG	1.409 (0.522–3.803)	0.499	1.451 (0.520–4.050)	0.477
Peak CK-MB	1.001 (1.000–1.002)	0.186	1.001 (1.000–1.002)	0.192
Peak troponin-I	1.001 (1.001–1.002)	<0.001	1.002 (1.001–1.002)	0.002
NT-ProBNP	1.000 (0.999–1.001)	0.001	1.001 (1.000–1.002)	0.026
Hs-CRP	0.998 (0.993–1.004)	0.550	0.997 (0.990–1.003)	0.325
Blood glucose	1.000 (0.999–1.002)	0.790	0.999 (0.997–1.001)	0.214
Total cholesterol	0.999 (0.995–1.002)	0.425	0.999 (0.995–1.004)	0.833
Triglyceride	0.999 (0.997–1.001)	0.445	0.999 (0.976–1.002)	0.527
HDL-cholesterol	0.979 (0.964–0.995)	0.008	0.980 (0.970–1.001)	0.051
LDL-cholesterol	1.002 (0.998–1.005)	0.397	1.002 (0.998–1.007)	0.353
Ticagrelor	1.228 (0.574–2.628)	0.596	1.436 (0.650–3.174)	0.371
Prasugrel	1.422 (0.527–3.839)	0.488	1.144 (0.398–3.288)	0.802
Cilostazole	1.238 (0.862–1.780)	0.248	1.293 (0.874–1.911)	0.198
ACEI	1.098 (0.796–1.514)	0.569	1.014 (0.660–1.559)	0.949
ARB	1.067 (0.766–1.484)	0.702	1.066 (0.691–1.645)	0.722
Beta-blocker	1.166 (0.783–1.737)	0.449	1.132 (0.731–1.753)	0.578
Lipid lowering agent	1.057 (0.722–1.546)	0.775	1.168 (0.768–1.776)	0.467
LM-IRA	1.451 (0.786–2.679)	0.234	1.004 (0.304–3.312)	0.995
LM-treated vessel	1.398 (0.821–2.381)	0.218	1.444 (0.522–3.993)	0.179
LAD-treated vessel	1.036 (0.752–1.429)	0.827	1.069 (0.743–1.538)	0.719
LCx-treated vessel	1.076 (0.784–1.478)	0.649	1.133 (0.791–1.622)	0.497
RCA-treated vessel	1.153 (0.842–1.580)	0.375	1.184 (0.812–1.725)	0.369

Table 3. *Cont.*

Variables	Unadjusted		Adjusted	
	HR (95% CI)	*p*	HR (95% CI)	*p*
ACC/AHA type B2/C lesion	1.263 (0.834–1.913)	0.270	1.105 (0.709–1.721)	0.680
IVUS	1.041 (0.695–1.559)	0.844	1.038 (0.681–1.582)	0.862
Time from admission to PCI	1.001 (0.998–1.003)	0.193	1.091 (1.000–1.271)	0.080
Stent diameter <3.0 mm	0.900 (0.647–1.253)	0.533	1.171 (0.820–1.671)	0.385
Stent length ≥30 mm	1.417 (1.026–1.957)	0.034	1.379 (0.968–1.966)	0.075
GRACE risk score	1.071 (1.012–1.031)	0.037	1.001 (0.993–1.010)	0.778

MACE, major adverse cardiac events; HR, hazard ratio; CI, confidence interval; C-PCI, culprit-only PCI, M-PCI, multivessel PCI; CR, complete revascularization; IR, incomplete revascularization; PCI, percutaneous coronary intervention; LVEF, left ventricular ejection fraction; CABG, coronary artery bypass graft; CK-MB, creatine kinase myocardial band; NT-ProBNP, N-terminal pro-brain natriuretic peptide; Hs-CRP, high-sensitivity C-reactive protein; HDL, high-density lipoprotein; LDL, low-density lipoprotein; ACEI, angiotensin converting enzyme inhibitor; ARB, angiotensin receptor blocker; LM, left main coronary artery; IRA, infarct-related artery; LAD, left anterior descending coronary artery; LCx, left circumflex coronary artery; RCA, right coronary artery; ACC/AHA, American College of Cardiology/American Heart Association; IVUS, intravascular ultrasound; GRACE, Global Registry of Acute Coronary Events.

4. Discussion

The main findings of this study are as follows: (1) the cumulative incidence rates of MACE, all-cause death, CD, re-MI, any repeat revascularization, TVR, non-TVR and ST were similar between the C-PCI and M-PCI groups, between the CR and IR groups, between the C-PCI and CR groups, and between the C-PCI and IR groups and (2) reduced LVEF (<40%), CPR on admission and peak troponin-I and NT-proBNP levels were significant independent predictors of MACE.

Patients with NSTEMI tend to have MVD and more complex disease than patients with STEMI [36]. Although the current guidelines recommend an early invasive strategy in patients with high-risk NSTEMI [4,5], the optimal treatment strategy for NSTEMI with MVD is still debatable. Recently, Rathod et al. [9] showed that single-stage CR appears to be superior to C-PCI in terms of long-term mortality (22.5% vs. 25.9, $p = 0.0005$) during a median of 4.1-year follow-up period in their 21,857 NSTEMI patients with MVD. This study has a large sample size, provides adequate power and is very valuable because it shows the mortality reduction capability of single-stage CR. However, about 24% of the enrolled patients received bare-metal stents (BMS) and the number of patients who received newer-generation DES is unclear. In the era of newer-generation DES, BMS is rarely used and 1G-DES is nearly replaced with a thinner and more biocompatible or biodegradable polymer-coated newer-generation DES with better clinical outcomes [30]. Furthermore, as mentioned, 2G-DES was beneficial in reducing mortality and TLR/TVR in patients with CKD [18]. The current guidelines also recommend newer-generation DES over BMS during PCI in patients with NSTE-acute coronary syndrome (ACS) and CKD [5]. Thus, their findings have some limitations in reflecting the current real-world practice. In the Impact of Different Treatment in Multivessel Non-ST-Elevation Myocardial Infarction (NSTEMI) Patients: One Stage Versus Multistaged PCI (SMILE) randomized trial [37], the 1-year rate of major adverse cardiovascular and cerebrovascular events was lower in the one-stage coronary revascularization group than that in the multistage PCI group (13.63% vs. 23.19%, $p = 0.004$). In their study [37], the number of patients who received BMS or plain old balloon angioplasty was approximately 18%. More recently, Liu et al. [6] demonstrated that immediate M-PCI was associated with worse long-term outcomes than stage M-PCI during index admission (log-rank $p < 0.001$). However, their study included about 40% of STEMI patients and the deployed stents were not confined to newer-generation DES. Similarly, other previous studies [7,8] also included patients who received BMS or 1G-DES. Additionally, studies concerning long-term outcomes according to different reperfusion strategies in patients with NSTEMI with MVD and CKD after PCI using newer-generation DES are limited.

Although CKD patients have frequent risk factors and comorbidities, many large-scale trials have excluded patients with CKD [17]. Hence, the long-term effects of revascularization therapy in these patients are not fully understood. A previous report [38] suggested that early revascularization could reduce the risk of 1-year mortality compared to initial medical therapy (odds ratio [OR], 0.46; p = 0.008) in 23,234 ACS patients. The most recent meta-analysis [39] demonstrated that PCI cannot improve short- ($\leq$1 month, OR, 0.65; p = 0.079) and medium-term (1 month to 1 year, OR, 0.70; p = 0.157) all-cause death compared with medical treatment in patients with AMI. The American guideline [4] recommends that an invasive strategy is reasonable in patients with NSTE-ACS with mild (stage 2) and moderate (stage 3) CKD (class IIa, level of evidence B). According to the European guideline [5], PCI should be considered for CABG in patients with NSTE-ACS and CKD with MVD whose surgical risk profile is high or the life expectancy is <1 year (class IIa, level of evidence B). Current evidence [40] does not recommend routine immediate M-PCI in AMI patients with cardiogenic shock. Therefore, the remaining issue concerns AMI patients with MVD without cardiogenic shock, which is considered an ongoing issue for interventional cardiologists [39]. As shown in Figure 1, patients with cardiogenic shock were excluded in our study. Patients with NSTEMI and cardiogenic shock have worse clinical outcomes than those with STEMI and cardiogenic shock [41] and PCI of the non-IRA may aggravate hemodynamic instability and jeopardize the viable myocardium in the milieu of AMI [6].

In our study, regarding baseline characteristics (Table 1), in the M-PCI group, the mean value of triglycerides, the number of LM as an IRA, the number of treated vessels (LM, LAD, LCx and RCA) and the mean time from admission to PCI were higher than that in the C-PCI group. The number of patients with hypertension, DM, previous PCI, previous CABG, LM as an IRA and $\geq$3-vessel disease was higher in the IR group than that in the CR group. Moreover, the mean value of LVEF was also lower in the IR group than that in the CR group (46.1% $\pm$ 12.5% vs. 49.7% $\pm$ 12.7%, p = 0.010). In the C-PCI group, the number of patients with previous PCI and the mean value of peak CK-MB were higher than that in the CR group. However, the number of patients with DM, LM as IRA and ACC/AHA type B2 lesions was higher in the IR group than that in the C-PCI group. Additionally, the mean value of LVEF was lower in the IR group than that in the C-PCI group (46.1% $\pm$ 12.5% vs. 48.3% $\pm$ 12.6%, p = 0.037, Table S1). Although baseline characteristics were significantly different between the four groups (C-PCI vs. M-PCI, CR vs. IR, C-PCI vs. CR and C-PCI vs. IR), the 2-year major clinical outcomes were not significantly different between these groups (Table 2). Although we could not precisely determine the etiologic factors for these results, one possible explanation may be related to the similar distribution of significant independent predictors for MACE (Table 3, reduced LVEF <40%, peak troponin-I and NT-proBNP levels) in these comparison groups. Recently, Kim et al. [42] reported that the cumulative incidences of major clinical outcomes were similar in the three comparison groups (C-PCI vs. M-PCI, CR vs. IR, or C-PCI vs. CR) except for non-TVR in 4588 patients with NSTEMI and MVD after newer-generation DES implantation. They mentioned that the higher incidence rate of non-TVR in the C-PCI group may be related to the initial selection of treatment strategies, that is, either C-PCI or M-PCI, during the index PCI. As this selection was based on the physician's preference, in the C-PCI group, regardless of whether the lesions were considered significantly invasive during the initial procedure, these lesions were not treated. As a result, the PCIs were possibly included as non-TVR in the C-PCI group. However, in their study [42], patients with cardiogenic shock were included and the enrolled patients were not confined to those with CKD. Because there are very limited studies that can be used to directly compare the results of our study, determining the value of this study in comparison to that of other studies and speculating the main cause of the results of this study compared to those of other studies are challenging.

Regarding patients with STEMI, Mehta et al. [43] demonstrated that CR was superior to C-PCI in patients with STEMI and MVD in reducing cardiovascular death or MI, as well as the risk of cardiovascular death, MI, or ischemia-driven revascularization in their randomized trial. However, in the more recent review [44], a strategy of staged PCI of obstructive non-culprit lesions should be considered the gold standard for the treatment of patient with STEMI and MVD. However, what is the optimal timing of staged PCI is not completely defined and the assessment of intermediate non-culprit lesions is still a major problem [44]. Moreover, they [44] also mentioned that there are no studies demonstrating that preventive PCI of vulnerable plaques or more intensive pharmacological treatment is associated with an improved clinical outcome.

Patients with CKD have a high prevalence of DM and an increased chance of having 3-vessel CAD, LM disease and coronary calcification [45]. As the severity of CKD progresses, the severity and extent of CAD also increases [46]. Therefore, patients with CKD undergoing PCI need to carefully consider diverse clinical options to minimize the risk of contrast-induced nephropathy and optimize clinical outcomes [47]. In real-world practice, despite the limitation in available data, CKD patients presenting with NSTEMI with MVD received the same approach as those with normal renal function [48]. With respect to these limitations of current practice in patients with NSTEMI with MVD and CKD, we believe that our results could be helpful to interventional cardiologists in terms of providing current real-world information regarding clinical outcomes among different multivessel reperfusion strategies in patients with NSTEMI and CKD. Furthermore, although the study population was insufficient to show meaningful results, more than 50 high-volume tertiary-care teaching hospitals in South Korea participated in this study.

This study had other limitations. First, because of the retrospective nature of this cohort study, there may have been some underreporting and/or missing data and selection bias. Second, CKD is strongly associated with an increased risk of bleeding in patients undergoing PCI [49]. However, because the value of this variable was incomplete due to missing values, we could not include this as a meaningful variable in our study. Therefore, this was a major limitation of this study. Third, the estimation of renal function was based on a single measurement of eGFR at the time of presentation to the hospital. Therefore, there is a possibility that eGFR may have worsened during the follow-up period. Unfortunately, we could not provide follow-up eGFR values because of the limitations of the registry data. Fourth, the variables that were not included in the data registry might have affected the study outcome. Fifth, although the time interval from symptom onset to PCI is an important determinant of major clinical outcomes, this variable included many missing values in the registry data. Therefore, we could not include this variable in the present study, which may have resulted in bias. Sixth, the 2-year follow-up period in this study was relatively short for estimating long-term clinical outcomes. Seventh, our study was focused on patients with CKD, so it is intuitive to have a primary or secondary outcome including for example need for renal replacement therapy during hospitalization, or occurrence of contrast-induced nephropathy. However, because these variables were not mandatory variables, we could not include these variables as the major outcomes in this study. This point was other important limitation of our study. Eighth, because limitations of medical insurance system in Korea, the use of fractional flow reserve/instant wave-free ratio was very restricted in this study (Table 1). Thus, in this study, the patients with intermediate stenotic lesions were not fully evaluated. Finally, this study enrolled patients who underwent PCI between May 2008 and June 2015 and this broad timeframe could have affected the clinical outcomes.

5. Conclusions

In the contemporary newer-generation DES era, our results suggest that C-PCI may be a better option for patients with NSTEMI with MVD and CKD rather than M-PCI, including CR and IR, with regard to procedure time and the risk of contrast-induced nephropathy. However, further well-designed, large-scale randomized studies are warranted to confirm these results.

Supplementary Materials: The following are available online at https://www.mdpi.com/article/10.3390/jcm10204629/s1, Table S1: Baseline clinical, laboratory, angiographic and procedural characteristics, Figure S1: Kaplan-Meier analyses for the MACE (A), all-cause death (B), cardiac death (C), recurrent MI (D), any repeat revascularization (E), TVR (F), non-TVR (G) and stent thrombosis (H) between the C-PCI group and the CR group and the C-PCI group and the IR group at 2 years. MACE, major adverse cardiac events; MI, myocardial infarction; TVR, target vessel revascularization; C-PCI, culprit-only PCI; M-PCI, multivessel PCI; CR, complete revascularization; IR, incomplete revascularization.

Author Contributions: Conceptualization, Y.H.K., A.-Y.H., M.-K.H. and Y.J.; Data curation, Y.H.K., A.-Y.H., S.-J.H. and S.-J.L.; Formal analysis, Y.H.K., A.-Y.H., S.-J.H. and S.-J.L.; Funding acquisition, M.H.J.; Project administration, Y.H.K., A.-Y.H., M.H.J., B.-K.K., S.-J.H., S.-J.L., C.-M.A., J.-S.K., Y.-G.K., D.C., M.-K.H. and Y.J.; Resources, M.H.J., B.-K.K., S.-J.H., S.-J.L., C.-M.A., J.-S.K., Y.-G.K., D.C., M.-K.H. and Y.J.; Supervision, Y.H.K., M.H.J., D.C., M.-K.H. and Y.J.; Validation, Y.H.K., A.-Y.H., M.H.J., B.-K.K., S.-J.H., S.-J.L., C.-M.A., J.-S.K., Y.-G.K., D.C., M.-K.H. and Y.J.; Visualization, Y.H.K., A.-Y.H., M.H.J., B.-K.K., S.-J.H., S.-J.L., C.-M.A., J.-S.K., Y.-G.K., D.C., M.-K.H. and Y.J.; Writing—original draft, Y.H.K. and A.-Y.H.; Writing—review & editing, Y.H.K., A.-Y.H., M.H.J., B.-K.K., S.-J.H., S.-J.L., C.-M.A., J.-S.K., Y.-G.K., D.C., M.-K.H. and Y.J. All authors have read and agreed to the published version of the manuscript.

Funding: This research was supported by a fund (2016-ER6304-02) by Research of Korea Centers for Disease Control and Prevention.

Institutional Review Board Statement: The study was conducted according to the guidelines of the Declaration of Helsinki and approved by the Chonnam National University Hospital Institutional Review Board (IRB) ethics committee (protocol code CNUH-2011-172 and 1 March 2011).

Informed Consent Statement: Informed written consent was obtained from all subjects involved in this study.

Data Availability Statement: Data is contained within the article or supplementary material.

Acknowledgments: This research was supported by a fund (2016-ER6304-02) by Research of Korea Centers for Disease Control and Prevention. Korea Acute Myocardial infarction Registry (KAMIR) investigators. Myung Ho Jeong, Youngkeun Ahn, Sung Chul Chae, Jong Hyun Kim, Seung-Ho Hur, Young Jo Kim, In Whan Seong, Donghoon Choi, Jei Keon Chae, Taek Jong Hong, Jae Young Rhew, Doo-Il Kim, In-Ho Chae, Junghan Yoon, Bon-Kwon Koo, Byung-Ok Kim, Myoung Yong Lee, Kee-Sik Kim, Jin-Yong Hwang, Myeong Chan Cho, Seok Kyu Oh, Nae-Hee Lee, Kyoung Tae Jeong, Seung-Jea Tahk, Jang-Ho Bae, Seung-Woon Rha, Keum-Soo Park, Chong Jin Kim, Kyoo-Rok Han, Tae Hoon Ahn, Moo-Hyun Kim, Ki Bae Seung, Wook Sung Chung, Ju-Young Yang, Chong Yun Rhim, Hyeon-Cheol Gwon, Seong-Wook Park, Young-Youp Koh, Seung Jae Joo, Soo-Joong Kim, Dong Kyu Jin, Jin Man Cho, Sang-Wook Kim, Jeong Kyung Kim, Tae Ik Kim, Deug Young Nah, Si Hoon Park, Sang Hyun Lee, Seung Uk Lee, Hang-Jae Chung, Jang-Hyun Cho, Seung Won Jin, Myeong-Ki Hong, Yangsoo Jang, Jeong Gwan Cho, Hyo-Soo Kim, and Seung-Jung Park.

Conflicts of Interest: The authors declared they do not have anything to disclose regarding conflict of interest with respect to this manuscript.

References

1. Sorajja, P.; Gersh, B.J.; Cox, D.A.; McLaughlin, M.G.; Zimetbaum, P.; Costantini, C.; Stuckey, T.; Tcheng, J.E.; Mehran, R.; Lansky, A.J.; et al. Impact of multivessel disease on reperfusion success and clinical outcomes in patients undergoing primary percutaneous coronary intervention for acute myocardial infarction. *Eur. Heart J.* **2007**, *28*, 1709–1716. [CrossRef]
2. Hassanin, A.; Brener, S.J.; Lansky, A.J.; Xu, K.; Stone, G.W. Prognostic impact of multivessel versus culprit vessel only percutaneous intervention for patients with multivessel coronary artery disease presenting with acute coronary syndrome. *EuroIntervention* **2015**, *11*, 293–300. [CrossRef]
3. Ferrara, L.A.; Russo, B.F.; Gente, R.; Esposito, G.; Rapacciuolo, A.; de Simone, G. STEMI and NSTEMI: A mono versus a multivessel disease? *Int. J. Cardiol.* **2013**, *168*, 2905–2906. [CrossRef]
4. Amsterdam, E.A.; Wenger, N.K.; Brindis, R.G.; Casey, D.E., Jr.; Ganiats, T.G.; Holmes, D.R., Jr.; Jaffe, A.S.; Jneid, H.; Kelly, R.F.; Kontos, M.C.; et al. 2014 AHA/ACC Guideline for the Management of Patients with Non-ST-Elevation Acute Coronary Syndromes: A report of the American College of Cardiology/American Heart Association Task Force on Practice Guidelines. *J. Am. Coll. Cardiol.* **2014**, *64*, e139–e228. [CrossRef]
5. Roffi, M.; Patrono, C.; Collet, J.P.; Mueller, C.; Valgimigli, M.; Andreotti, F.; Bax, J.J.; Borger, M.A.; Brotons, C.; Chew, D.P.; et al. 2015 ESC Guidelines for the management of acute coronary syndromes in patients presenting without persistent ST-segment elevation: Task Force for the Management of Acute Coronary Syndromes in Patients Presenting without Persistent ST-Segment Elevation of the European Society of Cardiology (ESC). *Eur. Heart J.* **2016**, *37*, 267–315.

6. Liu, E.S.; Hung, C.C.; Chiang, C.H.; Chang, C.H.; Cheng, C.C.; Kuo, F.Y.; Mar, G.Y.; Huang, W.C. Comparison of Different Timing of Multivessel Intervention during Index-Hospitalization for Patients with Acute Myocardial Infarction. *Front. Cardiovasc. Med.* **2021**, *8*, 639750. [CrossRef] [PubMed]
7. Hannan, E.L.; Samadashvili, Z.; Walford, G.; Jacobs, A.K.; Stamato, N.J.; Venditti, F.J.; Holmes, D.R., Jr.; Sharma, S.; King, S.B., 3rd. Staged versus one-time complete revascularization with percutaneous coronary intervention for multivessel coronary artery disease patients without ST-elevation myocardial infarction. *Cir. Cardiovasc. Interv.* **2013**, *6*, 12–20. [CrossRef] [PubMed]
8. Shishehbor, M.H.; Lauer, M.S.; Singh, I.M.; Chew, D.P.; Karha, J.; Brener, S.J.; Moliterno, D.J.; Ellis, S.G.; Topol, E.J.; Bhatt, D.L. In unstable angina or non-ST-segment acute coronary syndrome, should patients with multivessel coronary artery disease undergo multivessel or culprit-only stenting? *J. Am. Coll. Cardiol.* **2007**, *49*, 849–854. [CrossRef] [PubMed]
9. Rathod, K.S.; Koganti, S.; Jain, A.K.; Astroulakis, Z.; Lim, P.; Rakhit, R.; Kalra, S.S.; Dalby, M.C.; O'Mahony, C.; Malik, I.S.; et al. Complete Versus Culprit-Only Lesion Intervention in Patients with Acute Coronary Syndromes. *J. Am. Coll. Cardiol.* **2018**, *72*, 1989–1999. [CrossRef] [PubMed]
10. McNeice, A.; Nadra, I.J.; Robinson, S.D.; Fretz, E.; Ding, L.; Fung, A.; Aymong, E.; Chan, A.W.; Hodge, S.; Webb, J.; et al. The prognostic impact of revascularization strategy in acute myocardial infarction and cardiogenic shock: Insights from the British Columbia Cardiac Registry. *Cath. Cardiovasc. Interv.* **2018**, *92*, E356–E367. [CrossRef] [PubMed]
11. Mehran, R. Contrast-induced nephropathy remains a serious complication of PCI. *J. Interv. Cardiol.* **2007**, *20*, 236–240. [CrossRef]
12. Carande, E.J.; Brown, K.; Jackson, D.; Maskell, N.; Kouzaris, L.; Greene, G.; Mikhail, A.; Obaid, D.R. Acute Kidney Injury Following Percutaneous Coronary Intervention for Acute Coronary Syndrome: Incidence, Aetiology, Risk Factors and Outcomes. *Angiology* **2021**, 33197211040375.
13. Hanratty, C.G.; Koyama, Y.; Rasmussen, H.H.; Nelson, G.I.; Hansen, P.S.; Ward, M.R. Exaggeration of nonculprit stenosis severity during acute myocardial infarction: Implications for immediate multivessel revascularization. *J. Am. Coll. Cardiol.* **2002**, *40*, 911–916. [CrossRef]
14. Anavekar, N.S.; McMurray, J.J.; Velazquez, E.J.; Solomon, S.D.; Kober, L.; Rouleau, J.L.; White, H.D.; Nordlander, R.; Maggioni, A.; Dickstein, K.; et al. Relation between renal dysfunction and cardiovascular outcomes after myocardial infarction. *N. Engl. J. Med.* **2004**, *351*, 1285–1295. [CrossRef]
15. Manjunath, G.; Tighiouart, H.; Ibrahim, H.; MacLeod, B.; Salem, D.N.; Griffith, J.L.; Coresh, J.; Levey, A.S.; Sarnak, M.J. Level of kidney function as a risk factor for atherosclerotic cardiovascular outcomes in the community. *J. Am. Coll. Cardiol.* **2003**, *41*, 47–55. [CrossRef]
16. Szummer, K.; Lundman, P.; Jacobson, S.H.; Schön, S.; Lindbäck, J.; Stenestrand, U.; Wallentin, L.; Jernberg, T. Relation between renal function, presentation, use of therapies and in-hospital complications in acute coronary syndrome: Data from the SWEDEHEART register. *J. Intern. Med.* **2010**, *268*, 40–49. [CrossRef]
17. Strippoli, G.F.; Craig, J.C.; Schena, F.P. The number, quality, and coverage of randomized controlled trials in nephrology. *J. Am. Soc. Nephrol.* **2004**, *15*, 411–419. [CrossRef] [PubMed]
18. Crimi, G.; Gritti, V.; Galiffa, V.A.; Scotti, V.; Leonardi, S.; Ferrario, M.; Ferlini, M.; De Ferrari, G.M.; Oltrona Visconti, L.; Klersy, C. Drug eluting stents are superior to bare metal stents to reduce clinical outcome and stent-related complications in CKD patients, a systematic review, meta-analysis and network meta-analysis. *J. Interv. Cardiol.* **2018**, *31*, 319–329. [CrossRef] [PubMed]
19. Kim, Y.; Ahn, Y.; Cho, M.C.; Kim, C.J.; Kim, Y.J.; Jeong, M.H. Current status of acute myocardial infarction in Korea. *Korean J. Intern. Med.* **2019**, *34*, 1–10. [CrossRef]
20. Kim, J.H.; Chae, S.C.; Oh, D.J.; Kim, H.S.; Kim, Y.J.; Ahn, Y.; Cho, M.C.; Kim, C.J.; Yoon, J.H.; Park, H.Y.; et al. Multicenter Cohort Study of Acute Myocardial Infarction in Korea—Interim Analysis of the Korea Acute Myocardial Infarction Registry-National Institutes of Health Registry. *Circ. J.* **2016**, *80*, 1427–1436. [CrossRef]
21. Grech, E.D. ABC of interventional cardiology: Percutaneous coronary intervention. II: The procedure. *BMJ* **2003**, *326*, 1137–1140. [CrossRef]
22. Lee, S.W.; Park, S.W.; Hong, M.K.; Kim, Y.H.; Lee, B.K.; Song, J.M.; Han, K.H.; Lee, C.W.; Kang, D.H.; Song, J.K.; et al. Triple versus dual antiplatelet therapy after coronary stenting: Impact on stent thrombosis. *J. Am. Coll. Cardiol.* **2005**, *46*, 1833–1837. [CrossRef]
23. Chen, K.Y.; Rha, S.W.; Li, Y.J.; Poddar, K.L.; Jin, Z.; Minami, Y.; Wang, L.; Kim, E.J.; Park, C.G.; Seo, H.S.; et al. Triple versus dual antiplatelet therapy in patients with acute ST-segment elevation myocardial infarction undergoing primary percutaneous coronary intervention. *Circulation* **2009**, *119*, 3207–3214. [CrossRef] [PubMed]
24. Levey, A.S.; Stevens, L.A.; Schmid, C.H.; Zhang, Y.L.; Castro, A.F., 3rd; Feldman, H.I.; Kusek, J.W.; Eggers, P.; Van Lente, F.; Greene, T.; et al. A new equation to estimate glomerular filtration rate. *Ann. Intern. Med.* **2009**, *150*, 604–612. [CrossRef]
25. Salinero-Fort, M.A.; San Andrés-Rebollo, F.J.; de Burgos-Lunar, C.; Gómez-Campelo, P.; Chico-Moraleja, R.M.; López de Andrés, A.; Jiménez-García, R. Five-year incidence of chronic kidney disease (stage 3-5) and associated risk factors in a Spanish cohort: The MADIABETES Study. *PLoS ONE* **2015**, *10*, e0122030. [CrossRef] [PubMed]
26. Bangalore, S.; Guo, Y.; Samadashvili, Z.; Blecker, S.; Xu, J.; Hannan, E.L. Revascularization in Patients with Multivessel Coronary Artery Disease and Chronic Kidney Disease: Everolimus-Eluting Stents Versus Coronary Artery Bypass Graft Surgery. *J. Am. Coll. Cardiol.* **2015**, *66*, 1209–1220. [CrossRef] [PubMed]

27. Newby, L.K.; Jesse, R.L.; Babb, J.D.; Christenson, R.H.; De Fer, T.M.; Diamond, G.A.; Fesmire, F.M.; Geraci, S.A.; Gersh, B.J.; Larsen, G.C.; et al. ACCF 2012 expert consensus document on practical clinical considerations in the interpretation of troponin elevations: A report of the American College of Cardiology Foundation task force on Clinical Expert Consensus Documents. *J. Am. Coll. Cardiol.* **2012**, *60*, 2427–2463. [CrossRef] [PubMed]
28. Thiele, H.; Akin, I.; Sandri, M.; de Waha-Thiele, S.; Meyer-Saraei, R.; Fuernau, G.; Eitel, I.; Nordbeck, P.; Geisler, T.; Landmesser, U.; et al. One-Year Outcomes after PCI Strategies in Cardiogenic Shock. *N. Engl. J. Med.* **2018**, *379*, 1699–1710. [CrossRef]
29. Kim, M.C.; Jeong, M.H.; Ahn, Y.; Kim, J.H.; Chae, S.C.; Kim, Y.J.; Hur, S.H.; Seong, I.W.; Hong, T.J.; Choi, D.H.; et al. What is optimal revascularization strategy in patients with multivessel coronary artery disease in non-ST-elevation myocardial infarction? Multivessel or culprit-only revascularization. *Int. J. Cardiol.* **2011**, *153*, 148–153. [CrossRef]
30. Kim, Y.H.; Her, A.Y.; Jeong, M.H.; Kim, B.K.; Hong, S.J.; Kim, J.S.; Ko, Y.G.; Choi, D.; Hong, M.K.; Jang, Y. Impact of stent generation on 2-year clinical outcomes in ST-segment elevation myocardial infarction patients with multivessel disease who underwent culprit-only or multivessel percutaneous coronary intervention. *Cath. Cardiovasc. Interv.* **2020**, *95*, E40–E55. [CrossRef]
31. de Araújo Gonçalves, P.; Ferreira, J.; Aguiar, C.; Seabra-Gomes, R. TIMI, PURSUIT, and GRACE risk scores: Sustained prognostic value and interaction with revascularization in NSTE-ACS. *Eur. Heart J.* **2005**, *26*, 865–872. [CrossRef]
32. Lee, J.M.; Rhee, T.M.; Hahn, J.Y.; Kim, H.K.; Park, J.; Hwang, D.; Choi, K.H.; Kim, J.; Park, T.K.; Yang, J.H.; et al. Multivessel Percutaneous Coronary Intervention in Patients with ST-Segment Elevation Myocardial Infarction with Cardiogenic Shock. *J. Am. Coll. Cardiol.* **2018**, *71*, 844–856. [CrossRef] [PubMed]
33. Kim, Y.H.; Her, A.Y.; Jeong, M.H.; Kim, B.K.; Lee, S.Y.; Hong, S.J.; Shin, D.H.; Kim, J.S.; Ko, Y.G.; Choi, D.; et al. Impact of renin-angiotensin system inhibitors on long-term clinical outcomes in patients with acute myocardial infarction treated with successful percutaneous coronary intervention with drug-eluting stents: Comparison between STEMI and NSTEMI. *Atherosclerosis* **2019**, *280*, 166–173. [CrossRef] [PubMed]
34. Kim, Y.H.; Her, A.Y.; Jeong, M.H.; Kim, B.K.; Lee, S.Y.; Hong, S.J.; Ahn, C.M.; Kim, J.S.; Ko, Y.G.; Choi, D.; et al. One-year clinical outcomes between biodegradable-polymer-coated biolimus-eluting stent and durable-polymer-coated drug-eluting stents in STEMI patients with multivessel coronary artery disease undergoing culprit-only or multivessel PCI. *Atherosclerosis* **2019**, *284*, 102–109. [CrossRef]
35. Cutlip, D.E.; Windecker, S.; Mehran, R.; Boam, A.; Cohen, D.J.; van Es, G.A.; Steg, P.G.; Morel, M.A.; Mauri, L.; Vranckx, P.; et al. Clinical end points in coronary stent trials: A case for standardized definitions. *Circulation* **2007**, *115*, 2344–2351. [CrossRef] [PubMed]
36. Mahmud, E.; Ben-Yehuda, O. Percutaneous Coronary Intervention in Acute Coronary Syndrome: Completing the Job Saves Lives. *J. Am. Coll. Cardiol.* **2018**, *72*, 2000–2002. [CrossRef]
37. Sardella, G.; Lucisano, L.; Garbo, R.; Pennacchi, M.; Cavallo, E.; Stio, R.E.; Calcagno, S.; Ugo, F.; Boccuzzi, G.; Fedele, F.; et al. Single-Staged Compared with Multi-Staged PCI in Multivessel NSTEMI Patients: The SMILE Trial. *J. Am. Coll. Cardiol.* **2016**, *67*, 264–272. [CrossRef]
38. Huang, H.D.; Alam, M.; Hamzeh, I.; Virani, S.; Deswal, A.; Aguilar, D.; Rogers, P.; Kougias, P.; Birnbaum, Y.; Paniagua, D.; et al. Patients with severe chronic kidney disease benefit from early revascularization after acute coronary syndrome. *Int. J. Cardiol.* **2013**, *168*, 3741–3746. [CrossRef]
39. Yong, J.; Tian, J.; Zhao, X.; Yang, X.; Xing, H.; He, Y.; Song, X. Optimal treatment strategies for coronary artery disease in patients with advanced kidney disease: A meta-analysis. *Ther. Adv. Chronic Dis.* **2021**, *12*, 20406223211024367. [CrossRef]
40. Thiele, H.; Akin, I.; Sandri, M.; Fuernau, G.; de Waha, S.; Meyer-Saraei, R.; Nordbeck, P.; Geisler, T.; Landmesser, U.; Skurk, C.; et al. PCI Strategies in Patients with Acute Myocardial Infarction and Cardiogenic Shock. *N. Engl. J. Med.* **2017**, *377*, 2419–2432. [CrossRef]
41. Anderson, M.L.; Peterson, E.D.; Peng, S.A.; Wang, T.Y.; Ohman, E.M.; Bhatt, D.L.; Saucedo, J.F.; Roe, M.T. Differences in the profile, treatment, and prognosis of patients with cardiogenic shock by myocardial infarction classification: A report from NCDR. *Cir. Cardiovasc. Qual Outcomes* **2013**, *6*, 708–715. [CrossRef]
42. Kim, Y.H.; Her, A.Y.; Jeong, M.H.; Kim, B.K.; Hong, S.J.; Kim, S.; Ahn, C.M.; Kim, J.S.; Ko, Y.G.; Choi, D.; et al. Culprit-only versus multivessel or complete versus incomplete revascularization in patients with non-ST-segment elevation myocardial infarction and multivessel disease who underwent successful percutaneous coronary intervention using newer-generation drug-eluting stents. *Atherosclerosis* **2020**, *301*, 54–64. [PubMed]
43. Mehta, S.R.; Wood, D.A.; Storey, R.F.; Mehran, R.; Bainey, K.R.; Nguyen, H.; Meeks, B.; Di Pasquale, G.; López-Sendón, J.; Faxon, D.P.; et al. COMPLETE Trial Steering Committee and Investigators. Complete Revascularization with Multivessel PCI for Myocardial Infarction. *N. Engl. J. Med.* **2019**, *381*, 1411–1421. [CrossRef] [PubMed]
44. Montone, R.A.; Niccoli, G.; Crea, F.; Jang, I.K. Management of non-culprit coronary plaques in patients with acute coronary syndrome. *Eur. Heart J.* **2020**, *41*, 3579–3586. [CrossRef] [PubMed]
45. Chonchol, M.; Whittle, J.; Desbien, A.; Orner, M.B.; Petersen, L.A.; Kressin, N.R. Chronic kidney disease is associated with angiographic coronary artery disease. *Am. J. Nephrol.* **2008**, *28*, 354–360. [CrossRef] [PubMed]
46. Coskun, U.; Orta Kilickesmez, K.; Abaci, O.; Kocas, C.; Bostan, C.; Yildiz, A.; Baskurt, M.; Arat, A.; Ersanli, M.; Gurmen, T. The relationship between chronic kidney disease and SYNTAX score. *Angiology* **2011**, *62*, 504–508. [CrossRef] [PubMed]
47. Klein, E.C.; Kapoor, R.; Lewandowski, D.; Mason, P.J. Revascularization Strategies in Patients with Chronic Kidney Disease and Acute Coronary Syndromes. *Curr. Cardiol. Rep.* **2019**, *21*, 113. [CrossRef]

48. Charytan, D.M.; Wallentin, L.; Lagerqvist, B.; Spacek, R.; De Winter, R.J.; Stern, N.M.; Braunwald, E.; Cannon, C.P.; Choudhry, N.K. Early angiography in patients with chronic kidney disease: A collaborative systematic review. *Clin. J. Am. Soc. Nephrol.* **2009**, *4*, 1032–1043. [CrossRef]
49. Washam, J.B.; Kaltenbach, L.A.; Wojdyla, D.M.; Patel, M.R.; Klein, A.J.; Abbott, J.D.; Rao, S.V. Anticoagulant Use among Patients with End-Stage Renal Disease Undergoing Percutaneous Coronary Intervention: An Analysis From the National Cardiovascular Data Registry. *Circ. Cardiovasc. Interv.* **2018**, *11*, e005628. [CrossRef] [PubMed]

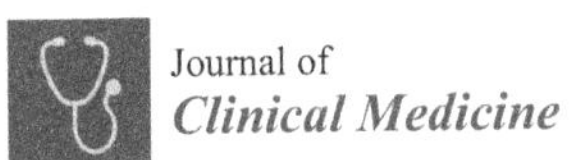

Journal of
Clinical Medicine

MDPI

Review

The Role of Uric Acid in Acute and Chronic Coronary Syndromes

Alessandro Maloberti [1,2,*], Marco Biolcati [1,2], Giacomo Ruzzenenti [1,2], Valentina Giani [1,2], Filippo Leidi [1,2], Massimiliano Monticelli [1,2], Michela Algeri [2], Sara Scarpellini [2], Stefano Nava [3], Francesco Soriano [3], Jacopo Oreglia [3], Alice Sacco [3], Nuccia Morici [3], Fabrizio Oliva [3], Federica Piani [4], Claudio Borghi [4] and Cristina Giannattasio [1,2]

1 School of Medicine and Surgery, University of Milano-Bicocca, 20126 Milan, Italy; marco.biolcati@ospedaleniguarda.it (M.B.); giacomo.ruzzenenti@ospedaleniguarda.it (G.R.); valentina.giani@ospedaleniguarda.it (V.G.); Filippo.leidi@ospedaleniguarda.it (F.L.); massimiliano.monticelli@ospedaleniguarda.it (M.M.); cristina.giannattasio@ospedaleniguarda.it (C.G.)

2 Cardiology 4, ASST GOM Niguarda Hospital, 20121 Milan, Italy; michela.algeri@ospedaleniguarda.it (M.A.); sara.scarpellini@ospedaleniguarda.it (S.S.)

3 Cardiology 1, ASST GOM Niguarda Hospital, 20121 Milan, Italy; stefano.nava@ospedaleniguarda.it (S.N.); francesco.soriano@ospedaleniguarda.it (F.S.); jacopo.oreglia@ospedaleniguarda.it (J.O.); alice.sacco@ospedaleniguarda.it (A.S.); nuccia.morici@ospedaleniguarda.it (N.M.); fabrizio.oliva@ospedaleniguarda.it (F.O.)

4 School of Medicine and Surgery, University of Bologna—IRCCS Policlinico S. Orsola, 40138 Bologna, Italy; federica.piani2@unibo.it (F.P.); claudio.borghi@unibo.it (C.B.)

* Correspondence: alessandro.maloberti@ospedaleniguarda.it; Tel.: +39-026-444-2141; Fax: +39-026-444-2566

Abstract: Uric acid (UA) is the final product of the catabolism of endogenous and exogenous purine nucleotides. While its association with articular gout and kidney disease has been known for a long time, new data have demonstrated that UA is also related to cardiovascular (CV) diseases. UA has been identified as a significant determinant of many different outcomes, such as all-cause and CV mortality, and also of CV events (mainly Acute Coronary Syndromes (ACS) and even strokes). Furthermore, UA has been related to the development of Heart Failure, and to a higher mortality in decompensated patients, as well as to the onset of atrial fibrillation. After a brief introduction on the general role of UA in CV disorders, this review will be focused on UA's relationship with CV outcomes, as well as on the specific features of patients with ACS and Chronic Coronary Syndrome. Finally, two issues which remain open will be discussed: the first is about the identification of a CV UA cut-off value, while the second concerns the possibility that the pharmacological reduction of UA is able to lower the incidence of CV events.

Keywords: uric acid; acute coronary syndrome; chronic coronary syndrome

Citation: Maloberti, A.; Biolcati, M.; Ruzzenenti, G.; Giani, V.; Leidi, F.; Monticelli, M.; Algeri, M.; Scarpellini, S.; Nava, S.; Soriano, F.; et al. The Role of Uric Acid in Acute and Chronic Coronary Syndromes. *J. Clin. Med.* **2021**, *10*, 4750. https://doi.org/10.3390/jcm10204750

Academic Editors: Atsushi Tanaka and Koichi Node

Received: 23 September 2021
Accepted: 13 October 2021
Published: 16 October 2021

Publisher's Note: MDPI stays neutral with regard to jurisdictional claims in published maps and institutional affiliations.

1. Introduction

Uric Acid (UA) is the final product of the catabolism of purine nucleotides from endogenous (cellular nucleoproteins) and exogenous origins (alimentary). Its biosynthesis, which principally involves the liver, also includes the gut, muscles and kidneys; urinary excretion is the main mechanism of UA elimination, while a small percentage thereof is removed by the intestine. At a pH of 7.4, the solubility limit of plasma UA is 6.8 mg/dL. Beyond this level, the conditions for urate crystal precipitation are created. Conditions which may raise UA levels include the increased production which occurs with a purine-rich diet, tumor lysis syndrome or specific drugs (chemotherapy and pyrazinamide), and also with a decrease in UA excretion, mainly in renal diseases. Genetics could also be a cause for hyperuricemia, as it happens in the gain of function of the enzyme phosphoribosyl-pyrophosphate synthetase, or in the deficit of hypoxantine-guanine phosphoribosyltransferase (completely in the Lesch-Nyhan syndrome, partially in the Kelley-Seegmiller syndrome) [1].

The association of UA with articular gout and kidney disease has been known for a long time, while new data has demonstrated that UA is also related to cardiovascular (CV) diseases. [1] In fact, UA was identified as a significant determinant of many different outcomes in the CV area, such as all-cause and CV mortality [2], and also of CV events (mainly Acute Coronary Syndrome—ACS) and stroke [3,4]. Furthermore, UA is correlated with the development of Heart Failure (HF) [5], and with a higher mortality in this group of patients [6], as well as with the onset of atrial fibrillation [7]. All of these significant findings led the latest European Guidelines of Arterial Hypertension to introduce UA among CV risk factors that should be assessed in order to stratify a patient's risk [8].

Hyperuricemia represents an epidemiological problem, especially if CV comorbidities are present. Its prevalence ranges from 6% in healthy subjects [9] to 14% in hypertensives [10], with a significant increase to 23% among patients with ACS and Chronic Coronary Syndrome (CCS) [11,12]. After a brief introduction on UA's general role in CV events, this review focuses on UA's relationship with CV outcomes, as well as on specific features of patients with ACS and CCS. Despite the important number of publications on this topic, two issues remain open: the first is about the identification of a CV UA cut-off value, while the second concerns the possibility that the pharmacological reduction of UA is able to lower the incidence of CV events. These two fundamental points will also be discussed in this research paper.

2. Uric Acid and Cardiovascular Events

The connection between UA and CV events was demonstrated for the first time in 1967 by Kannel et al. [13] in the Framingham study, which included 5127 subjects with a 12-year follow-up, in which an increased risk of Myocardial Infarction (MI) was identified in subjects with hyperuricemia. Since this pivotal work, many other later publications confirmed this association, and hyperuricemia was recognized as an independent CV risk factor, and also when added to the traditional ones [1]. In fact, one of the biggest meta-analyses on this issue, including 29 prospective studies (for a total of 958,410 individuals), found a Hazard Ratio (HR) of 1.13 (95% CI 1.05–1.21) for MI, and of 1.27 (95% CI 1.16–1.39) for CV mortality in hyperuricemic patients [14].

The mechanisms by which UA could determine CV events have not been definitively identified. However, UA certainly acts at multiple levels, as shown in Figure 1.

First, the oxidative stress determined by the two final biochemical reactions is involved: during the conversion of hypoxanthine into xanthine (and hence into UA) determined by the xanthine oxidase enzyme, the generated superoxide anions increase oxidative stress, a well-known atherosclerotic risk factor [15,16]. In addition, concurrent processes induced by xanthine oxidase include the oxidative role of NADH and the nitrate reduction activity [17], which are two other factors which are able to induce oxidative stress. This leads to the "xanthine oxidase theory", according to which the decrease of UA through the inhibition of the enzyme, instead of an increased renal elimination of UA, is most beneficial in terms of CV risk reduction.

Oxidative stress represents a fundamental pathway in diseases related to hyperuricemia (hypertension and Diabetes Mellitus—DM), and in the development of heart and vessels organ damage. In fact, UA has been linked to the development of arterial hypertension [18], DM [19], and metabolic syndrome [20], which in turn increase the rate of CV events. The molecular paths possibly explaining the relationship between UA and hypertension include the activation of the renin-angiotensin-aldosterone system [21] and an impairment in endothelial function due to a reduction of nitric oxide levels [22]. Regarding metabolic derangement, UA is involved in the deamination of adenosine monophosphate, resulting in increased fat accumulation, which is one of the steps at the basis of hyperinsulinemia, and consequently of insulin resistance [23]. In addition, UA can block oxide nitric-mediated insulin release, and increases the oxidative damage in pancreatic B-cells [24].

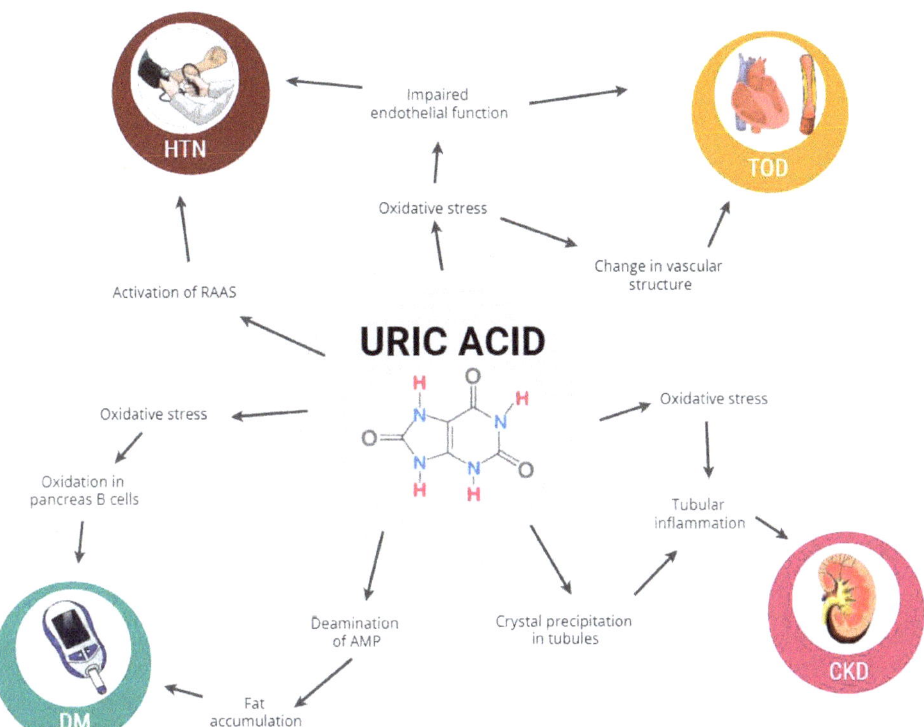

Figure 1. Mechanisms contributing to the relationship between uric acid and cardiovascular diseases. HTN = Arterial Hypertension; DM = Diabetes Mellitus; CKD = Chronic Kidney Disease; TOD = Target Organ Damage.

One of the most important mechanisms through which UA is probably related to CV events is renal damage, a well-known CV risk factor. UA can affect kidneys by depositing crystals in renal tubules during hyperuricosuria [25], resulting, together with increased oxidative stress, in tubule-interstitial inflammation with afferent arteriopathy of the arteriole and hyperplasia/hypertrophy of the tunica muscularis [26]. In fact, UA is definitely related to the reduction of the glomerular filtration rate, as well as to microalbuminuria [27]. However, the link between UA and kidney damage is certainly a two-way correlation, as the loss of renal function results in the decreased excretion capacity of UA with increased plasma levels [28].

Finally, UA also appears to be linked to heart and vessel damages. In particular, the relationship with pulse wave velocity, which is the most widely used measurement of arterial stiffness, suggests a possible association between UA and changes in vascular structure and function [29].

Another relevant aspect in the relation between UA and CV diseases is the role of gender. Some studies describe a link with target organ damage only in females [11], while CV outcomes (all-cause mortality, CV mortality and ACS) seem to be related to UA only in females in some studies [30] and only in males in others [31]. Some possible explanations include the existence of gender differences in the gene functions controlling the biochemical pathways of UA [32], but also the role of hormones in women and their involvement in UA metabolism. In fact, hyperuricemia has been associated with a higher left ventricular mass index during post-menopause, but not in pre-menopause [33].

3. Uric Acid and Acute Coronary Syndrome

As was already mentioned, hyperuricemia appears to be associated with fatal and non-fatal ACS in the general population [4]. In patients experiencing an ACS, it is a common finding (reported in 23% of the total subjects [11]). Moreover, in patients admitted for an ACS, UA seems to be related to in-hospital [11] and long term [34] all-cause and CV mortality, and also to higher rates of in-hospital adverse events (such as atrial fibrillation or bleeding [35]) and to longer inpatient stays.

In particular, many studies found an association between UA levels at admission and specific HF-related issues, such as the Killip class, the use of intra-aortic balloon pump and cardiogenic shock, and a reduced left ventricular ejection fraction at admission [11,36]. This last point raises an interesting question, i.e., whether UA in ACS is a determinant of worse presentation or simply a marker of a poorer condition. In other words, is UA a significant determinant or just an innocent bystander in the context of an ACS? To date, the answer is not totally clear, and both supporting and non-supporting data has been published (Table 1). Furthermore, most knowledge on this issue is derived from cross-sectional and prospective studies, while only a few Randomized Clinical Trials have been published (and will be discussed further on).

Some studies identify UA as a determinant of a more severe coronary artery involvement, a larger infarct size [37], a greater risk of acute plaque complications (such as the formation of a completely obstructing thrombus) [38] and a higher prevalence of challenging revascularization procedures, which could remain incomplete [39]. It is also possible that the UA increase in HF is merely an epiphenomenon of the cardiac damage, and is not the triggering cause, as it could secondarily rise due to increased purine metabolism caused by hypoxia and tissue catabolism [40], enhanced purine release from ischemic cells (both from the heart and from peripheral hypoperfused tissue) and the reduced clearance deriving from ACS-related impaired renal function. Furthermore, a hyperactivation in xanthine oxidase activity was also found in acute decompensated HF [41]. Finally, patients with HF-related issues during ACS make use of diuretics more frequently; the latter are a well-known iatrogenic cause of hyperuricemia [42].

If the assumption that UA acutely increases during hospitalization due to secondary hemodynamic effects is true, a decrease in its values from admission to discharge should be expected. However, data on longitudinal UA changes in ACS subjects are still lacking.

4. Uric Acid and Chronic Coronary Syndrome

Hyperuricemia is a significant epidemiological problem in CCS, and has been strongly connected to CV mortality and CV events in this specific subgroup of patients [43–47]. The most important issue in these subjects is the possible relationship between UA levels and the extent and severity of Coronary Artery Disease (CAD). As was also shown in Table 2, most of the publications on this topic show that UA correlates with CAD, as defined as both the number of vessels involved [48] and specific scores, such as Gensan [49] or Syntax [50]. However, other studies did not identify this association [9,51,52]. This heterogeneity may be explained by differences in the sample selection (never revascularized, newly diagnosed patients versus individuals with previous MI and/or previous coronary revascularization) and in the assessment of the CAD. In this realm, studies that assessed CAD only in terms of the number of damaged vessels, without taking into account more sensitive scores [51,52], did not find any significant correlation. Furthermore, other surveys which considered newly diagnosed and never treated subjects more frequently found a positive association [53,54]; by contrast, when patients presented a positive anamnesis for previous MI/revascularization [9] or a strong risk factor (such as DM [55]), the association lacked. Taken together, these findings lead to the hypothesis that UA could act on coronary arteries only in an early phase of the atherosclerosis disease, through the various mechanisms seen in Section 2. In other words, when CAD progresses to a more advanced stage, other factors (such as previous MI, previous myocardial revascularization, DM) may overshadow the effects of UA and limit the possibility of finding a significant association with CAD. Thus, in a group of patients with very high CV risk, the presence/absence of hyperuricemia may not change further the overall risk profile.

Gender could be another factor influencing the UA–CAD association. Only two studies carried out a separate analysis in males and females, finding a connection only in the latter [56]. In addition, a piece of research based on non-menopausal females only confirmed the association with the severity of CAD [57].

Table 1. Summary of the available data on the association between uric acid and Acute Coronary Syndrome.

Study	Type of Study	Supporting Data	Non-Supporting Data	Reference
Bos et al.	Prospective cohort study	Significant association between baseline UA and risk of both CAD and stroke, only slightly attenuated by adjustment for other CV risk factors		[4]
Centola et al.	Prospective cohort study	High admission levels of UA are independently associated with in-hospital adverse outcomes and mortality of ACS patients		[11]
Mehmet ed al.	Prospective cohort study	Elevated UA levels on admission are independently associated with impaired coronary flow after primary PCI and both short-term and long term outcomes in patients who undergo primary PCI for the management of STEMI		[34]
Nadkar et al.	Case control study	UA levels are higher in patients with acute MI and correlate with Killip class.		[36]
Kobayashi et al.	Prospective cohort study	High UA levels are the primary predictor of 2-year cardiac mortality.		[37]
Lazzeri et al.	Prospective cohort study	UA levels are associated to greater risk of acute plaque complications		[38]
Okazaki et al.	Case control study		Plasma XOR activity was extremely high in patients with severely decompensated AHF, in association with a high lactate value and leading eventually to hyperuricaemia	[40]
Maloberti et al.	Prospective cohort study		Diuretic-related hyperuricemia carry a similar risk of CV events and all-cause mortality when compared with individuals that present hyperuricemia in absence of diuretic therapy	[42]

XOR: Xanthine Oxido-Reductase. AHF: Acute Heart Failure. CAD: Coronary Artery Disease. CV: cardiovascular. UA: Uric acid. ACS: Acute Coronary Syndromes. PCI: Percutaneous Coronary Intervention. STEMI: ST-Elevated Myocardial Infarction.

Table 2. Summary of the available data on the association between uric acid and Chronic Coronary Syndrome.

Study	Type of Study	Supporting Data	Non-Supporting Data	Reference
Okura et al.	Population based cohort study	Elevated UA is an independent predictor of CV events and all-cause mortality combined in patients with CCS		[43]
Tian et al.	Population based cohort study	UA levels were associated with the presence and severity of CAD; UA may be involved in the progression of CCS.		[48]
Duran et al.	Population based cohort study	UA was significantly associated with number of diseased vessels and is an independent risk factor for multivessel disease.		[49]
Karabağ et al.	Population based cohort study	UA was to be associated with high Syntax Score and long-term mortality in patients with MVD		[50]
Tasić et al.	Population based cohort study		Asymptomatic hyperuricemia is not significantly associated with the severity of CAD	[51]
Zand et al.	Case control study		UA is not an independent risk factor for premature CAD but is weakly correlated with the extent of the disease	[52]
Verdoia et al.	Population based cohort study		Among diabetic patients, higher UA is not independently associated with the extent of CAD or with platelet aggregation.	[55]
Maloberti et al.	Population based cohort study		UA do not play a role in determining coronary arteries disease as well as LV diastolic dysfunction in CCS subjects	[12]

CCS: Chronic Coronary Syndrome. MVD: Multi Vessel Disease.

5. The First Open Question: The Cardiovascular Cut-Off

The commonly-used cut-offs of 6 mg/dL in women and 7 mg/dL in men were established on evidence regarding gouty patients, rather than CV events in asymptomatic hyperuricemia. These thresholds are based on the UA saturation point (6.8 mg/dl at a pH of 7.4) which determines its precipitation in joints and kidneys, leading to the classic form of gout. However, previous evidence suggests that UA could act negatively on the CV system even at lower serum levels [1], as crystal precipitation is just one of the possible causes determining the relationship between UA and CV events.

Despite the large number of published studies, the identification of a CV UA cut-off value is still a matter of discussion. Among others, recently published results from an Italian multicenter, retrospective, observational cohort study brought new light on the CV cut-off question. The URRAH project (Uric acid Right for heArt Health) entailed data collection on outpatients (mainly hypertensives) and the general population, with a total of 23,475 subjects and a follow-up period of 20 years. Regarding all-cause mortality, a threshold of 4.7 mg/dL was detected, while 5.6 mg/dL emerged as the most suitable cut-off for CV mortality [58]. In both cases, the addition of the UA to the CV risk scores determined a significant increase of the area under the curve, leading to a re-classification of 33% of outpatients and 40% of the general population subjects. Concerning the specific analysis on MI, similar thresholds emerged: according to gender, cut-offs of 5.27 mg/dL in women and 5.49 mg/dL in men were identified [59]. In addition, a further threshold of 4.89 mg/dL was found to be predictive of fatal HF in another specific analysis [5]. These data come from population studies, while, despite our specific focus, no paper has ever been published about CCS. In acute events, subjects with UA > 7.5 mg/dL reported a significant subsequent mortality, but with low sensibility and specificity (0.64 and 0.66 respectively) [60]. In spite of the differences according to the considered outcome, all of these values emerged as being much lower than the conventional hyperuricemia cut-offs (Figure 2). That a lower cut-off should be used when evaluating the relationship between UA and CV outcomes is, to date, undoubted. However, what is already known is insufficient to recommend a single UA threshold for CV risk. While waiting for further results on this issue, a more suitable cut-off must be chosen on an individual basis strongly, depending on the patient's CV risk and previous CV events.

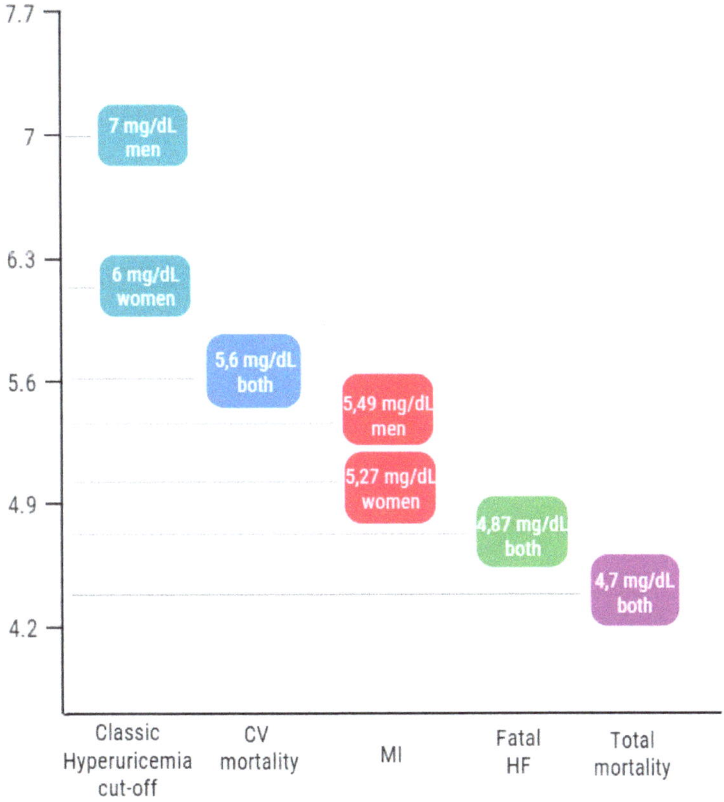

Figure 2. Summary of the different uric acid cut-offs according to cardiovascular diseases. CV = Cardiovascular; MI = Myocardial Infarction; HF = Heart Failure.

Another interesting point is the identification, in some studies, of a J-curve in the relationship between UA levels and CV events, meaning not only that high levels of UA raise the risk but also that too-low values could be harmful [61,62]. For example, according to the largest of these works (which included 127,771 subjects), an increased risk was detected in individuals with hyperuricemia, and also in subjects with circulating UA levels below 4 mg/dL. This occurrence showed differences in terms of its statistical correlation depending on gender: while women showed a linear trend in the link between UA and all-cause mortality, a J-shaped association was found in men, in which a lower-cut off of 3.4 mg/dL was identified as a significant threshold of adverse outcomes [62]. This evidence can be possibly interpreted as being due to the fact that, besides the potential pro-oxidative role, UA also has anti-oxidant properties which contribute to scavenging reactive oxygen species, chelating transition metals, and preventing the degradation of superoxide dismutase [63].

6. The Second Open Question: Are Uric-Acid-Lowering Therapies Effective in Reducing the Risk of Cardiovascular Events?

Currently, the therapies for the reduction of UA levels are exclusively recommended in patients with hyperuricemia associated with gouty arthritis or gouty nephropathy; these include xanthine oxidase inhibitors (Allopurinol and Febuxostat) and uricosurics (Probenecid and Lenisurad). Xanthine oxidase inhibitors were the first registered drugs, and Febuxostat showed the greatest inhibiting effectiveness with a complete selectivity for xanthine oxidase, while allopurinol also works on other enzymes involved in purine metabolism. Instead, Probenecid and Lenisurad increase the urinary excretion of UA acting on a specific renal transporter. Many other molecules are under development [64], but they still require further studies before becoming available. The reduction of UA achieved by these drugs has been demonstrated to reduce the amount of gout exacerbation and the disease severity [65], but whether it leads also to a decrease in CV morbidity and mortality is still a matter of debate. Currently, few large and randomized studies using CV events as a primary outcome have been published, and most of the evidence is based on pre-clinical investigations or studies on humans with surrogate end-points. For example, allopurinol was found to be able to lower blood pressure [66] and reduce subclinical organ damage (in particular intima-media thickness [67] and left ventricular mass index [68]), and this could theoretically lead to a possible reduction of CV events. Furthermore, experimental evidence suggests that allopurinol improves mechano-energetic uncoupling in the myocardium, thus decreasing myocardial oxygen consumption [69], and might be beneficial to patients with cardiac ischemia and angina. Possible explanations include the prevention of oxygen wastage for the avoidance of its consumption, due to the inhibition of xanthine-oxidase, and an improvement in microvascular function thanks to its positive effects on endothelial function [70]. However, there are currently no data regarding the possible link between these effects and the reduction in UA determined by allopurinol [71].

Some observational studies reported a decrease of CV events in patients treated with hypouricemic drugs [72], but, as is well known, this kind of design implies a high probability of bias; thus, these preliminary results need to be confirmed by double-blinded Randomized Clinical Trials (RCT) in order to exclude the presence of confounding factors (Table 3).

Two RCTs limited to individuals with gout have been published, showing opposite results. The CARES (Cardiovascular safety of Febuxostat and Allopurinol in patients with gout and cardiovascular comorbidities) study randomized 6190 patients with gout and previous CV events to Allopurinol vs. Febuxostat [73]. The subjects treated with Febuxostat reported a greater number of CV events, which worried the scientific community and consequently induced national agencies for drugs safety worldwide to warn about its use in patients with prior MI. In 2018, the FAST (Febuxostat versus Allopurinol Streamlined Trial) study, performed on 6128 gouty patients without prior CV events randomized to Allopurinol versus Febuxostat, found the non-inferiority of the latter with respect to the primary CV endpoint (a composite of hospitalization for non-fatal CV events and CV death) [74]. An extensive discussion about the differences between the two RCTs is beyond the purpose of this review, as a focused paper has been published on this topic [75]. However, the CARES trial presents many important biases; foremost, and also valid for the FAST trial, is that the absence of a control group disallows us to conclude whether Allopurinol reduces CV risk or Febuxostat raises it. Secondly, more than 50% of the individuals discontinued the therapy within the first year from enrolment, and although this trend was comparable between the two groups, no information about the following administered drugs was provided. As the patients were symptomatic for gout, it is likely that another drug had been prescribed (e.g., shifting Allopurinol to Febuxostat or vice-versa, or introducing a uricosuric). Similarly, no data were supplied on specific therapies about the other CV risk factors (hypertension, DM and dyslipidemia) which could underlie the differences in the CV events. In conclusion, these studies are not sufficient to demonstrate the superiority of one approach over the other in patients with gout, and, furthermore, they did not take into consideration asymptomatic patients with hyperuricemia.

For this latter group, one study is on-going and another one has been already published. The FREED (Febuxostat for cerebral and caRdiorenovascular events PrEvEntion StuDy) trial [76] compared Febuxostat with other treatments in 1,070 subjects without gout but with high CV risk or previous CV events. The main findings include the absence of differences in CV events and mortality, but with a significant reduction in renal events (defined as new-onset microalbuminuria or its progression) in the Febuxostat-treated patients. The on-going ALL-HEART (ALLopurinol and Cardiovascular Outcomes in Patients with Ischemic HEART Disease) study [77] already randomized 5,938 patients with CCS to Allopurinol versus placebo; its results are particularly awaited because they will determine whether Allopurinol improves major CV outcomes in patients with CCS, thereby changing the paradigm of secondary CV prevention strategies. Until it is concluded, the treatment of hyperuricemic individuals without gout is clinically not recommended.

Unfortunately, no information about the efficacy of UA reduction in primary CV prevention is available because of the lack of studies on asymptomatic hyperuricemia in individuals without prior CV events.

Eventually, regarding ACS, one specific but small and non-randomized study is available [78]; it enrolled 50 patients that started allopurinol for clinical indications within 14 days from ACS admission, and another 50 individuals that were not in therapy as a control group. During the 2-year follow-up period, inflammatory biomarkers were significantly lowered in the allopurinol group, as well as the number of CV events (10% vs. 30% for allopurinol and the control group, respectively). However, a larger sample is needed in the subset of ACS patients to confirm this possible benefit.

Table 3. Studies on the relationship between drugs acting on UA and their effects on CV diseases.

Study	No of Participants	Drugs Compared	Outcomes	Results	Reference
CARES	6198	Febuxostat vs. Allopurinol	4-component MACE (CV death, non-fatal MI, nonfatal stroke and unstable angina with urgent coronary revascularization)	Febuxostat is associated to a greater number of CV events	[73]
FAST	6128	Febuxostat vs. Allopurinol	Composite of hospitalization for non-fatal MI or biomarker-positive ACS; non-fatal stroke; CV death	Febuxostat is non-inferior to allopurinol	[74]
FREED	1070	Febuxostat vs. Other treatments	Composite of cerebral or cardiorenovascular events, all deaths	Febuxostat is associated to a redu-ction in renal events.	[76]

Table 3. *Cont.*

Study	No of Participants	Drugs Compared	Outcomes	Results	Reference
ALL-HEART	5938	Allopurinol vs. placebo	Composite of non-fatal MI, non-fatal stroke or CV death	On going	[77]
Huang et al.	100	Allopurinol vs. placebo	CV events	Allopurinol reduces inflammatory biomarkers and CV events	[78]

MACE: Major Adverse Cardiovascular Events.

7. Conclusions

Although many findings have been published in favor of a role of UA in CV diseases (particularly in ACS and CCS), several points remain not completely understood in this complicated relationship. From a pathophysiological point of view, the question of whether hyperuricemia contributes directly to the genesis of ACS and CCS, or if it is just an innocent bystander determined by an increased catabolism in ischemic myocardium is still a matter of debate. Furthermore, the lack of an unequivocally accepted UA CV cut-off does not allow us to define a clear threshold of CV events' risk and their fatality. While waiting for further results on this issue, a more suitable cut-off must be chosen on an individual basis, strongly depending on the patients' CV risk and previous CV events. Finally, there is currently no strong evidence about a certain benefit deriving from a pharmacological treatment of hyperuricemia in terms of the reduction of CV morbidity and mortality. The on-going ALL-HEART trial will provide us with an important answer, by determining whether allopurinol reduces CV events in patients with CCS, and it could perhaps change the role of UA in secondary CV prevention strategies. In conclusion, more studies should be performed in order to clarify the involvement of this molecule in the spectrum of CV disease and its possible role as a target in CV prevention strategies.

Author Contributions: Conceptualization, A.M., M.B., V.G., F.L. and M.M.; writing—original draft preparation, A.M., M.B., V.G., F.L. and M.M.; writing—review and editing, A.M., M.B., V.G., F.L. and M.M.; visualization, all authors; supervision A.M. and C.G.; All authors have read and agreed to the published version of the manuscript.

Funding: This work was funded by the Italian Ministry of University and Research (MIUR)—Department of Excellence project PREMIA (PREcision MedIcine Approach: bringing biomarker research to the clinic)—A. De Gasperis Cardiology and Cardiac Surgery Foundation.

Conflicts of Interest: The authors declare no conflict of interest.

References

1. Maloberti, A.; Giannattasio, C.; Bombelli, M.; Desideri, G.; Cicero, A.F.G.; Muiesan, M.L.; Rosei, E.A.; Salvetti, M.; Ungar, A.; Rivasi, G.; et al. Hyperuricemia and risk of cardiovascular outcomes: The experience of the URRAH (Uric Acid Right for Heart Health) project. *High Blood Press. Cardiovasc. Prev.* **2020**, *27*, 121–128. [CrossRef] [PubMed]
2. Meisinger, C.; Koenig, W.; Baumert, J.; Doring, A. Uric acid levels are associated with all cause and cardiovascular disease mortality independent of systemic inflammation in men from the general population: The MONICA/KORA cohort study. *Arterioscler. Thromb. Vasc. Biol.* **2008**, *28*, 1186–1192. [CrossRef] [PubMed]
3. Fang, J.; Alderman, M.H. Serum uric acid and cardiovascular mortality the NHANES I epidemiologic follow-up study, 1971–1992. National Health and nutrition examination survey. *JAMA* **2000**, *283*, 2404–2410. [CrossRef] [PubMed]
4. Bos, M.J.; Koudstaal, P.J.; HofmaN, A.; Witteman, J.C.; Breteler, M.M. Uric acid is a risk factor for myocardial infarction and stroke: The Rotterdam study. *Stroke* **2006**, *37*, 1503–1507. [CrossRef]
5. Muiesan, M.L.; Salvetti, M.; Virdis, A.; Masi, S.; Casiglia, E.; Tikhonoff, V.; Barbagallo, C.M.; Bombelli, M.; Cicero, A.F.G.; Cirillo, M.; et al. Serum uric acid, predicts heart failure in a large Italian cohort: Search for a cut-off value the URic acid Right for heArt Health study. *J. Hypertens.* **2021**, *39*, 62–69. [CrossRef]
6. Tamariz, L.; Harzand, A.; Palacio, A.; Verma, S.; Jones, J.; Hare, J. Uric acid as a predictor of all-cause mortality in heart failure: A meta-analysis. *Congest. Heart Fail.* **2011**, *17*, 25–30. [CrossRef]

7. Tamariz, L.; Agarwal, S.; Soliman, E.Z.; Chamberlain, A.M.; Prineas, R.; Folsom, A.R.; Ambrose, M.; Alonso, A. Association of serum uric acid with incident atrial fibrillation (from the Atherosclerosis Risk in Communities [ARIC] study). *Am. J. Cardiol.* **2011**, *108*, 1272–1276. [CrossRef]
8. Williams, B.; Mancia, G.; Spiering, W.; Rosei, E.A.; Azizi, M.; Burnier, M.; Clement, D.L.; Coca, A.; De Simone, G.; Dominiczak, A.; et al. 2018 ESC/ESH Guidelines for the management of arterial hypertension. *Eur. Heart J.* **2018**, *39*, 3021–3104. [CrossRef]
9. Maloberti, A.; Qualliu, E.; Occhi, L.; Sun, J.; Grasso, E.; Tognola, C.; Tavecchia, G.; Cartella, I.; Milani, M.; Vallerio, P.; et al. Hyperuricemia prevalence in healthy subjects and its relationship with cardiovascular target organ damage. *Nutr. Metab. Cardiovasc. Dis.* **2021**, *31*, 178–185. [CrossRef]
10. Maloberti, A.; Maggioni, S.; Occhi, L.; Triglione, N.; Panzeri, F.; Nava, S.; Signorini, S.; Falbo, R.; Casati, M.; Grassi, G.; et al. Sex-related relationships between uric acid and target organ damage in hypertension. *J. Clin. Hypertens.* **2018**, *20*, 193–200. [CrossRef]
11. Centola, M.; Maloberti, A.; Castini, D.; Persampieri, S.; Sabatelli, L.; Ferrante, G.; Lucreziotti, S.; Morici, N.; Sacco, A.; Oliva, F.; et al. Impact of admission serum acid uric levels on in-hospital outcomes in patients with acute coronary syndrome. *Eur. J. Intern. Med.* **2020**, *82*, 62–67. [CrossRef]
12. Maloberti, A.; Bossi, I.; Tassistro, E.; Rebora, P.; Racioppi, A.; Nava, S.; Soriano, F.; Piccaluga, E.; Piccalò, G.; Oreglia, J.; et al. Uric acid in chronic coronary syndromes: Relationship with coronary artery disease severity and left ventricular diastolic parameter. *Nutr. Metab. Cardiovasc. Dis.* **2021**, *31*, 1501–1508. [CrossRef]
13. Kannel, W.B.; Castelli, W.P.; McNamara, P.M. The coronary profile: 12-year follow-up in the Framingham study. *J. Occup. Med.* **1967**, *9*, 611–619. [PubMed]
14. Li, M.; Hu, X.; Fan, Y.; Li, K.; Zhang, X.; Hou, W.; Tang, Z. Hyperuricemia and the risk for coronary heart disease morbidity and mortality a systematic review and dose-response meta-analysis. *Sci. Rep.* **2016**, *6*, 19520. [CrossRef]
15. Glantzounis, G.K.; Tsimoyiannis, E.C.; Kappas, A.M.; Galaris, D.A. Uric acid and oxidative stress. *Curr. Pharm. Des.* **2005**, *11*, 4145–4151. [CrossRef] [PubMed]
16. Kattoor, A.J.; Pothineni, N.V.K.; Palagiri, D.; Mehta, J.L. Oxidative stress in atherosclerosis. *Curr. Atheroscler. Rep.* **2017**, *19*, 42. [CrossRef] [PubMed]
17. Berry, C.E.; Hare, J.M. Xanthine oxidoreductase and cardiovascular disease: Molecular mechanisms and pathophysiological implications. *J. Physiol.* **2004**, *555*, 589–606. [CrossRef]
18. Bombelli, M.; Ronchi, I.; Volpe, M.; Facchetti, R.; Carugo, S.; Dell'oro, R.; Cuspidi, C.; Grassi, G.; Mancia, G. Prognostic value of serum uric acid: New-onset in and out-of-office hypertension and long-term mortality. *J. Hypertens.* **2014**, *32*, 1237–1244. [CrossRef]
19. Taniguchi, Y.; Hayashi, T.; Tsumura, K.; Endo, G.; Fujii, S.; Okada, K. Serumuric acid and the risk for hypertension and type 2 diabetes in Japanesemen: The Osaka Health Survey. *J. Hypertens.* **2001**, *19*, 1209–1215. [CrossRef]
20. Pugliese, N.R.; Mengozzi, A.; Virdis, A.; Casiglia, E.; Tikhonoff, V.; Cicero, A.F.G.; Ungar, A.; Rivasi, G.; Salvetti, M.; Barbagallo, C.M.; et al. The importance of including uric acid in the definition of metabolic syndrome when assessing the mortality risk. *Clin. Res. Cardiol.* **2021**, *110*, 1073–1082. [CrossRef]
21. Perlstein, T.S.; Gumieniak, O.; Hopkins, P.N.; Murphey, L.J.; Brown, N.J.; Williams, G.H.; Hollenberg, N.K.; Fisher, N.D. Uric acid and the state of the intrarenal renin-angiotensin system in humans. *Kidney Int.* **2004**, *66*, 1465–1470. [CrossRef]
22. Kato, M.; Hisatome, I.; Tomikura, Y.; Kotani, K.; Kinugawa, T.; Ogino, K.; Ishida, K.; Igawa, O.; Shigemasa, C.; Somers, V.K. Status of endothelial dependent vasodilation in patients with hyperuricemia. *Am. J. Cardiol.* **2005**, *96*, 1576–1578. [CrossRef]
23. Lanaspa, M.A.; Sanchez-Lozada, L.G.; Choi, Y.J.; Cicerchi, C.; Kanbay, M.; Roncal-Jimenez, C.A.; Ishimoto, T.; Li, N.; Marek, G.; Duranay, M.; et al. Uric acid induces hepatic steatosis by generation of mitochondrial oxidative stress: Potential role in fructose-dependent and -independent fatty liver. *J. Biol. Chem.* **2012**, *287*, 40732–40744. [CrossRef]
24. Scott, F.W.; Trick, K.D.; Stavric, B.; Braaten, J.T.; Siddiqui, Y. Uric acid-induced decrease in rat insulin secretion. *Proc. Soc. Exp. Biol. Med.* **1981**, *166*, 123–128. [CrossRef] [PubMed]
25. Spencer, H.W.; Yarger, W.E.; Robinson, R.R. Alterations of renal function during dietary-induced hyperuricemia in the rat. *Kidney Int.* **1976**, *9*, 489–500. [CrossRef]
26. Sanchez-Lozada, L.G.; Tapia, E.; Lopez-Molina, R.; Nepomuceno, T.; Soto, V.; Avila-Casado, C.; Nakagawa, T.; Johnson, R.J.; Herrera-Acosta, J.; Franco, M. Effects of acute and chronic L-arginine treatment in experimental hyperuricemia. *Am. J. Physiol.* **2007**, *292*, 1238–1244. [CrossRef] [PubMed]
27. Russo, E.; Viazzi, F.; Pontremoli, R.; Barbagallo, C.M.; Bombelli, M.; Casiglia, E.; Cicero, A.F.G.; Cirillo, M.; Cirillo, P.; Desideri, G.; et al. Association of uric acid with kidney function and albuminuria: The Uric Acid Right for heArt Health (URRAH) Project. *J. Nephrol.* **2021**. [CrossRef] [PubMed]
28. Fathallah-Shaykh, S.A.; Cramer, M.T. Uric acid and the kidney. *Pediatr. Nephrol.* **2014**, *29*, 999–1008. [CrossRef]
29. Rebora, P.; Andreano, A.; Triglione, N.; Piccinelli, E.; Palazzini, M.; Occhi, L.; Grassi, G.; Valsecchi, M.G.; Giannattasio, C.; Maloberti, A. Association between uric acid and pulse wave velocity in hypertensive patients and in the general population: A systematic review and meta-analysis. *Blood Press.* **2020**, *29*, 220–231. [CrossRef]
30. Braga, F.; Pasqualetti, S.; Ferraro, S.; Panteghini, M. Hyperuricemia as risk factor for coronary heart disease incidence and mortality in the general population: A systematic review and meta-analysis. *Clin. Chem. Lab. Med.* **2016**, *54*, 7–15. [CrossRef]

31. Storhaug, H.M.; Norvik, J.V.; Toft, I.; Eriksen, B.O.; Løchen, M.L.; Zykova, S.; Solbu, M.; White, S.; Chadban, S.; Jenssen, T. Uric acid is a risk factor for ischemic stroke and all-cause mortality in the general population: A gender specific analysis from The Tromsø Study. *BMC Cardiovasc. Disord.* **2013**, *13*, 115. [CrossRef] [PubMed]
32. Kolz, M.; Johnson, T.; Sanna, S.; Teumer, A.; Vitart, V.; Perola, M.; Mangino, M.; Albrecht, E.; Wallace, C.; Farrall, M.; et al. Meta-analysis of 28,141 individuals identifies common variants within five new loci that influence uric acid concentrations. *PLoS Genet.* **2009**, *5*, e1000504. [CrossRef] [PubMed]
33. Yu, S.; Yang, H.; Guo, X.; Zheng, L.; Sun, Y. Hyperuricemia is independently associated with left ventricular hypertrophy in post-menopausal women but not in pre-menopausal women in rural Northeast China. *Gynecol. Endocrinol.* **2015**, *31*, 736–741. [CrossRef] [PubMed]
34. Kaya, M.G.; Uyarel, H.; Akpek, M.; Kalay, N.; Ergelen, M.; Ayhan, E.; Isik, T.; Cicek, G.; Elcik, D.; Sahin, O.; et al. Prognostic value of uric acid in patients with ST-elevated myocardial infarction undergoing primary coronary intervention. *Am. J. Cardiol.* **2012**, *109*, 486–491. [CrossRef] [PubMed]
35. Basar, N.; Sen, N.; Ozcan, F.; Erden, G.; Kanat, S.; Sokmen, E.; Isleyen, A.; Yuzgecer, H.; Ozlu, M.F.; Yildirimkaya, M.; et al. Elevated serum uric acid predicts angiographic impaired reperfusion and 1-year mortality in ST-segment elevation myocardial infarction patients undergoing percutaneous coronary intervention. *J. Investig. Med.* **2011**, *59*, 931–937. [CrossRef]
36. Nadkar, M.Y.; Jain, V.I. Serum uric acid in acute myocardial infarction. *J. Assoc. Physicians India* **2008**, *56*, 759–762.
37. Kobayashi, N.; Asai, K.; Tsurumi, M.; Shibata, Y.; Okazaki, H.; Shirakabe, A.; Goda, H.; Uchiyama, S.; Tani, K.; Takano, M.; et al. Impact of accumulated serum uric acid on coronary culprit lesion morphology determined by optical coherence tomography and cardiac outcomes in patients with acute coronary syndrome. *Cardiology* **2018**, *141*, 190–198. [CrossRef]
38. Lazzeri, C.; Valente, S.; Chiostri, M.; Picariello, C.; Gensini, G.F. Uric acid in the early risk stratification of ST-elevation myocardial infarction. *Intern. Emerg. Med.* **2012**, *7*, 33–39. [CrossRef]
39. Akpek, M.; Kaya, M.G.; Uyarel, H.; Yarlioglues, M.; Kalay, N.; Gunebakmaz, O.; Dogdu, O.; Ardic, I.; Elcik, D.; Sahin, O.; et al. The association of serum uric acid levels on coronary flow in patients with STEMI undergoing primary PCI. *Atherosclerosis* **2011**, *219*, 334–341. [CrossRef]
40. Okazaki, H.; Shirakabe, A.; Matsushita, M.; Shibata, Y.; Sawatani, T.; Uchiyama, S.; Tani, K.; Murase, T.; Nakamura, T.; Takayasu, T.; et al. Plasma xanthine oxidoreductase activity in patients with decompensated acute heart failure requiring intensive care. *ESC Heart Fail.* **2019**, *6*, 336–343. [CrossRef]
41. Doehner, W.; Jankowska, E.A.; Springer, J.; Lainscak, M.; Anker, S.D. Uric acid and xanthine oxidase in heart failure—Emerging data and therapeutic implications. *Int. J. Cardiol.* **2016**, *213*, 15–19. [CrossRef]
42. Maloberti, A.; Bombelli, M.; Facchetti, R.; Barbagallo, C.M.; Bernardino, B.; Rosei, E.A.; Casiglia, E.; Cicero, A.F.G.; Cirillo, M.; Cirillo, P.; et al. Relationships between diuretic-related hyperuricemia and cardiovascular events: Data from the URic acid Right for heArt Health study. *J. Hypertens.* **2021**, *39*, 333–340. [CrossRef] [PubMed]
43. Okura, T.; Higaki, J.; Kurata, M.; Irita, J.; Miyoshi, K.; Yamazaki, T.; Hayashi, D.; Kohro, T.; Nagai, R. Elevated serum uric acid is an independent predictor for cardiovascular events in patients with severe coronary artery stenosis: Subanalysis of the Japanese Coronary Artery Disease (JCAD) Study. *Circ. J.* **2009**, *73*, 885–891. [CrossRef] [PubMed]
44. Spoon, D.B.; Lerman, A.; Rule, A.D.; Prasad, A.; Lennon, R.J.; Holmes, D.R.; Rihal, C.S. The association of serum uric acid levels with outcomes following percutaneous coronary intervention. *J. Interv. Cardiol.* **2010**, *23*, 277–283. [CrossRef] [PubMed]
45. Silbernagel, G.; Hoffmann, M.M.; Grammer, T.B.; Boehm, B.O.; Marz, W. Uric acid is predictive of cardiovascular mortality and sudden cardiac death in subjects referred for coronary angiography. *Nutr. Metab. Cardiovasc. Dis.* **2013**, *23*, 46–52. [CrossRef]
46. Ndrepepa, G.; Braun, S.; King, L.; Fusaro, M.; Tada, T.; Cassese, S.; Hadamitzky, M.; Haase, H.U.; Schömig, A.; Kastrati, A. Uric acid and prognosis in angiography-proven coronary artery disease. *Eur. J. Clin. Investig.* **2013**, *43*, 256–266. [CrossRef]
47. Bickel, C.; Rupprecht, H.J.; Blankenberg, S.; Rippin, G.; Hafner, G.; Daunhauer, A.; Hofmann, K.P.; Meyer, J. Serum uric acid as an independent predictor of mortality in patients with angiographically proven coronary artery disease. *Am. J. Cardiol.* **2002**, *89*, 12–17. [CrossRef]
48. Tian, T.T.; Li, H.; Chen, S.J.; Wang, Q.; Tian, Q.W.; Zhang, B.B.; Zhu, J.; He, G.W.; Lun, L.M.; Xuan, C. Serum uric acid as an independent risk factor for the presence and severity of early-onset coronary artery disease: A case-control study. *Dis. Markers* **2018**, *2018*, 1236837. [CrossRef] [PubMed]
49. Duran, M.; Kalay, N.; Akpek, M.; Orscelik, O.; Elcik, D.; Ocak, A.; Inanc, M.T.; Kasapkara, H.A.; Oguzhan, A.; Eryol, N.K.; et al. High levels of serum uric acid predict severity of coronary artery disease in patients with acute coronary syndrome. *Angiology* **2012**, *63*, 448–452. [CrossRef]
50. Karabağ, Y.; Rencuzogullari, I.; Çağdaş, M.; Karakoyun, S.; Yesin, M.; Atalay, E.; Çağdaş, Ö.S.; Gürsoy, M.O.; Burak, C.; Tanboğa, H.I. Association of serum uric acid levels with SYNTAX score II and long term mortality in the patients with stable angina pectoris who undergo percutaneous coronary interventions due to multivessel and/or unprotected left main disease. *Int. J. Cardiovasc. Imaging* **2019**, *35*, 1–7. [CrossRef]
51. Tasić, I.; Kostić, S.; Stojanović, N.M.; Skakić, V.; Cvetković, J.; Djordjević, A.; Karadzić, M.; Djordjević, D.; Andonov, S.; Stoičkov, V.; et al. Significance of asymptomatic hyperuricemia in patients after coronary events. *Scand. J. Clin. Lab. Investig.* **2018**, *78*, 312–317. [CrossRef]
52. Zand, S.; Shafiee, A.; Boroumand, M.; Jalali, A.; Nozari, Y. Serum uric Acid is not an independent risk factor for premature coronary artery disease. *Cardiorenal Med.* **2013**, *3*, 246–253. [CrossRef] [PubMed]

53. Gaubert, M.; Marlinge, M.; Alessandrini, M.; Laine, M.; Bonello, L.; Fromonot, J.; Cautela, J.; Thuny, F.; Barraud, J.; Mottola, G.; et al. Uric acid levels are associated with endothelial dysfunction and severity of coronary atherosclerosis during a first episode of acute coronary syndrome. *Purinergic Signal.* **2018**, *14*, 191–199. [CrossRef]
54. Barbieri, L.; Verdoia, M.; Schaffer, A.; Marino, P.; Suryapranata, H.; De Luca, G. Impact of sex on uric acid levels and its relationship with the extent of coronary artery disease: A single-centre study. *Atherosclerosis* **2015**, *241*, 241–248. [CrossRef]
55. Verdoia, M.; Barbieri, L.; Schaffer, A.; Cassetti, E.; Nardin, M.; Bellomo, G.; Aimaretti, G.; Marino, P.; Sinigaglia, F.; De Luca, G. Impact of diabetes on uric acid and its relationship with the extent of coronary artery disease and platelet aggregation: A single-centre cohort study. *Metabolism* **2014**, *63*, 640–646. [CrossRef]
56. Zhang, J.W.; He, L.J.; Cao, S.J.; Yang, Q.; Yang, S.W.; Zhou, Y.J. Association of serum uric acid and coronary artery disease in premenopausal women. *PLoS ONE* **2014**, *9*, e106130. [CrossRef] [PubMed]
57. Demir, Ş.; Karakoyun, G.; Kanadasi, M. Elevated high sensitivity C-reactive protein and uric acid levels in coronary artery ectasia. *Acta Biochim. Pol.* **2014**, *61*, 687–691. [CrossRef] [PubMed]
58. Virdis, A.; Masi, S.; Casiglia, E.; Tikhonoff, V.; Cicero, A.F.G.; Ungar, A.; Rivasi, G.; Salvetti, M.; Barbagallo, C.M.; Bombelli, M.; et al. Identification of the uric acid thresholds predicting an increased total and cardiovascular mortality over 20 years. *Hypertension* **2020**, *75*, 302–308. [CrossRef]
59. Casiglia, E.; Tikhonoff, V.; Virdis, A.; Masi, S.; Barbagallo, C.M.; Bombelli, M.; Bruno, B.; Cicero, A.F.G.; Cirillo, M.; Cirillo, P.; et al. Serum uric acid and fatal myocardial infarction: Detection of prognostic cut-off values: The URRAH (Uric Acid Right for Heart Health) study. *J. Hypertens.* **2020**, *38*, 412–419. [CrossRef]
60. Kojima, S.; Sakamoto, T.; Ishihara, M.; Kimura, K.; Miyazaki, S.; Yamagishi, M.; Tei, C.; Hiraoka, H.; Sonoda, M.; Tsuchihashi, K.; et al. Prognostic usefulness of serum uric acid after acute myocardial infarction (the Japanese Acute Coronary Syndrome Study). *Am. J. Cardiol.* **2005**, *96*, 489–495. [CrossRef]
61. Bae, E.; Cho, H.J.; Shin, N.; Kim, S.M.; Yang, S.H.; Kim, D.K.; Kim, Y.L.; Kang, S.W.; Yang, C.W.; Kim, N.H.; et al. Lower serum uric acid level predicts mortality in dialysis patients. *Medicine* **2016**, *95*, e3701. [CrossRef] [PubMed]
62. Browne, L.D.; Jaouimaa, F.Z.; Walsh, C.; Perez-Ruiz, F.; Richette, P.; Burke, K.; Stack, A.G. Serum uric acid and mortality thresholds among men and women in the Irish health system: A cohort study. *Eur. J. Intern. Med.* **2021**, *84*, 46–55. [CrossRef]
63. Hink, H.U.; Santanam, N.; Dikalov, S.; McCann, L.; Nguyen, A.D.; Parthasarathy, S.; Harrison, D.G.; Fukai, T. Peroxidase properties of extracellular superoxide dismutase role of uric acid in modulating in vivo activity. *Arterioscler. Thromb. Vasc. Biol.* **2002**, *22*, 1402–1408. [CrossRef]
64. Stamp, L.K.; Merriman, T.R.; Singh, J.A. Expert opinion on emerging urate-lowering therapies. *Expert Opin. Emerg. Drugs* **2018**, *23*, 201–209. [CrossRef]
65. Clebak, K.T.; Morrison, A.; Croad, J.R. Gout: Rapid evidence review. *Am. Fam. Physician* **2020**, *102*, 533–538.
66. Beattie, C.J.; Fulton, R.L.; Higgins, P.; Padmanabhan, S.; McCallum, L.; Walters, M.R.; Dominiczak, A.F.; Touyz, R.M.; Dawson, J. Allopurinol initiation and change in blood pressure in older adults with hypertension. *Hypertension* **2014**, *64*, 1102–1107. [CrossRef] [PubMed]
67. Higgins, P.; Walters, M.R.; Murray, H.M.; McArthur, K.; McConnachie, A.; Lees, K.R.; Dawson, J. Allopurinol reduces brachial and central blood pressure, and carotid intima-media thickness progression after ischaemic stroke and transient ischaemic attack: A randomised controlled trial. *Heart* **2014**, *100*, 1085–1092. [CrossRef]
68. Kao, M.P.; Ang, D.S.; Gandy, S.J.; Nadir, M.A.; Houston, J.G.; Lang, C.C.; Struthers, A.D. Allopurinol benefits left ventricular mass and endothelial dysfunction in chronic kidney disease. *J. Am. Soc. Nephrol.* **2011**, *22*, 1382–1389. [CrossRef]
69. Cappola, T.P.; Kass, D.A.; Nelson, G.S.; Berger, R.D.; Rosas, G.O.; Kobeissi, Z.A.; Marbán, E.; Hare, J.M. Allopurinol improves myocardial efficiency in patients with idiopathic dilated cardiomyopathy. *Circulation* **2001**, *104*, 2407–2411. [CrossRef] [PubMed]
70. Noman, A.; Ang, D.S.; Ogston, S.; Lang, C.C.; Struthers, A.D. Effect of high-dose allopurinol on exercise in patients with chronic stable angina: A randomised, placebo controlled crossover trial. *Lancet* **2010**, *375*, 2161–2167. [CrossRef]
71. Rajendra, N.S.; Ireland, S.; George, J.; Belch, J.J.; Lang, C.C.; Struthers, A.D. Mechanistic insights into the therapeutic use of high-dose allopurinol in angina pectoris. *J. Am. Coll. Cardiol.* **2011**, *58*, 820–828. [CrossRef] [PubMed]
72. Grimaldi-Bensouda, L.; Alpérovitch, A.; Aubrun, E.; Danchin, N.; Rossignol, M.; Abenhaim, L.; Richette, P. Impact of allopurinol on risk of myocardial infarction. *Ann. Rheum. Dis.* **2015**, *74*, 836–842. [CrossRef] [PubMed]
73. Pontremoli, R. The role of urate-lowering treatment on cardiovascular and renal disease: Evidence from CARES, FAST, ALL-HEART, and FEATHER studies. *Curr. Med. Res. Opin.* **2017**, *33*, 27–32. [CrossRef]
74. Mackenzie, I.S.; Ford, I.; Nuki, G.; Hallas, J.; Hawkey, C.J.; Webster, J.; Ralston, S.H.; Walters, M.; Robertson, M.; De Caterina, R.; et al. Long-term cardiovascular safety of febuxostat compared with allopurinol in patients with gout (FAST): A multicentre, prospective, randomised, open-label, non-inferiority trial. *Lancet* **2020**, *396*, 1745–1757. [CrossRef]
75. Katsiki, N.; Borghi, C. The future of febuxostat after the Cardiovascular Safety of Febuxostat and Allopurinol in Patients with Gout and Cardiovascular Morbidities (CARES) trial: Who CARES? *Expert Opin. Pharmacother.* **2018**, *19*, 1853–1856. [CrossRef]
76. Kojima, S.; Matsui, K.; Ogawa, H.; Jinnouchi, H.; Hiramitsu, S.; Hayashi, T.; Yokota, N.; Kawai, N.; Tokutake, E.; Uchiyama, K.; et al. Rationale, design, and baseline characteristics of a study to evaluate the effect of febuxostat in preventing cerebral, cardiovascular, and renal events in patients with hyperuricemia. *J. Cardiol.* **2017**, *69*, 169–175. [CrossRef]

77. Mackenzie, I.S.; Ford, I.; Walker, A.; Hawkey, C.; Begg, A.; Avery, A.; Taggar, J.; Wei, L.; Struthers, A.D.; MacDonald, T.M. Multicentre, prospective, randomised, open-label, blinded end point trial of the efficacy of allopurinol therapy in improving cardiovascular outcomes in patients with ischaemic heart disease: Protocol of the ALL-HEART study. *BMJ Open* **2016**, *6*, e013774. [CrossRef]
78. Huang, Y.; Zhang, C.; Xu, Z.; Shen, J.; Zhang, X.; Du, H.; Zhang, K.; Zhang, D. Clinical Study on efficacy of allopurinol in patients with acute coronary syndrome and its functional mechanism. *Hellenic J. Cardiol.* **2017**, *58*, 360–365. [CrossRef] [PubMed]

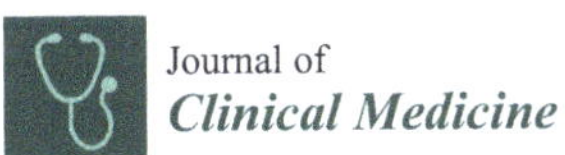
Journal of
Clinical Medicine

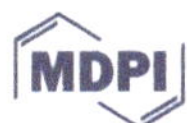

Article

Gender Differences in the Impact of Plasma Xanthine Oxidoreductase Activity on Coronary Artery Spasm

Ken Watanabe [1], Tetsu Watanabe [1,*], Yoichiro Otaki [1], Takayo Murase [2], Takashi Nakamura [3], Shigehiko Kato [1], Harutoshi Tamura [1], Satoshi Nishiyama [1], Hiroki Takahashi [1], Takanori Arimoto [1] and Masafumi Watanabe [1]

1 Department of Cardiology, Pulmonology and Nephrology, Yamagata University School of Medicine, Yamagata 990-9585, Japan; k.watanabe0418@med.id.yamagata-u.ac.jp (K.W.); y-otaki@med.id.yamagata-u.ac.jp (Y.O.); sg-kato@med.id.yamagata-u.ac.jp (S.K.); htamura@med.id.yamagata-u.ac.jp (H.T.); mnisiyam@med.id.yamagata-u.ac.jp (S.N.); hitakaha@med.id.yamagata-u.ac.jp (H.T.); t-arimoto@med.id.yamagata-u.ac.jp (T.A.); m-watanabe@med.id.yamagata-u.ac.jp (M.W.)
2 Radioisotope and Chemical Analysis Center, Sanwa Kagaku Kenkyusho Co., Ltd., Inabe 511-0406, Japan; ta_murase@skk-net.com
3 Pharmaceutical Research Laboratories, Pharmacological Study Group, Sanwa Kagaku Kenkyusho Co., Ltd., Inabe 511-0406, Japan; ta_nakamura@mb4.skk-net.com
* Correspondence: tewatana@med.id.yamagata-u.ac.jp; Tel.: +81-23-628-5302; Fax: +81-23-628-5305

Abstract: Xanthine oxidoreductase (XOR) is the rate-limiting enzyme in uric acid (UA) production that plays a pivotal role in generating oxidative stress. Gender differences in the impact of plasma XOR activity on coronary artery spasm (CAS) remain unclear. We investigated plasma XOR activity in 132 patients suspected of having CAS (male, n = 78; female, n = 54) and who underwent an intracoronary acetylcholine provocation test. Plasma XOR activity was significantly lower in female patients compared with male patients. CAS was provoked in 36 male patients and 17 female patients, and both had significantly higher plasma XOR activity than those without. Multivariate logistic regression analysis showed that this activity was independently associated with the incidence of CAS in both sexes after adjusting for confounding factors. The optimal cut-off values for predicting CAS were lower in female patients than in male patients. Multivariate analysis demonstrated that female patients with high XOR activity exhibited a higher incidence of CAS than male patients. Plasma XOR activity was an independent predictor of the incidence of CAS in both sexes. The impact of plasma XOR activity on CAS was stronger in female patients than in male patients.

Keywords: xanthine oxidoreductase; coronary artery spasm; gender differences

Citation: Watanabe, K.; Watanabe, T.; Otaki, Y.; Murase, T.; Nakamura, T.; Kato, S.; Tamura, H.; Nishiyama, S.; Takahashi, H.; Arimoto, T.; et al. Gender Differences in the Impact of Plasma Xanthine Oxidoreductase Activity on Coronary Artery Spasm. *J. Clin. Med.* **2021**, *10*, 5550. https://doi.org/10.3390/jcm10235550

Academic Editors: Atsushi Tanaka and Koichi Node

Received: 28 October 2021
Accepted: 25 November 2021
Published: 26 November 2021

1. Introduction

Coronary artery spasm (CAS) is an important cause of acute coronary syndrome (ACS) and sudden death [1]. Patients with CAS are associated with poor prognosis compared with those without CAS in ACS patients [2]. It has been reported that women have higher mortality rates than men after myocardial infarction [3]. It was reported that female patients with CAS had more frequently diffuse spasm by acetylcholine tests than male patients [4].

Decreased nitric oxide (NO) bioavailability due to increased reactive oxygen species (ROS) is one of the most important causes of CAS [5]. Uric acid (UA) is the end-product of purine metabolism that can induce inflammation and ROS production in vascular endothelial cells, leading to a number of cardiovascular diseases [6,7]. It has been demonstrated that serum UA is independently correlated with CAS [8].

Xanthine oxidoreductase (XOR) is a pivotal enzyme in the production of UA that is accompanied by the generation of ROS [9]. Increased levels of XOR have been recognized as a high risk factor for cardiovascular diseases, such as heart failure and coronary artery disease, including CAS [10–13]. It is well known that gender differences exist in the impact of serum UA levels on cardiovascular risk [14]. However, little is known about the gender differences in plasma XOR activity. The aim of this study, therefore, was to investigate gender differences in the impact of plasma XOR activity on CAS.

2. Materials and Methods

2.1. Study Subjects

We investigated plasma XOR activity in 132 patients (male, n = 78; female, n = 54) suspected of having CAS due to episodes of chest pain that occurred during rest, not exertion, in the early morning or late at night. All patients underwent an intracoronary acetylcholine provocation test in our hospital between June 2008 and October 2016. Intracoronary infusion of acetylcholine was performed according to the CAS guidelines of the Japanese Circulation Society [15]. Before performing the acetylcholine test, we obtained the control coronary angiography. Acetylcholine was injected into the right coronary artery at a dose of 20 or 50 μg and into the left coronary artery at a dose of 20, 50, or 100 μg each over a period of 20 s. Provoked CAS was defined as total or subtotal occlusion (≥90%) with accompanying symptoms of chest pain and/or ischemic ST-segment changes on the electrocardiogram. Vasoactive medications, including calcium channel blockers, nitrates, nicorandil, and other vasodilators, were withdrawn for at least three days before initiating the study. We excluded patients who had significant coronary artery stenosis (≥50%) and/or were taking XOR inhibitors. The diagnoses of hypertension, dyslipidemia, and diabetes mellitus were based on medical records or history of medical therapy. Smoking included both current and past smokers. Clinical data, including age, sex, and medications at discharge, were obtained from medical records. The study protocol was approved by the Institutional Ethics Committee of Yamagata University School of Medicine, and all patients provided written informed consent.

2.2. XOR Activity Assay

Blood samples were collected in the early morning within 24 h after admission. Following centrifugation at 3000× g for 15 min at 4 °C, and the obtained plasma was stored at −80 °C until analysis. The XOR activity assay was performed using stable isotope-labeled substrate and liquid chromatography-triple quadrupole mass spectrometry (Sanwa Kagaku Kenkyusho Co., Ltd., Nagoya, Japan) [16].

Other biochemistry parameters were measured using routine laboratory methods. The estimated glomerular filtration rate (GFR) was calculated by using the Japanese equation, as previously reported [17].

2.3. Statistical Analysis

The results are expressed as the mean ± standard deviation for continuous variables and percentages for categorical variables. Skewed values are presented as median and interquartile range (IQR). Correlations between plasma XOR activity, age, body mass index (BMI), and UA were analyzed using a single linear regression analysis. We used t-tests and chi-squared tests to compare continuous and categorical variables, respectively. If the data were not normally distributed, the Mann–Whitney U-test was employed. Logistic regression analysis was performed to determine variables independently associated with CAS. Multivariate analysis using a forward stepwise multiple regression model was performed to identify the independent predictors of CAS. Receiver-operating characteristic (ROC) curves for plasma XOR activity were constructed to determine the optimal cut-off values for sensitivity and specificity. Statistical significance was set at $p < 0.05$. All statistical analyses were performed using a standard software package (JMP version 12; SAS Institute, Cary, NC, USA).

3. Results

3.1. Comparisons of Clinical Characteristics between Males and Females

A comparison of clinical characteristics between male and female patients is shown in Table 1. As seen from the table, male patients were significantly younger, had higher rates of smoking, and higher levels of triglycerides and lower levels of high-density lipoprotein cholesterol (HDL-C) than the female patients. Serum UA levels and plasma XOR activity were significantly lower in female patients than in male patients. Gender differences in the distribution of plasma XOR activity are shown in Figure 1. There were no significant differences in BMI, medication use, prevalence of hypertension, dyslipidemia, and diabetes mellitus between male and female patients. There was a negative correlation between plasma XOR activity and age, and a positive correlation between plasma XOR activity and BMI in male patients. However, there was no correlation between plasma XOR activity, age, and BMI in female patients. In both sexes, there was no significant correlation between plasma XOR activity and levels of serum UA (Figure 2).

Table 1. Comparison of clinical characteristics between male and female patients.

Variables	Male $n = 78$	Female $n = 54$	p Value
Age (years old)	62 ± 13	68 ± 8	0.003
BMI (kg/m^2)	23.6 ± 3.3	23.8 ± 3.9	0.728
Hypertension, *n* (%)	50 (64)	31 (57)	0.438
Dyslipidemia, *n* (%)	32 (41)	31 (57)	0.064
Diabetes mellitus, *n* (%)	12 (15)	7 (13)	0.695
Smoking, *n* (%)	43 (55)	18 (33)	0.013
Blood examination			
Triglycerides (mg/dL)	128 (93–188)	100 (76–132)	0.006
LDL-C (mg/dL)	102 ± 28	107 ± 26	0.239
HDL-C (mg/dL)	50 ± 9	62 ± 18	<0.001
HbA1c (%)	5.7 ± 0.8	5.7 ± 0.6	0.729
eGFR (mL/min/1.73 m^2)	79 ± 22	72 ± 17	0.045
UA (mg/dL)	6.1 ± 1.3	4.7 ± 1.1	<0.001
XOR (pmol/h/mL)	51.7 (34.7–101.8)	30.3 (22.8–42.7)	<0.001
hs-CRP (mg/dL)	0.053 (0.021–0.133)	0.032 (0.018–0.087)	0.052
Medications			
ACEIs and/or ARBs, *n* (%)	37 (47)	18 (33)	0.104
CCBs, *n* (%)	52 (67)	40 (74)	0.360
Statins, *n* (%)	33 (42)	24 (44)	0.808
Antiplatelet drugs, *n* (%)	41 (53)	25 (46)	0.479
Nitrates, *n* (%)	27 (35)	12 (22)	0.121
Nicorandils, *n* (%)	27 (35)	15 (28)	0.446

Data are expressed as mean ± SD, number (percentage), or median (interquartile range). ACEIs, angiotensin-converting enzyme inhibitors; ARBs, angiotensin II receptor blockers; BMI, body mass index; CCBs, calcium-channel blockers; eGFR, estimated glomerular filtration rate; HbA1c, hemoglobin A1c; HDL-C, high-density lipoprotein cholesterol; hs-CRP, high-sensitivity C-reactive protein; LDL-C, low-density lipoprotein cholesterol; UA, uric acid; XOR, xanthine oxidoreductase.

3.2. Gender Differences in the Impact of Plasma XOR Activity on CAS

CAS was provoked in 36 male and 17 female patients. In both sexes, patients with CAS had significantly higher plasma XOR activity than those without CAS (Figure 3). Univariate and multivariate logistic regression analyses were performed to determine the factors that predict the incidence of CAS. In male patients, multivariate logistic regression analysis showed that plasma XOR activity was independently associated with the incidence of CAS after adjustment for HDL-C and high-sensitivity C-reactive protein (Table 2). Similarly, in female patients, plasma XOR activity was significantly associated with the incidence of CAS after adjustment for age and smoking (Table 3)

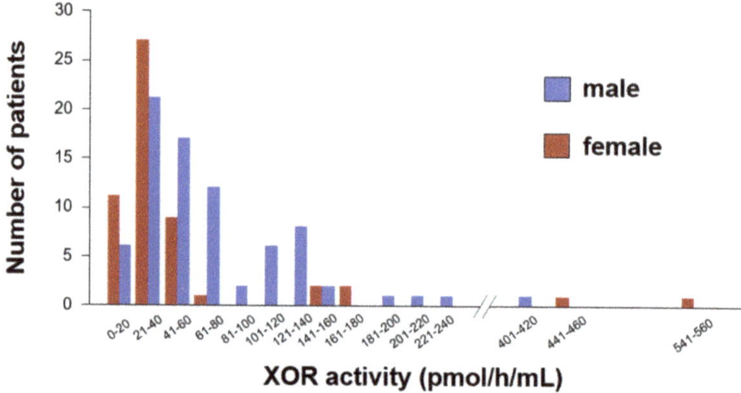

Figure 1. Gender differences in the distribution of plasma XOR activity.

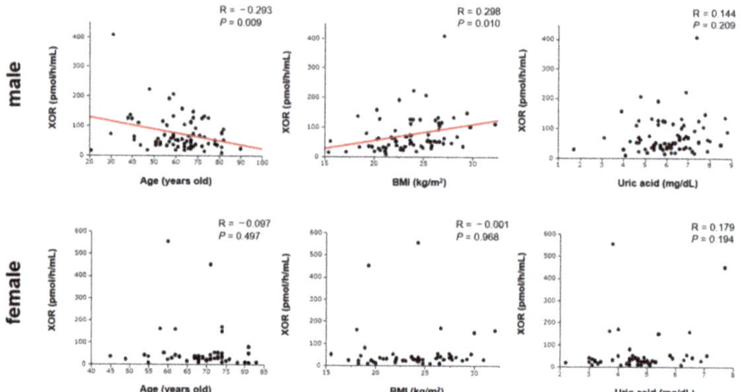

Figure 2. Correlations between plasma XOR activity, age, BMI, and serum UA levels in male and female patients.

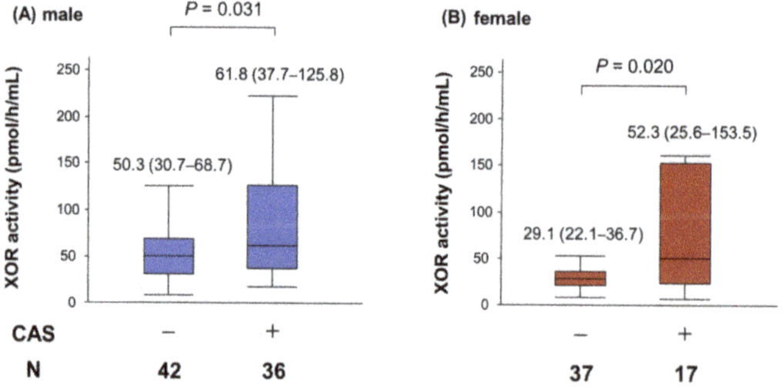

Figure 3. Gender differences in the impact of plasma XOR activity on CAS. (**A**) The comparison of plasma XOR activity between male patients with and without CAS. (**B**) The comparison of plasma XOR activity between female patients with and without CAS.

Table 2. Univariate and multivariate logistic regression analysis for predicting the incidence of CAS in male patients.

	Univariate			Multivariate		
Variables	OR	95% CI	p-Value	OR	95% CI	p-Value
Age †	0.903	0.570–1.418	0.656			
BMI †	1.236	0.778–2.008	0.371			
Hypertension	1.231	0.486–3.167	0.662			
Dyslipidemia	2.000	0.806–5.076	0.135			
Diabetes mellitus	0.333	0.069–1.231	0.102			
Smoking	0.680	0.274–1.666	0.399			
Triglycerides †	1.480	0.931–2.515	0.099			
LDL-C †	1.215	0.775–1.931	0.396			
HDL-C †	0.642	0.384–1.024	0.063	0.495	0.264–0.849	0.010
HbA1c †	0.799	0.473–1.263	0.344			
eGFR †	0.940	0.589–1.478	0.788			
UA †	0.886	0.557–1.390	0.596			
XOR †	2.125	1.194–4.286	0.008	2.821	1.426–6.616	0.001
hs-CRP †	1.654	0.997–3.246	0.052	1.742	1.012–3.523	0.049

BMI, body mass index; CAS, coronary artery spasm; CI, confidence interval; eGFR, estimated glomerular filtration rate; HbA1c, hemoglobin A1c; HDL-C, high-density lipoprotein cholesterol; hs-CRP, high-sensitivity C-reactive protein; LDL-C, low-density lipoprotein cholesterol; UA, uric acid; XOR, xanthine oxidoreductase. † Per 1-SD increase.

Table 3. Univariate and multivariate logistic regression analysis for predicting the incidence of CAS in female patients.

	Univariate			Multivariate		
Variables	OR	95% CI	p Value	OR	95% CI	p Value
Age †	1.745	0.945–3.570	0.076	1.742	0.989–5.522	0.054
BMI †	0.886	0.485–1.598	0.687			
Hypertension	0.952	0.305–3.018	0.933			
Dyslipidemia	1.336	0.428–4.351	0.620			
Diabetes mellitus	0.304	0.015–1.987	0.236			
Smoking	2.160	0.660–7.140	0.201	3.493	0.880–15.151	0.075
Triglycerides †	1.155	0.638–2.047	0.620			
LDL-C †	1.144	0.634–2.050	0.646			
HDL-C †	0.797	0.421–1.430	0.452			
HbA1c †	0.977	0.521–1.728	0.939			
eGFR †	0.967	0.527–1.725	0.910			
UA †	1.416	0.801–2.598	0.232			
XOR †	6.365	1.613–54.975	0.001	9.251	1.974–85.363	<0.001
hs-CRP †	0.995	0.496–1.742	0.986			

BMI, body mass index; CAS, coronary artery spasm; CI, confidence interval; eGFR, estimated glomerular filtration rate; HbA1c, hemoglobin A1c; HDL-C, high-density lipoprotein cholesterol; hs-CRP, high-sensitivity C-reactive protein; LDL-C, low-density lipoprotein cholesterol; UA, uric acid; XOR, xanthine oxidoreductase. † Per 1-SD increase.

Since the results of this study indicated that there were gender differences in plasma XOR activity, we performed ROC analysis to evaluate the best cut-off value for predicting CAS in each sex. As shown in Figure 4, the ROC analysis demonstrated that plasma XOR activity of 91.6 pmol/h/mL was the threshold value for predicting the incidence of CAS in male patients. The ROC analysis also revealed that plasma XOR activity of 52.3 pmol/h/mL was the threshold value for predicting the incidence of CAS in female patients, which was lower than that in male patients. On the other hand, as shown in Figure 5, multivariate analysis demonstrated that female patients with high XOR activity ($\geq$52.3 pmol/h/mL; OR 22.6, $p < 0.001$) exhibited a higher incidence of CAS than male patients ($\geq$91.6 pmol/h/mL; OR 8.2, $p < 0.001$).

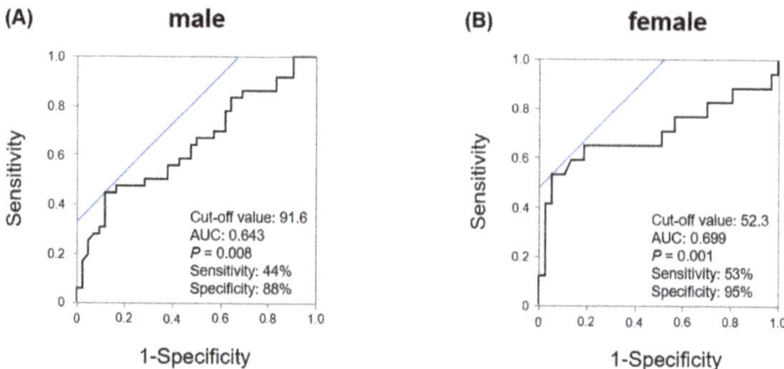

Figure 4. ROC curves to predict the incidence of CAS. (**A**) ROC curves for the threshold values in male patients. (**B**) ROC curves for the threshold values in female patients.

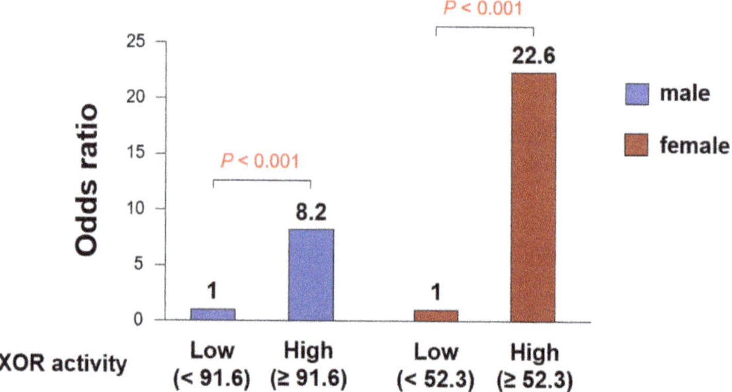

Figure 5. Association between plasma XOR activity and the incidence of CAS in each gender.

Among patients without provoked CAS, there were four patients (male, $n = 3$; female, $n = 1$) with typical chest pain and/or ischemic electrocardiogram changes who might develop a coronary microvascular spasm. Three male patients and one female patient had low XOR activity according to the ROC curve analysis.

4. Discussion

The main findings of the present study were as follows: (1) there was a gender difference in the distribution of plasma XOR activity, (2) the optimal cut-off values for predicting CAS were lower in women than in men, (3) high plasma XOR activity was an independent predictive factor for the incidence of CAS in both sexes, and (4) high plasma XOR activity was largely associated with the incidence of CAS in female patients than in male patients.

In the present study, although plasma XOR activity was significantly lower in female patients than in male patients, there was a stronger association between increased plasma XOR activity and the incidence of CAS in female patients. Although the mechanisms of CAS are multifactorial, it has been documented that genetic risk, gene–environment interactions, and mutations in the endothelial nitric oxide synthase (eNOS) gene contribute to CAS, especially in female patients [18,19]. These results indicate that eNOS malfunction is associated with CAS in female patients rather than in male patients. In endothelial cells, eNOS oxidizes L-arginine to L-citrulline and NO, which plays an important role in blood vessel relaxation. XOR-derived ROS can inactivate NO and contribute to eNOS uncoupling. Once uncoupled, eNOS itself generates ROS at the expense of NO, leading to endothelial dysfunction [20,21]. Therefore, it is possible that XOR-derived ROS mediated eNOS downregulation and might affect the high rates of CAS in female patients rather than in males.

Although there is no established consensus on gender differences in plasma XOR activity, Furuhashi et al. reported that males had significantly higher plasma XOR activity than females [22]. Consistent with this report, we observed significantly higher levels of plasma XOR activity in male patients in the present study. Furthermore, it has been reported that plasma XOR activity is correlated with metabolic parameters, insulin resistance, and levels of liver enzymes and adipokines [23]. Adipose tissue is one of the major sources of XOR, which is particularly enhanced in visceral fat in obesity [24]. Males were found to have more visceral adipose tissue, whereas females had more subcutaneous adipose tissue. Sex differences in visceral and subcutaneous fat distribution can possibly explain the positive correlation between plasma XOR activity and BMI in male patients but not in female patients. In addition, differences in sex hormones, including estrogen, may contribute to reduced insulin resistance in female patients [25]. These reports support the results of the present study, in which plasma XOR activity differed between genders.

In the present study, univariate and multivariate logistic regression analyses showed that elderly female patients tended to have a higher risk of CAS. It has been reported that women have lower UA levels because of the uricosuric effect of estrogen [26]. On the other hand, postmenopausal women are at risk of elevated UA levels and cardiovascular disease [27]. However, there is limited information on the association between sex hormones and plasma XOR activity. Considering that visceral fat mass is increased in postmenopausal women [28], elderly female patients could have higher plasma XOR activity, which can contribute to the incidence of CAS. In the present study, despite male patients having a negative correlation between age and plasma XOR activity ($R = -0.293$, $p = 0.009$), there was no significant correlation between them in female patients ($R = -0.097$, $p = 0.487$). Although visceral fat mass usually decreases with aging, elderly female patients might have more stored visceral fat, leading to relatively higher levels of plasma XOR activity compared to elderly male patients.

To our knowledge, this is the first study to investigate gender differences in the impact of plasma XOR activity on CAS. Our results suggest that plasma XOR activity is more associated with the incidence of CAS in women than in men. Decreasing XOR activity could be a novel therapeutic target for CAS, especially in female patients. Further studies are needed to examine whether XOR inhibitors are effective for the treatment of CAS.

The current study had several limitations. First, since this was an observational study, the causal relationship between plasma XOR activity and CAS and its impact on gender differences could not be assessed. Second, as we enrolled patients who were suspected of having CAS, gender differences in plasma XOR activity could not be generalized. Finally, because this study enrolled only patients from Japan from a single center, the results might have been affected due to racial bias.

5. Conclusions

Plasma XOR activity was an independent predictor of CAS incidence in both sexes. The impact of plasma XOR activity on CAS was stronger in female patients than in male patients.

Author Contributions: Conceptualization, K.W. and T.W.; methodology, T.M. and T.N.; validation, S.K., H.T. (Hiroki Takahashi) and S.N.; formal analysis, H.T. (Harutoshi Tamura) and T.A.; investigation, K.W.; data curation, K.W. and Y.O.; writing—original draft preparation, K.W.; writing—review and editing, T.W.; visualization, K.W.; supervision, M.W. All authors have read and agreed to the published version of the manuscript.

Funding: This work was in part supported by the consigned research fund from Japan society for promotion of science KAKENHI (grant no. 21K16015).

Institutional Review Board Statement: The study was conducted according to the guidelines of the Declaration of Helsinki and approved by the Institutional Ethics Committee of Yamagata University School of Medicine.

Informed Consent Statement: Written informed consent has been obtained from the patient(s) to publish this paper.

Acknowledgments: This work was supported in part by a consigned research fund from Sanwa Kagaku Kenkyusho Co., Ltd.

Conflicts of Interest: Takayo Murase and Takashi Nakamura are employees of Sanwa Kagaku Kenkyusho. There are no conflict of interest between Sanwa Kagaku Kenkyusho and the others. The authors declare no conflict of interest.

References

1. Satoh, S.; Omura, S.; Inoue, H.; Mori, T.; Takenaka, K.; Numaguchi, K.; Mori, E.; Aso, A.; Nakamura, T.; Hiyamuta, K. Clinical impact of coronary artery spasm in patients with no significant coronary stenosis who are experiencing acute coronary syndrome. *J. Cardiol.* **2013**, *61*, 404–409. [CrossRef] [PubMed]
2. Wakabayashi, K.; Suzuki, H.; Honda, Y.; Wakatsuki, D.; Kawachi, K.; Ota, K.; Koba, S.; Shimizu, N.; Asano, F.; Sato, T.; et al. Provoked coronary spasm predicts adverse outcome in patients with acute myocardial infarction: A novel predictor of prognosis after acute myocardial infarction. *J. Am. Coll. Cardiol.* **2008**, *52*, 518–522. [CrossRef] [PubMed]
3. Vaccarino, V.; Parsons, L.; Every, N.R.; Barron, H.V.; Krumholz, H.M. Sex-based differences in early mortality after myocardial infarction. National Registry of Myocardial Infarction 2 Participants. *N. Engl. J. Med.* **1999**, *341*, 217–225. [CrossRef]
4. Sato, K.; Kaikita, K.; Nakayama, N.; Horio, E.; Yoshimura, H.; Ono, T.; Ohba, K.; Tsujita, K.; Kojima, S.; Tayama, S.; et al. Coronary vasomotor response to intracoronary acet.t.tylcholine injection, clinical features, and long-term prognosis in 873 consecutive patients with coronary spasm: Analysis of a single-center study over 20 years. *J. Am. Heart Assoc.* **2013**, *2*, e000227. [CrossRef] [PubMed]
5. Kawano, H.; Node, K. The role of vascular failure in coronary artery spasm. *J. Cardiol.* **2011**, *57*, 2–7. [CrossRef]
6. Ando, K.; Takahashi, H.; Watanabe, T.; Daidoji, H.; Otaki, Y.; Nishiyama, S.; Arimoto, T.; Shishido, T.; Miyashita, T.; Miyamoto, T.; et al. Impact of Serum Uric Acid Levels on Coronary Plaque Stability Evaluated Using Integrated Backscatter Intravascular Ultrasound in Patients with Coronary Artery Disease. *J. Atheroscler. Thromb.* **2016**, *23*, 932–939. [CrossRef]
7. Saito, Y.; Tanaka, A.; Node, K.; Kobayashi, Y. Uric acid and cardiovascular disease: A clinical review. *J. Cardiol.* **2021**, *78*, 51–57. [CrossRef] [PubMed]
8. Nishino, M.; Mori, N.; Yoshimura, T.; Nakamura, D.; Lee, Y.; Taniike, M.; Makino, N.; Kato, H.; Egami, Y.; Shutta, R.; et al. Higher serum uric acid and lipoprotein(a) are correlated with coronary spasm. *Heart Vessel.* **2014**, *29*, 186–190. [CrossRef]
9. Chen, C.; Lu, J.M.; Yao, Q. Hyperuricemia-Related Diseases and Xanthine Oxidoreductase (XOR) Inhibitors: An Overview. *Med. Sci. Monit. Int. Med. J. Exp. Clin. Res.* **2016**, *22*, 2501–2512. [CrossRef]
10. Spiekermann, S.; Landmesser, U.; Dikalov, S.; Bredt, M.; Gamez, G.; Tatge, H.; Reepschläger, N.; Hornig, B.; Drexler, H.; Harrison, D.G. Electron spin resonance characterization of vascular xanthine and NAD(P)H oxidase activity in patients with coronary artery disease: Relation to endothelium-dependent vasodilation. *Circulation* **2003**, *107*, 1383–1389. [CrossRef]
11. Otaki, Y.; Watanabe, T.; Kinoshita, D.; Yokoyama, M.; Takahashi, T.; Toshima, T.; Sugai, T.; Murase, T.; Nakamura, T.; Nishiyama, S.; et al. Association of plasma xanthine oxidoreductase activity with severity and clinical outcome in patients with chronic heart failure. *Int. J. Cardiol.* **2017**, *228*, 151–157. [CrossRef] [PubMed]
12. Okazaki, H.; Shirakabe, A.; Matsushita, M.; Shibata, Y.; Sawatani, T.; Uchiyama, S.; Tani, K.; Murase, T.; Nakamura, T.; Takayasu, T.; et al. Plasma xanthine oxidoreductase activity in patients with decompensated acute heart failure requiring intensive care. *ESC Heart Fail.* **2019**, *6*, 336–343. [CrossRef] [PubMed]
13. Watanabe, K.; Shishido, T.; Otaki, Y.; Watanabe, T.; Sugai, T.; Toshima, T.; Takahashi, T.; Yokoyama, M.; Kinoshita, D.; Murase, T.; et al. Increased plasma xanthine oxidoreductase activity deteriorates coronary artery spasm. *Heart Vessel.* **2019**, *34*, 1–8. [CrossRef] [PubMed]
14. Fang, J.; Alderman, M.H. Serum uric acid and cardiovascular mortality the NHANES I epidemiologic follow-up study, 1971–1992. National Health and Nutrition Examination Survey. *JAMA* **2000**, *283*, 2404–2410. [CrossRef] [PubMed]
15. JCS Joint Working Group. Guidelines for diagnosis and treatment of patients with vasospastic angina (Coronary Spastic Angina) (JCS 2013). *Circ. J. Off. J. Jpn. Circ. Soc.* **2014**, *78*, 2779–2801.
16. Murase, T.; Nampei, M.; Oka, M.; Miyachi, A.; Nakamura, T. A highly sensitive assay of human plasma xanthine oxidoreductase activity using stable isotope-labeled xanthine and LC/TQMS. *J. Chromatogr. B Anal. Technol. Biomed. Life Sci.* **2016**, *1039*, 51–58. [CrossRef] [PubMed]
17. Matsuo, S.; Imai, E.; Horio, M.; Yasuda, Y.; Tomita, K.; Nitta, K.; Yamagata, K.; Tomino, Y.; Yokoyama, H.; Hishida, A. Revised equations for estimated GFR from serum creatinine in Japan. *Am. J. Kidney Dis. Off. J. Natl. Kidney Found.* **2009**, *53*, 982–992. [CrossRef] [PubMed]

18. Nakayama, M.; Yasue, H.; Yoshimura, M.; Shimasaki, Y.; Kugiyama, K.; Ogawa, H.; Motoyama, T.; Saito, Y.; Ogawa, Y.; Miyamoto, Y.; et al. T-786–>C mutation in the 5′-flanking region of the endothelial nitric oxide synthase gene is associated with coronary spasm. *Circulation* **1999**, *99*, 2864–2870. [CrossRef]
19. Murase, Y.; Yamada, Y.; Hirashiki, A.; Ichihara, S.; Kanda, H.; Watarai, M.; Takatsu, F.; Murohara, T.; Yokota, M. Genetic risk and gene-environment interaction in coronary artery spasm in Japanese men and women. *Eur. Heart J.* **2004**, *25*, 970–977. [CrossRef]
20. Yang, Y.M.; Huang, A.; Kaley, G.; Sun, D. eNOS uncoupling and endothelial dysfunction in aged vessels. *Am. J. Physiol. Heart Circ. Physiol.* **2009**, *297*, H1829–H1836. [CrossRef]
21. Gielis, J.F.; Lin, J.Y.; Wingler, K.; Van Schil, P.E.; Schmidt, H.H.; Moens, A.L. Pathogenetic role of eNOS uncoupling in cardiopulmonary disorders. *Free Radic. Biol. Med.* **2011**, *50*, 765–776. [CrossRef] [PubMed]
22. Furuhashi, M.; Matsumoto, M.; Tanaka, M.; Moniwa, N.; Murase, T.; Nakamura, T.; Ohnishi, H.; Saitoh, S.; Shimamoto, K.; Miura, T. Plasma Xanthine Oxidoreductase Activity as a Novel Biomarker of Metabolic Disorders in a General Population. *Circ. J. Off. J. Jpn. Circ. Soc.* **2018**, *82*, 1892–1899. [CrossRef] [PubMed]
23. Furuhashi, M.; Matsumoto, M.; Murase, T.; Nakamura, T.; Higashiura, Y.; Koyama, M.; Tanaka, M.; Moniwa, N.; Ohnishi, H.; Saitoh, S.; et al. Independent links between plasma xanthine oxidoreductase activity and levels of adipokines. *J. Diabetes Investig.* **2019**, *10*, 1059–1067. [CrossRef]
24. Tsushima, Y.; Nishizawa, H.; Tochino, Y.; Nakatsuji, H.; Sekimoto, R.; Nagao, H.; Shirakura, T.; Kato, K.; Imaizumi, K.; Takahashi, H.; et al. Uric acid secretion from adipose tissue and its increase in obesity. *J. Biol. Chem.* **2013**, *288*, 27138–27149. [CrossRef] [PubMed]
25. Geer, E.B.; Shen, W. Gender differences in insulin resistance, body composition, and energy balance. *Gend. Med.* **2009**, *6* (Suppl. 1), 60–75. [CrossRef]
26. Adamopoulos, D.; Vlassopoulos, C.; Seitanides, B.; Contoyiannis, P.; Vassilopoulos, P. The relationship of sex steroids to uric acid levels in plasma and urine. *Acta Endocrinol.* **1977**, *85*, 198–208. [CrossRef]
27. Feig, D.I.; Kang, D.H.; Johnson, R.J. Uric acid and cardiovascular risk. *N. Engl. J. Med.* **2008**, *359*, 1811–1821. [CrossRef] [PubMed]
28. Kozakowski, J.; Gietka-Czernel, M.; Leszczynska, D.; Majos, A. Obesity in menopause—Our negligence or an unfortunate inevitability? *Prz. Menopauzalny Menopause Rev.* **2017**, *16*, 61–65. [CrossRef] [PubMed]

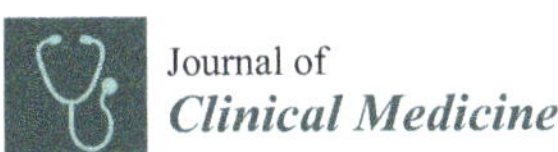
Journal of
Clinical Medicine

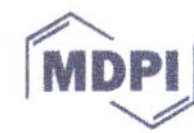

Article

Coronary Microvascular Vasodilatory Function: Related Clinical Features and Differences According to the Different Coronary Arteries and Types of Coronary Spasm

Hiroki Teragawa *, Chikage Oshita, Yuko Uchimura, Ryota Akazawa and Yuichi Orita

Department of Cardiovascular Medicine, JR Hiroshima Hospital, Hiroshima 732-0057, Japan; chikage-ooshita@jrhh.or.jp (C.O.); yuuko-uchimura@jrhh.or.jp (Y.U.); ryota-akazawa@jrhh.or.jp (R.A.); yuichi-orita@jrhh.or.jp (Y.O.)

* Correspondence: hiroki-teragawa@jrhh.or.jp; Tel.: +81-82-262-1171; Fax: +81-82-262-1499

Abstract: Background: In the clinical setting; the microvascular vasodilatory function test (MVFT) with a pressure wire has been used in ischaemia patients with non-obstructive coronary arteries (INOCA), including vasospastic angina (VSA) and microvascular angina (MVA). The exact factors that affect the microvascular vasodilatory function (MVF) in such patients are still unknown. We aimed to identify the factors, including clinical parameters and lesion characteristics, affecting the MVF in such patients. Methods: A total of 53 patients who underwent coronary angiography, spasm provocation tests (SPTs) and MVFTs were enrolled. In the MVFT, the coronary flow reserve (CFR) and index of microcirculatory resistance (IMR) were measured. Of the 53 patients, MVFT data in the left anterior descending coronary artery (LAD) were obtained from 49 patients, and the clinical parameters were checked in all of them. Based on the results of the SPT, coronary spasms were divided into focal spasm, diffuse spasm, and microvascular spasm (MVS). To assess the lesion characteristics influencing MVF, MVFT data were compared according to the types of coronary spasm and coronary vessels in 73 vessels of the 53 patients. Results: In 49 patients who underwent the MVFT in the LAD, the IMR was higher in active smokers (n = 7) than in former smokers (n = 15) and never smokers (n = 27, $p < 0.01$). In the 73 coronary arteries in this study, the type of coronary spasm did not correlate with the CFR or IMR, whereas a higher IMR were more frequently observed in cases of focal spasm than in cases of diffuse spasm (p = 0.03). In addition, the IMR was higher in the right coronary artery (RCA) than in the LAD (p = 0.02). Conclusion: These results indicate that the smoking status affected the MVF in patients with INOCA, suggesting the possibility of improvement in the MVF by smoking cessation in such patients. In addition, in the assessment of MVF, it may be important to take into account which coronary artery or types of coronary spasm are being evaluated.

Keywords: vasospastic angina; microvascular spasm; microvascular vasodilatory function

Citation: Teragawa, H.; Oshita, C.; Uchimura, Y.; Akazawa, R.; Orita, Y. Coronary Microvascular Vasodilatory Function: Related Clinical Features and Differences According to the Different Coronary Arteries and Types of Coronary Spasm. *J. Clin. Med.* **2022**, *11*, 130. https://doi.org/10.3390/jcm11010130

Academic Editors: Koichi Node, Atsushi Tanaka and Mahboob Alam

Received: 28 November 2021
Accepted: 23 December 2021
Published: 27 December 2021

1. Introduction

The assessment and treatment of epicardial coronary stenosis are well established [1]. However, in the clinical setting, many patients develop ischaemia with non-obstructive coronary arteries (INOCA) [2]. INOCA has several endotypes, such as vasospastic angina (VSA), microvascular spasm (MVS), microvascular vasodilatory dysfunction (MVD) and a combination of VSA and MVD [3–5]. INOCA is not always benign [4,6], and an effective treatment for it has not yet been determined. A recent expert consensus document has strengthened the importance of treatment according to the endotypes of INOCA [5]. Thus, the diagnosis of INOCA and the differentiation of its endotypes are more important than ever.

Non-invasive imaging techniques such as transthoracic Doppler echocardiography and positron emission tomography with coronary computed tomographic angiography can effectively diagnose INOCA [5]. However, these methods have some clinical limitations due to local expertise and availability or variability in assessing these modalities. Thus, an invasive method using guidewire-based coronary flow reserve (CFR) and/or microcirculatory resistance measurements is widely recommended [1] because an established protocol is followed, and the inter-observer variability is low.

In the clinical setting, it has been demonstrated that several factors, such as ageing, smoking, hypertension, dyslipidaemia and diabetes mellitus, are associated with MVD [5,7–10]. In any event, it would be beneficial to elucidate the clinical indicators associated with these MVDs so that we could intervene in their treatment. Other clinical questions are whether or not microvascular vasodilatory function (MVF) varies with the type of coronary spasm or with each coronary artery. Recently, it has been reported that the prognosis in patients with VSA and MVD is worse than those without MVD [4]. Thus, it is also clinically important to elucidate the relationship between the type of coronary spasm and MVF. Furthermore, MVF testing (MVFT) has been often measured in the left anterior descending coronary artery (LAD) [4,11], but it is not known whether it varies by coronary artery. This study aimed to investigate the relationship between the MVF and clinical parameters and whether the function varies according to the lesion characteristics of the coronary artery, including the types of coronary spasm.

2. Materials and Methods

2.1. Study Population

This was a retrospective study of 66 patients with chest pain on whom we performed coronary angiography (CAG) and a spasm provocation test (SPT) between March 2020 and October 2021 at our institution (Figure 1). In two patients with moderate tandem lesions, another pressure guidewire was used. In one patient with VSA, coronary angioscopy was performed. MVFT was not performed on 10 patients because of either their intolerance to lengthy procedures (n = 4) or the judgement of the doctor-in-charge (n = 6). Thus, 53 patients who underwent both SPT and MVFT with a pressure wire were enrolled. The patient selection process and the number of analysed patients who underwent each procedure are presented in Figure 1. We excluded patients who had moderate coronary stenosis (% stenosis $\geq$ 30%) or moderate chronic kidney disease (CKD) with an estimated glomerular filtration rate (eGFR) of <45 mL/min/1.73 m^2 or a history of heart failure or percutaneous coronary interventions. The ethics committee of JR Hiroshima Hospital approved this study (2021-37). Informed consent was obtained from all patients.

2.2. Coronary Function Test (CFT)

The methods used for the SPT at our institution have been previously described [12]. In brief, an SPT is performed after a standard diagnostic CAG employing the percutaneous brachial approach using a 5-Fr sheath diagnostic Judkins-type catheter. After the initial CAG, 50, 100 and 200 µg of acetylcholine (ACh) were infused into the left coronary artery (LCA) for 20 s at 3-min intervals [13]. CAG was performed immediately after coronary spasms were induced or the maximum ACh infusion was completed. If a coronary spasm was induced but improved spontaneously, a right coronary artery (RCA) SPT was then performed without the intracoronary injection of nitroglycerin (NTG) into the LCA. Once the SPT for the RCA was finished, CAG was repeated after an NTG injection into the LCA. If a prolonged coronary spasm was provoked by ACh infusion into the LCA or it induced haemodynamic instability, an intracoronary injection of 0.3 mg of NTG was administered. After spasm provocation in the LCA, 20, 50 and 80 µg of ACh were infused into the RCA for 20 s at a 3-min interval. CAG was performed immediately after coronary spasms were induced or the maximum ACh infusion was completed. After an intracoronary injection of 0.3 mg of NTG, the final CAG of the RCA was performed. We could not determine (NA) when the subsequent SPT was negative after an inevitable use of NTG.

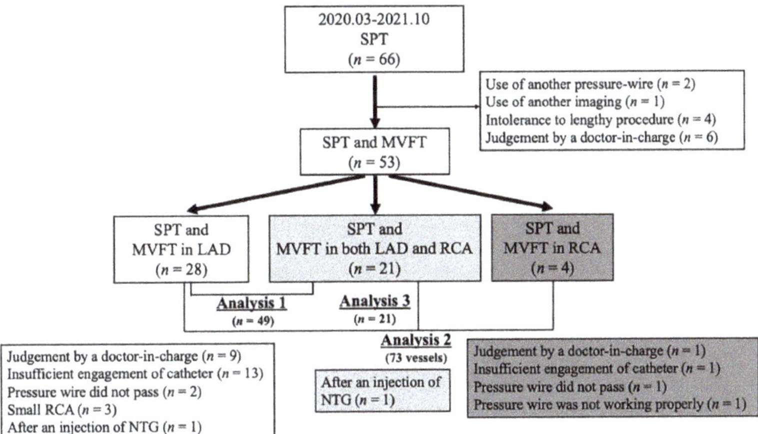

Figure 1. This is a figure of the study flowchart. Analysis 1 examined the relationship between the clinical parameters and IMR in 49 patients in whom MVFT data could be obtained in the LAD. Analysis 2 examined the relationship between MVFT data and lesion characteristics in 73 coronary vessels. Analysis 3 compared MVFT data between LAD and RCA in 21 patients in whom MVFT data could be obtained in both the LAD and RCA. LAD, left anterior descending coronary artery; MVFT, microvascular vasodilatory function test; NTG, nitroglycerin; RCA, right coronary artery; SPT, spasm provocation test.

The methods employed for the MVFT were as described in previous papers [11,14]. A pressure–temperature sensor-tipped PressureWire X Cabled Guidewire (Abbot Laboratories, Abbot Park, IL, USA) was used. Parameters were assessed using the CoroFlow software program (Coroventis, Uppsala, Sweden). The PressureWire was safely advanced in the LAD and RCA distally. To derive the resting mean transit time (Tmn), a thermodilution curve was obtained with three injections of 3-mL saline at room temperature. Hyperaemia was induced by intravenous infusion of adenosine triphosphate (160 µg/kg/min) through the peripheral vein. The hyperaemic proximal aortic pressure (Pa), distal arterial pressure (Pd) and hyperaemic Tmn were measured during maximal hyperaemia. The fractional flow reserve (FFR) was calculated as the lowest average of three consecutive beats during stable hyperaemia. CFR was calculated using the formula resting T_{mn}/hyperaemic T_{mn}. The index of microcirculatory resistance (IMR) was calculated using the formula Pd $\times$ T_{mn} during hyperaemia. To avoid the occurrence of pressure drift in the measurement of these parameters, we routinely calibrated the aortic pressure in the catheter and the pressure obtained by the PressureWire before measuring these parameters in each coronary artery. In addition, we confirmed that there was no pressure drift between the pressure obtained from the withdrawal of the PressureWire and the aortic pressure.

2.3. Definitions of CFT

The method used for measuring the diameter of the coronary artery has been described previously [12]. We selected spastic and atherosclerotic segments for quantitative analysis. The average value of three measurements was used for analysis. Changes in the coronary artery diameter in response to the ACh and NTG infusions were expressed as percentage changes from baseline angiographic measurements. Lesions with >20% stenosis were defined as atherosclerotic lesions. As previously reported [15,16], we investigated whether a myocardial bridge, defined as the systolic narrowing of the coronary artery diameter by >20% compared with that in diastole, was present. We also checked the frequency of a dominant RCA (an RCA with both the posterior descending artery and the posterolateral branch) [17].

Coronary spasm was defined as >90% narrowing of the epicardial coronary arteries on angiography during SPT, the presence of characteristic chest pain and/or ST-segment deviation identified via electrocardiography (ECG) [18,19]. A focal spasm was defined as a transient vessel narrowing of >90% within the borders of one isolated coronary segment as defined by the American Heart Association [20]. A diffuse spasm was defined as a 90% diffuse vasoconstriction observed in ≥2 adjacent coronary segments of the coronary arteries [21]. MVS was defined as the absence of angiographic coronary spasm accompanied by characteristic chest pain and ST-T ECG changes during SPT [5,22]. MVD was defined as the presence of IMR values of ≥25 units or CFR values of <2.0 [1,5].

2.4. Definitions of Clinical Parameters

We classified the patients according to smoking status as active smokers, former smokers (had stopped smoking for at least 1 month) or never smokers. Hypertension was defined as a systolic blood pressure of ≥140 mmHg, a diastolic blood pressure of ≥90 mmHg or the use of antihypertensive medication. We measured the levels of triglycerides, low-density lipoprotein cholesterol, fasting blood glucose, haemoglobin A1C, creatinine, C-reactive protein and N-terminal pro-brain natriuretic peptide. The eGFR (mL/min/1.73 m^2) was calculated using the standard formula, and the presence of CKD was defined using standard criteria [23]. Dyslipidaemia was defined as a low-density lipoprotein cholesterol level of ≥120 mg/dL or the use of medications for dyslipidaemia. Diabetes mellitus was defined as a fasting blood sugar level of ≥126 mg/dL, haemoglobin A1C level of ≥6.5% or use of anti-diabetic medications. Metabolic syndrome (MtS) was also defined using standard criteria [24]. The left ventricular ejection fraction (LVEF) was measured via echocardiography. The left ventricular mass index (LVMI) was calculated using the formula of Devereux and Reichek [25,26]. As demonstrated previously [27], the flow-mediated dilation (FMD) and NTG-mediated dilation (NMD) of the brachial artery, which are objective measures of the endothelium-dependent and endothelium-nondependent functions, respectively, were evaluated using the UNEXEF device (UNEX Corp, Nagoya, Japan). Finally, peripheral endothelial function was measured via reactive hyperaemia peripheral artery tonometry (RH-PAT) using the Endo-PAT2000 device (Itamar Medical, Caesarea, Israel). The reactive hyperaemia index (RHI) was calculated as demonstrated previously [28].

2.5. Statistical Analyses

Continuous data are expressed as median values with interquartile ranges. The relationship between the IMR and clinical parameters was assessed using the Wilcoxon signed-rank test or Spearman's rank correlation coefficient. Multiple comparisons in nonparametric methods were used to compare the IMR between the groups for smoking. The relationship between MVFT data and lesion characteristics was evaluated using the Wilcoxon signed-rank test or χ^2 analysis. Logistic regression analysis was employed to determine the presence of MVD. In the 21 patients with MVFT data from both LAD and RCA, data were displayed using the Bland–Altman plots and data comparisons were performed using the Wilcoxon signed-rank test. All statistical analyses were conducted using JMP Ver. 16 (SAS Institute Inc., Cary, NC, USA). A p value of <0.05 was considered significant.

3. Results

A total of 53 patients (median age, 69 years; 24 men and 29 women) underwent CAG, SPT and MVFT. Of them, 21 experienced an MVFT in both the LAD and the RCA, 28 underwent an MVFT only in the LAD and 4 patients underwent an MVFT only in the RCA (Figure 1). The reasons for the non-performance of the MVFT in both coronary arteries were as follows: judgement by the treating physician (n = 10 vessels), insufficient engagement of the catheter during the insertion of the pressure wire or injection of saline (n = 1 vessel, LAD; n = 13 vessels, RCA), difficulty in inserting the pressure wire into the distal coronary artery (n = 3 vessels), a small RCA (n = 3 vessels, SPT was also not performed), and NTG administration during coronary spasm in another coronary artery (n = 2 vessels). Thus, subsequent analyses of the relationship between the clinical parameters and IMR were conducted on 49 patients in whom MVFT data could be obtained in the LAD (Analysis 1). The relationship between MVFT data and lesion characteristics was determined in 73 coronary vessels (Analysis 2). Finally, comparisons of MVFT data between LAD and RCA of the same patient were performed in 21 patients in whom MVFT data could be obtained in both the LAD and RCA (Analysis 3).

3.1. Relationship between Patients' Characteristics and MVFT Data (Analysis 1)

The characteristics of 49 patients in whom MVFT data could be obtained in the LAD are presented in Table 1. The factors shown in Table 1, except for smoking status, were not associated with either the CFR or the IMR. The values of LVMI, FMD, RHI and presences of a myocardial bridge or VSA did not affect the CFR and IMR. The CFR correlated negatively with the IMR ($p < 0.01$). With regard to the smoking status, the IMR values were 50.2 (34.8, 54.6), 21.3 (16.1, 34.8) and 25.0 (14.9, 34.0) in active smokers (n = 7), former smokers (n = 15) and never smokers (n = 27, $p < 0.01$), respectively, whereas those that were not associated with the CFR were 1.8 (1.3, 2.8) in active smokers, 2.4 (2.1, 4.5) in former smokers and 2.5 (2.1, 3.3) in never smokers (p = 0.12, Figure 2).

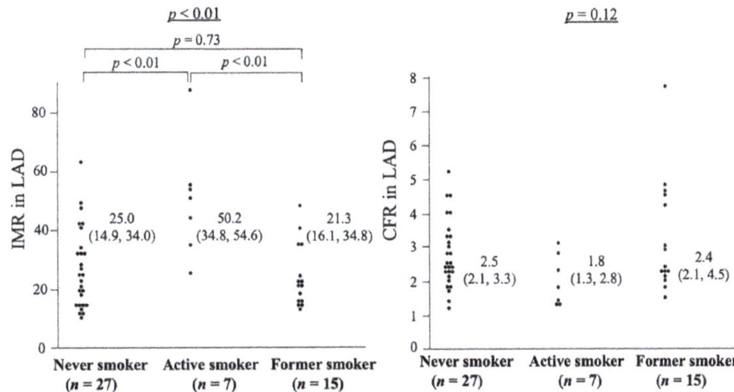

Figure 2. This is a figure of IMR and CFR regarding the smoking status in 49 patients who had MVFT in LAD (Analysis 1). The **left** panel shows the relationship between smoking status and IMR: active smokers had significantly higher IMR than never smokers and former smokers. The **right** panel shows the association between smoking status and CFR, which is not significant among the three groups. CFR, coronary flow reserve; IMR, index of microcirculatory resistance, LAD, left anterior descending coronary artery; MVFT, microvascular vasodilatory function test.

Table 1. Patients' characteristics of 49 patients who had MVFT in LAD.

Factors	Numbers or Values	Relationship between Factors and CFR, *p* Value	Relationship between Factors and IMR, *p* Value
Age (years)	69 (53, 76)	0.54	0.65
Men/Women	22/27	0.16	0.54
Body mass index	23.5 (21.8, 25.7)	0.13	0.37
Coronary risk factors			
Smoker (active/former/never)	7/15/27	0.12	<0.01
Hypertension	28 (57%)	0.65	0.15
Dyslipidaemia	26 (53%)	0.94	0.35
Diabetes mellitus	6 (13%)	0.92	0.36
Presence of MtS	7 (14%)	0.08	0.39
Presence of CKD	9 (18%)	1.00	0.53
Blood chemical data			
LDL-cholesterol (mg/dL)	100 (88, 123)	0.71	0.16
Triglyceride (mg/dL)	99 (82, 156)	0.24	0.77
Fasting blood sugar (mg/dL)	99 (90, 109)	0.32	0.43
Haemoglobin A1C (%)	5.9 (5.6, 6.2)	0.42	0.56
CRP (mg/dL)	0.05 (0.03, 0.11)	0.78	0.99
eGFR (mL/min/1.73 m^2)	67.0 (61.4, 74.7)	0.73	0.25
NT-proBNP (pg/mL)	92 (45, 195)	0.17	0.12
Echocardiography			
LVEF (%)	66 (62, 70)	0.22	0.86
LVMI (g/m^2)	80 (68, 94)	0.48	0.29
Peripheral endothelial function			
FMD (%)	3.5 (2.3, 5.3)	0.55	0.82
NMD (%)	15.8 (10.3, 18.1)	0.14	0.16
RHI	1.57 (1.43, 2.10)	0.71	0.69
CAG SPT MVFT			
Myocardial bridge	13 (27%)	0.18	0.28
VSA	31 (63%)	0.58	0.33
MVS	9 (18%)	0.43	0.35
Baseline Pd/Pa in LAD	0.96 (0.95, 0.98)	0.84	0.65
FFR in LAD	0.92 (0.89, 0.94)	0.94	0.84
CFR in LAD	2.4 (2.0, 3.3)	(−)	<0.01
IMR in LAD	25.0 (16.1, 40.3)	<0.01	(−)

Numbers were expressed as the numbers (percentage) and values were expressed as the median with interquartile ranges. CAG, coronary angiography; CFR, coronary flow reserve; CKD, chronic kidney disease; CRP, C-reactive protein; eGFR, estimated glomerular filtration rate; FFR, fractional flow reserve; FMD, flow-mediated dilation; IMR, index of microcirculatory resistance; LAD, left anterior descending coronary artery; LDL, low-density lipoprotein; LVEF, left ventricular ejection fraction; LVMI, left ventricular mass index; MtS, metabolic syndrome; MVFT, microvascular vasodilatory function test; MVS, microvascular spasm; NMD, nitroglycerin-mediated dilation; NT-proBNP, N-terminal pro-brain natriuretic peptide; RHI, index of reactive hyperemia; SPT, spasm provocation test; VSA, vasospastic angina. (−) means that the test was not performed because they were for the same indexes.

3.2. Relationship between MVFT Data and Lesion Characteristics (Analysis 2)

In 28, 21 and 4 patients had MVFT data in the LAD, in both the LAD and the RCA and, in the RCA, respectively; thus, a total of 73 sets of MVFT data for all coronary vessels were analysed (Table 2). Atherosclerosis (% stenosis < 30%) did not affect the CFR or IMR, while it reduced the baseline Pd/Pa ($p = 0.04$) and FFR ($p = 0.01$). In the vessel analyses, the baseline Pd/Pa, FFR and IMR in the RCA ($n = 24$) were significantly higher than those in the LAD ($n = 49$). The presence of MVD was higher in the RCA than in the LAD ($p = 0.01$). The CFR value did not significantly differ between the LAD and RCA. The types of coronary spasm did not significantly differ between the RCA and LAD ($p = 0.07$). Regarding the types of spasm, FFR values was different in the 4 groups ($p = 0.03$), however, the baseline Pd/Pa, CFR and IMR were not different in the 4 groups. The frequency of MVD was different in the four groups (p = 0.046). In the comparisons of MVFT data between focal and diffuse spasms, the FFR (p = 0.03), IMR (p = 0.03) and presence of MVD (p < 0.01) were higher in focal spasms than in diffuse spasms. Logistic regression analysis revealed that focal spasm and the measurement in the RCA were factors associated with MVD (Table 3).

Table 2. Relationship between MVFT and lesion characteristics.

Lesion Characteristics		No.	Baseline Pd/Pa	p Value	FFR	p Value	CFR	p Value	IMR	p Value	*MVD*	p Value
Atherosclerosis	(+)	26	0.97 (0.95, 0.98)	0.04	0.92 (0.85, 0.96)	0.01	2.4 (1.9, 3.5)	0.88	25.1 (20.9, 41.9)	0.72	15 (57%)	0.14
	(−)	47	0.98 (0.96, 1.00)		0.94 (0.92, 0.99)		2.5 (2.0, 3.3)		28.8 (19.5, 41.2)		35 (74%)	
Vessels	LAD	49	0.96 (0.95, 0.98)	<0.01	0.92 (0.89, 0.94)	<0.01	2.4 (2.0, 3.3)	0.83	25.0 (16.1, 40.3)	0.01	29 (59%)	0.01
	RCA	24	1.02 (1.00, 1.03)		1.00 (0.96, 1.02)		2.7 (1.8, 3.3)		36.6 (25.3, 46.1)		21 (88%)	
Types of spasm	Focal spasm	24	0.97 (0.95, 1.00)	0.15	0.94 * (0.91, 0.99)	0.03	2.4 (1.8, 3.2)	0.09	33.4 * (25.1, 48.4)	0.15	21 * (88%)	0.05
	Diffuse spasm	15	0.96 (0.94, 0.98)		0.92 (0.87, 0.94)		2.8 (2.1, 4.5)		23.0 (16.1, 35.0)		7 (47%)	
	MVS	12	0.97 (0.95, 1.00)		0.94 (0.90, 0.97)		2.3 (1.7, 2.6)		31.6 (13.8, 40.1)		8 (67%)	
	None	22	0.98 (0.95, 1.02)		0.96 (0.92, 1.01)		2.9 (2.3, 3.9)		25.3 (21.8, 44.2)		14 (64%)	

Numbers were expressed as the numbers (percentage) and values were expressed as the median with interquartile ranges. CFR, coronary flow reserve; FFR, fractional flow reserve; IMR, index of microcirculatory resistance; LAD, left anterior descending coronary artery; MVFT, microvascular vasodilatory function test; MVS, microvascular spasm; Pa, aortic pressure; Pd, distal pressure; RCA, right coronary artery. * p < 0.05 vs. diffuse spasm.

Table 3. Logistic regression analyses of lesion characteristics of the presence of MVD.

Factors	Estimate	95% CI	χ^2	p Value
Atherosclerosis	−0.36	−0.99–0.25	1.34	0.25
Vessels				
RCA	0.90	0.20–1.75	5.37	0.02
Types of spasm				
Focal spasm	1.41	0.41–2.63	6.49	0.01
Diffuse spasm	−0.77	−1.77–0.20	2.40	0.12
MVS	−0.04	−1.16–1.13	0.01	0.93
				R^2 = 0.19

CI, confidence interval; MVD, microvascular vasodilatory dysfunction; MVS, microvascular spasm; RCA, right coronary artery.

3.3. Relationship between MVFT Data in the LAD and RCA (Analysis 3)

The data of 21 patients in whom SPT and MVFT were performed in both LAD and RCA are presented in Table 4 and Figure 3. The baseline Pd/Pa, FFR and IMR values in the RCA were significantly higher than those in the LAD (p < 0.01, p < 0.01 and p < 0.05, respectively), whereas the CFR values did not significantly differ between the LAD and RCA (p = 0.27). A higher IMR in the RCA than in the LAD was detected in 12 out of 21 patients (57%). A dominant RCA was detected in 17 out of 21 patients (81%). No significant relationship was observed between a higher IMR in the RCA than in the LAD and a dominant RCA (p = 0.75). The types of spasm types between LAD and RCA matched in only 7 of 21 cases (33%). MVD was detected in 14 out of 21 LAD (67%) and 17 out of 21 RCA (81%) and there was a coincidence in 14 out of 21 patients (67%). Out of seven patients with disparities in the presence of MVD between the LAD and the RCA, the types of spasm in the LAD and the RCA were different in 5 out of 7 patients (71%). Figure 4 presents a representative case (Case 11) with normal MVF in the LAD with MVS (CFR, 4.0; IMR, 13.7) and MVD in the RCA without any types of spasm (CFR, 2.0; IMR, 32).

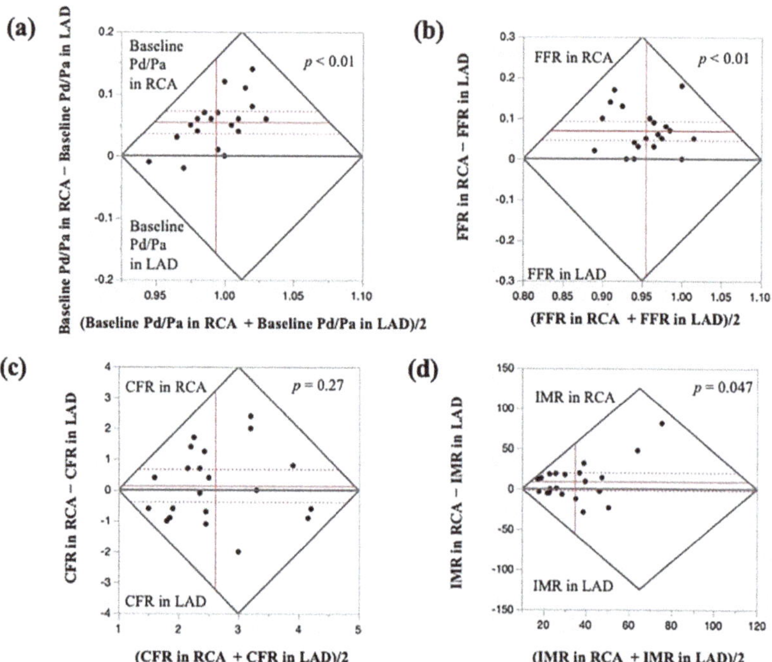

Figure 3. Comparison of MVFT data in the LAD and RCA. The Bland–Altman plots show the baseline Pd/Pa (**a**), FFR (**b**), CFR (**c**) and IMR (**d**) in the LAD and RCA. The baseline Pd/Pa, FFR and IMR were significantly higher in the RCA than in the LAD, whereas no significant difference was observed in the CFR values between the LAD and RCA. CFR, coronary flow reserve; FFR, fractional flow reserve; IMR, index of microcirculatory resistance; LAD, left anterior descending coronary artery; MVFT, microvascular vasodilatory function test; RCA, right coronary artery.

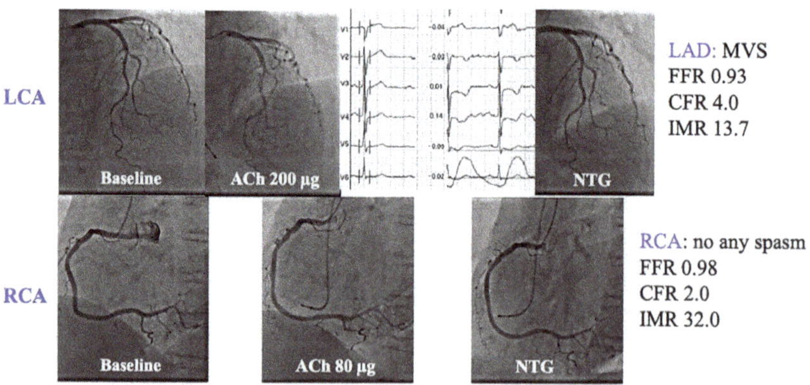

Figure 4. A representative case (Case 11 in Table 4).

Table 4. Data in patients who performed MVFT in both LAD and RCA.

Case No.	Age (Years)	Gender	Diagnosis	LAD								RCA								IMR in RCA> in LAD	Dominant RCA
				Athero-sclerosis	Epi-Spasm	Type of Spasm	Baseline Pd/Pa	FFR	CFR	IMR	MVD	Athero-sclerosis	Epi-Spasm	Type of Spasm	Baseline Pd/Pa	FFR	CFR	IMR	MVD		
1	72	M	VSA	1	0	MVS	0.95	0.83	2	35	1	0	0	None	1.00	1.00	4.4	44	1	1	1
2	78	F	VSA	0	1	Focal	0.96	0.93	3.5	25	1	1	0	None	1.00	0.93	4.3	20	0	0	0
3	50	F	MVS	0	0	MVS	0.96	0.94	1.8	40.5	1	0	0	None	1.02	1.02	2.5	54.3	1	1	1
4	73	F	VSA	0	1	Focal	0.94	0.86	3.3	41.2	1	0	1	Focal	1.06	0.99	3.3	28.8	1	0	1
5	66	M	VSA	1	1	Diffuse	0.96	0.92	2.5	25.5	1	0	1	Diffuse	1.07	0.96	2.1	26.3	1	1	1
6	82	M	VSA	1	1	Focal	0.95	0.91	1.4	32	1	1	1	Focal	1.09	1.09	1.8	25.2	1	0	1
7	71	M	VSA	0	1	Diffuse	0.96	0.92	2.2	40.2	1	0	1	Focal	1.03	1.01	1.6	87.7	1	1	0
8	71	F	VSA	0	1	Focal	1	0.99	2	27	1	0	0	None	1.06	1.04	2.7	46.6	1	1	1
9	42	M	VSA	0	1	Focal	0.96	0.94	1.8	21.2	1	0	0	None	1.02	1.00	3.05	38.7	1	1	1
10	73	F	VSA	1	1	Diffuse	0.99	0.95	3	11.3	0	1	0	None	1.00	1.00	1.9	23.2	1	1	1
11	79	F	MVS	0	0	MVS	0.98	0.93	4	13.7	0	1	0	None	1.06	0.98	2	32	1	1	1
12	72	F	VSA	0	1	Focal	0.99	0.95	2.3	34.8	1	1	1	Focal	1.09	0.98	1.4	116.2	1	1	1
13	83	M	VSA	0	1	Focal	0.95	0.95	1.5	47.6	1	0	0	None	1.02	1.02	2.9	44.8	1	0	1
14	55	F	MVS	0	0	MVS	0.95	0.93	2.2	12.2	0	0	0	None	1.02	0.96	4.2	25.5	1	1	0
15	28	F	VSA	0	1	Diffuse	0.95	0.91	2.4	24.5	0	0	NA	NA	1.01	1.01	2.3	19	0	0	1
16	58	M	VSA	1	1	Diffuse	0.95	0.88	4.6	16.1	0	0	1	Diffuse	0.94	0.90	3.7	35	1	1	1
17	74	F	MVS	0	0	MVS	1.00	1.00	2.3	62.2	1	0	0	MVS	1.00	1.00	2.7	38.8	1	0	1
18	47	F	VSA	0	1	Focal	0.98	0.94	1.8	19.5	1	0	1	Diffuse	0.96	0.94	1.2	16.2	1	0	0
19	54	F	VSA	0	1	Diffuse	0.98	0.94	1.4	53.0	1	0	0	None	1.03	1.02	3.1	24.2	0	0	1
20	29	M	VSA	1	1	Diffuse	0.98	0.84	4.5	23.0	0	0	0	None	1.04	0.98	3.9	22.9	0	0	1
21	74	M	MVD	1	0	None	0.95	0.85	2.3	23.1	0	1	0	None	0.98	0.95	1.3	54.6	1	1	1
	71 (52, 74)	M/F 9/12	VSA/ MVS/ MVD 16/4/1	7 (33%)	15 (71%)		0.96 (0.95, 0.98)	0.93 (0.90, 0.95	2.3 (1.8, 3.2)	25.5 (20.4, 40.4)	14 (67%)	6 (29%)	7 (33%)		1.02 * (1.00, 1.05)	1.00 * (0.96, 1.02	2.7 (1.9, 3.5)	32.0 # (23.7, 45.7)	17 (81%)	12 (57%)	17 (81%)

Numbers were expressed as the numbers and values were expressed as the median with interquartile ranges. CFR, coronary flow reserve; FFR, fractional flow reserve; IMR, index of microcirculatory resistance; LAD, left anterior descending coronary artery; MVD, microvascular vasodilatory dysfunction; MVFT, microvascular vasodilatory function test; MVS, microvascular spasm; Pa, aortic pressure; Pd, distal pressure, RCA; right coronary artery. * $p < 0.01$ vs. the same values in the LAD, # $p < 0.05$ vs. the same value in the LAD.

A 79-year-old woman complained of chest pain at rest. LAD SPT revealed no inductions of epicardial coronary spasm (upper panels). With chest pain and precordial inverted T waves during SPT in the LAD, MVS was considered in the LAD. Contrarily, the SPT for the RCA showed no inductions of angiographic and electrocardiographic changes. The MVFT revealed normal CFR and IMR in the LAD with MVS. There was reduced CFR and increased IMR in the RCA without any types of spasm. This patient might have different MVFs in the RCA and LAD.

CFR, coronary flow reserve; IMR, index of microcirculatory resistance; MVF, microvascular vasodilatory function; MVFT, microvascular vasodilatory function test; MVS, microvascular spasm; SPT, spasm provocation test.

4. Discussion

In this study, we investigated MVF in patients who underwent SPT and MCFT to evaluate their chest symptoms. We found that (1) smoking status, especially active smoking may increase IMR; (2) the focal spasm type and RCA may affect IMR and (3) the baseline Pd/Pa, FFR and IMR in the RCA were higher than those in the LAD, although the CFR did not significantly differ between the two vessels.

Factors such as ageing, smoking, hypertension, dyslipidaemia and diabetes mellitus are associated with MVD [5,7–10]. In this study, smoking status, especially active smoking, was associated with an increased IMR, which is in agreement with the results of other studies [7,9]. However, other factors were not associated with the MVFT data. In general, smoking has been known to increase oxidative stress, leading to vascular inflammation, impaired prostacyclin production, and vascular dysfunction [29,30]. Moreover, 60% of our patients had VSA, and smoking is one of the major risk factors for VSA [31]. This population and the small sample size may have contributed to the slight difference in the results. In addition, since this study was cross-sectional, it is unclear from the results whether smoking cessation improves MVD. However, considering the fact that there was no significant difference in the MVFT data between former smokers and never smokers, smoking cessation may be a valuable treatment for MVD.

The present study demonstrated that the IMR value in the RCA was higher than that in the LAD, which is in agreement with the results reported by Murai et al. [10]. They speculated that the spatial heterogeneity of myocardial flow in different vascular beds caused the IMR to be higher in the RCA. The metabolic difference between the left and right ventricles may cause a difference in the myocardial flow between the LAD and the RCA. In the present study, we checked the presence of a dominant RCA, which could lead to more spatial heterogeneity of myocardial blood flow in the RCA. We could not demonstrate such a relationship, neither can we draw a definite conclusion owing to the small number of study participants. On the other hand, our results indicate that the distal pressures of the RCA at rest and during hyperaemia, indicated by baseline Pd/Pa and FFR, were significantly higher than those of the LAD. These findings are due to the lower anatomical position of the pressure wire tip in the distal RCA than in the distal LAD [32–34]. Furthermore, our results reveal no statistically significant difference between the CFR values in the LAD and RCA. This suggests that the increased IMR in the RCA may often be caused by the differences in the distal LAD and RCA pressures used in the formula for calculating IMR rather than by a real difference in the MVF. Other methods for assessing the MVF using a Doppler flow guidewire may be needed to confirm our results. Finally, methodological issues may also be the cause. Although we thoroughly checked for calibration before measuring each coronary artery and for drift after measurement, we still could not deny the possibility that a systematic error occurred. In summary, the difference in the IMR between the LAD and the RCA may be due to (1) the spatial heterogeneity in myocardial blood flow between the LAD and the RCA due to the differences in the perfused myocardial territory and/or metabolism in the left and right ventricles, (2) the anatomical differences in the distal pressure and (3) other factors, such as a systematic error. However, in our representative case (Figure 4), the CFR also significantly differs between the LAD and the RCA, indicating the presence of diverse MVFs. In such cases, calcium-channel blockers seem to be the first choice because of the presence of MVS; however, to evaluate the drug efficacy and prognosis in such cases, careful observation and data collection, such as from a multicentre registry, will be needed in the future.

Regarding the relationship between MVF and VSA, the presence of MVD has been noted in patients with VSA [4,35,36], partially owing to the increased coronary perivascular adipose tissue in VSA patients [37]. In this study, we could not find any relationship in terms of CFR and IMR between VSA and non-VSA patients, partly because of the difference in patients' characteristics and a small number of studied patients. However, we demonstrated the relationship between focal spasm and MVD. With regard to the types of spasm and CFR, a previous study revealed that the CFR was reduced in diffuse spasm [38]. Although there are differences in the drugs used to induce coronary spasms, the definitions of diffuse spasms and the methods for assessing the CFR may influence the results. It has been demonstrated that VSA patients with focal spasms had a poorer prognosis than those with diffuse spasm [21]. It was also demonstrated that VSA patients with MVD had a poorer prognosis than those without [4]. The results of these studies may suggest the close link between focal spasm and MVD. Another possible explanation was the insufficient microvascular vasodilation due to the standard dose of NTG, especially in focal spasm. Suda et al. demonstrated that the intracoronary infusion of fasudil, a Rho-kinase inhibitor, improved the IMR [4], and these data could support the fact that the IMR was increased due to inadequate microvascular vasodilatation in the case of focal spasm. In the case of focal spasm, it might be better to use a more sufficient dose of NTG or other coronary dilators that dilate the microvascular blood vessels and take a little time to assess the MVF. Finally, some attention has been focused on the MVF in patients with MVS [4,35], showing that MVD is not always present in MVS. Our results also did not indicate a significantly higher frequency of MVD in MVS. However, the number of analysed patients was insufficient. Thus, further studies with a larger sample size may be needed to confirm our results.

Our results show that MVF, especially IMR, may vary from vessel to vessel, depending on coronary artery anatomy, or on the function of each coronary artery itself. Although it takes time to perform CFT, it may suggest that it is more important to evaluate each coronary artery rather than on a patient-by-patient basis. Again, owing to the small number of cases, it reiterates the fact that large multicentre registries and prospective consecutive case studies are needed.

This study has some limitations. First, the sample size of present study was relatively small, especially in the subgroup analyses, such as the active smokers ($n = 7$). This may have introduced some type II errors. Second, this was a retrospective study conducted in one institution, with a non-consecutive design. Thus, further prospective studies with more participants or a multicentre registry study will be needed to confirm our results. Third, routine CFT was performed using a 5-Fr catheter, and in some patients, it was not possible to engage the catheter in the ostium of the coronary artery, especially the RCA. Since we excluded patients, whose data were not completely available, the results obtained from the RCA may have varied, leading to the difference in coronary MVF between the RCA and the LAD. Further studies using a 6-Fr guiding catheter will be needed to further investigate our results. Fourth, the median IMR in this study was approximately 25, which was overall higher than those from the usual INOCA studies [4]. The frequency of hypertension, time off coronary dilation drugs, blood pressure during the test, and NTG and ATP load were considered as possible causes, but nothing definite was found; there may be an effect of RCA vessels and frequency of focal spasm, but the exact mechanism was not elucidated. Finally, we performed MVFT in the LAD and RCA but not in the left circumflex coronary artery (LCX) as we had no information on the MVF in the LCX.

5. Conclusions

Our results indicated that smoking status might be associated with an increased IMR, although there have been no clinically confident markers suggestive of MVD. The results suggest that smoking cessation might be one of the possible treatments for such MVD in our patients. The results also indicate that the IMR may be elevated during RCA and in focal spasm. It may be important to carefully examine the vessel that is being measured and to take measures such as adding sufficient coronary dilator and taking some time before measuring the IMR in case of focal spasm. However, the sample size of this study was small, and the investigation needs to be repeated with a larger sample size.

Author Contributions: H.T., C.O., Y.U., R.A. and Y.O. were involved in patient enrolment and the collection of clinical data. H.T. wrote the whole manuscript, and C.O., Y.U., R.A. and Y.O. checked the manuscript before submission. All authors have read and agreed to the published version of the manuscript.

Funding: This research received no external funding.

Institutional Review Board Statement: This study was conducted according to the guidelines of the Declaration of Helsinki and was approved by the Institutional Review Board of the JR Hiroshima Hospital (protocol code: 2021-37; date of approval: 5 November 2021).

Informed Consent Statement: Informed consent was obtained from all patients who underwent SPT and MVFT before the procedure. The opt-out method was adopted due to the retrospective design of the study.

Data Availability Statement: Date sharing is not applicable.

Acknowledgments: The authors thank Akemi Seno for her secretary help, the entire staff of the cardiac catheterisation room and the entire nursing staff of the Cardiovascular Medicine Ward, JR Hiroshima Hospital.

Conflicts of Interest: The authors declare no conflict of interest.

References

1. Knuuti, J.; Wijns, W.; Saraste, A.; Capodanno, D.; Barbato, E.; Funck-Brentano, C.; Prescott, E.; Storey, R.F.; Deaton, C.; Cuisset, T.; et al. 2019 ESC Guidelines for the diagnosis and management of chronic coronary syndromes. *Eur. Heart J.* **2020**, *41*, 407–477. [CrossRef]
2. Reeh, J.; Therming, C.B.; Heitmann, M.; Hojberg, S.; Sorum, C.; Bech, J.; Husum, D.; Dominguez, H.; Sehestedt, T.; Hermann, T.; et al. Prediction of obstructive coronary artery disease and prognosis in patients with suspected stable angina. *Eur. Heart J.* **2019**, *40*, 1426–1435. [CrossRef] [PubMed]
3. Marinescu, M.A.; Loffler, A.I.; Ouellette, M.; Smith, L.; Kramer, C.M.; Bourque, J.M. Coronary microvascular dysfunction, microvascular angina, and treatment strategies. *JACC Cardiovasc. Imaging* **2015**, *8*, 210–220. [CrossRef]
4. Suda, A.; Takahashi, J.; Hao, K.; Kikuchi, Y.; Shindo, T.; Ikeda, S.; Sato, K.; Sugisawa, J.; Matsumoto, Y.; Miyata, S.; et al. Coronary functional abnormalities in patients with angina and nonobstructive coronary artery disease. *J. Am. Coll. Cardiol.* **2019**, *74*, 2350–2360. [CrossRef] [PubMed]
5. Kunadian, V.; Chieffo, A.; Camici, P.G.; Berry, C.; Escaned, J.; Maas, A.; Prescott, E.; Karam, N.; Appelman, Y.; Fraccaro, C.; et al. An EAPCI expert consensus document on ischaemia with non-obstructive coronary arteries in collaboration with European society of cardiology working group on coronary pathophysiology & microcirculation endorsed by coronary vasomotor disorders international study group. *Eur. Heart J.* **2020**, *41*, 3504–3520. [CrossRef]
6. Murthy, V.L.; Naya, M.; Taqueti, V.R.; Foster, C.R.; Gaber, M.; Hainer, J.; Dorbala, S.; Blankstein, R.; Rimoldi, O.; Camici, P.G.; et al. Effects of sex on coronary microvascular dysfunction and cardiac outcomes. *Circulation* **2014**, *129*, 2518–2527. [CrossRef] [PubMed]
7. Zeiher, A.M.; Schachinger, V.; Minners, J. Long-term cigarette smoking impairs endothelium-dependent coronary arterial vasodilator function. *Circulation* **1995**, *92*, 1094–1100. [CrossRef]
8. Pepine, C.J.; Anderson, R.D.; Sharaf, B.L.; Reis, S.E.; Smith, K.M.; Handberg, E.M.; Johnson, B.D.; Sopko, G.; Bairey Merz, C.N. Coronary microvascular reactivity to adenosine predicts adverse outcome in women evaluated for suspected ischemia results from the National Heart, Lung and Blood Institute WISE (Women's Ischemia Syndrome Evaluation) study. *J. Am. Coll. Cardiol.* **2010**, *55*, 2825–2832. [CrossRef]
9. Mygind, N.D.; Michelsen, M.M.; Pena, A.; Frestad, D.; Dose, N.; Aziz, A.; Faber, R.; Host, N.; Gustafsson, I.; Hansen, P.R.; et al. Coronary microvascular function and cardiovascular risk factors in women with angina pectoris and no obstructive coronary artery disease: The iPOWER Study. *J. Am. Heart Assoc.* **2016**, *5*, e003064. [CrossRef]
10. Murai, T.; Lee, T.; Yonetsu, T.; Iwai, T.; Takagi, T.; Hishikari, K.; Masuda, R.; Iesaka, Y.; Isobe, M.; Kakuta, T. Variability of microcirculatory resistance index and its relationship with fractional flow reserve in patients with intermediate coronary artery lesions. *Circ. J.* **2013**, *77*, 1769–1776. [CrossRef]

11. Kobayashi, Y.; Fearon, W.F.; Honda, Y.; Tanaka, S.; Pargaonkar, V.; Fitzgerald, P.J.; Lee, D.P.; Stefanick, M.; Yeung, A.C.; Tremmel, J.A. Effect of sex differences on invasive measures of coronary microvascular dysfunction in patients with angina in the absence of obstructive coronary artery disease. *JACC Cardiovasc. Interv.* **2015**, *8*, 1433–1441. [CrossRef] [PubMed]
12. Teragawa, H.; Oshita, C.; Ueda, T. History of gastroesophageal reflux disease in patients with suspected coronary artery disease. *Heart Vessel.* **2019**, *34*, 1631–1638. [CrossRef] [PubMed]
13. Sueda, S.; Kohno, H.; Ochi, T.; Uraoka, T. Overview of the acetylcholine spasm provocation test. *Clin. Cardiol.* **2015**, *38*, 430–438. [CrossRef] [PubMed]
14. Lee, J.M.; Jung, J.H.; Hwang, D.; Park, J.; Fan, Y.; Na, S.H.; Doh, J.H.; Nam, C.W.; Shin, E.S.; Koo, B.K. Coronary flow reserve and microcirculatory resistance in patients with intermediate coronary stenosis. *J. Am. Coll. Cardiol.* **2016**, *67*, 1158–1169. [CrossRef]
15. Saito, Y.; Kitahara, H.; Shoji, T.; Tokimasa, S.; Nakayama, T.; Sugimoto, K.; Fujimoto, Y.; Kobayashi, Y. Relation between severity of myocardial bridge and vasospasm. *Int. J. Cardiol.* **2017**, *248*, 34–38. [CrossRef]
16. Teragawa, H.; Oshita, C.; Ueda, T. The myocardial bridge: Potential influences on the coronary artery vasculature. *Clin. Med. Insights Cardiol.* **2019**, *13*, 1179546819846493. [CrossRef]
17. Parikh, N.I.; Honeycutt, E.F.; Roe, M.T.; Neely, M.; Rosenthal, E.J.; Mittleman, M.A.; Carrozza, J.P., Jr.; Ho, K.K. Left and codominant coronary artery circulations are associated with higher in-hospital mortality among patients undergoing percutaneous coronary intervention for acute coronary syndromes: Report from the national cardiovascular database cath percutaneous coronary intervention (CathPCI) registry. *Circ. Cardiovasc. Qual. Outcomes* **2012**, *5*, 775–782. [CrossRef]
18. JCS Joint Working Group. Guidelines for diagnosis and treatment of patients with vasospastic angina (Coronary Spastic Angina) (JCS 2013). *Circ. J.* **2014**, *78*, 2779–2801. [CrossRef]
19. Beltrame, J.F.; Crea, F.; Kaski, J.C.; Ogawa, H.; Ong, P.; Sechtem, U.; Shimokawa, H.; Bairey Merz, C.N.; Coronary Vasomotion Disorders International Study Group. International standardization of diagnostic criteria for vasospastic angina. *Eur. Heart J.* **2017**, *38*, 2565–2568. [CrossRef]
20. Austen, W.G.; Edwards, J.E.; Frye, R.L.; Gensini, G.G.; Gott, V.L.; Griffith, L.S.; McGoon, D.C.; Murphy, M.L.; Roe, B.B. A reporting system on patients evaluated for coronary artery disease. Report of the Ad Hoc committee for grading of coronary artery disease, council on cardiovascular surgery, American heart association. *Circulation* **1975**, *51*, 5–40. [CrossRef]
21. Sato, K.; Kaikita, K.; Nakayama, N.; Horio, E.; Yoshimura, H.; Ono, T.; Ohba, K.; Tsujita, K.; Kojima, S.; Tayama, S.; et al. Coronary vasomotor response to intracoronary acetylcholine injection, clinical features, and long-term prognosis in 873 consecutive patients with coronary spasm: Analysis of a single-center study over 20 years. *J. Am. Heart Assoc.* **2013**, *2*, e000227. [CrossRef]
22. Ong, P.; Camici, P.G.; Beltrame, J.F.; Crea, F.; Shimokawa, H.; Sechtem, U.; Kaski, J.C.; Bairey Merz, C.N.; Coronary Vasomotion Disorders International Study Group. International standardization of diagnostic criteria for microvascular angina. *Int. J. Cardiol.* **2018**, *250*, 16–20. [CrossRef]
23. Matsuo, S.; Imai, E.; Horio, M.; Yasuda, Y.; Tomita, K.; Nitta, K.; Yamagata, K.; Tomino, Y.; Yokoyama, H.; Hishida, A.; et al. Revised equations for estimated GFR from serum creatinine in Japan. *Am. J. Kidney Dis.* **2009**, *53*, 982–992. [CrossRef]
24. National Cholesterol Education Program. Third report of the national cholesterol education program (NCEP) expert panel on detection, evaluation, and treatment of high blood cholesterol in adults (Adult Treatment Panel III) final report. *Circulation* **2002**, *106*, 3143–3421. [CrossRef]
25. Devereux, R.B.; Reichek, N. Echocardiographic determination of left ventricular mass in man. Anatomic validation of the method. *Circulation* **1977**, *55*, 613–618. [CrossRef]
26. Devereux, R.B.; Lutas, E.M.; Casale, P.N.; Kligfield, P.; Eisenberg, R.R.; Hammond, I.W.; Miller, D.H.; Reis, G.; Alderman, M.H.; Laragh, J.H. Standardization of M-mode echocardiographic left ventricular anatomic measurements. *J. Am. Coll. Cardiol.* **1984**, *4*, 1222–1230. [CrossRef]
27. Teragawa, H.; Oshita, C.; Orita, Y. Clinical significance of prolonged chest pain in vasospastic angina. *World J. Cardiol.* **2020**, *12*, 450–459. [CrossRef]
28. Tanaka, A.; Shimabukuro, M.; Machii, N.; Teragawa, H.; Okada, Y.; Shima, K.R.; Takamura, T.; Taguchi, I.; Hisauchi, I.; Toyoda, S.; et al. Secondary analyses to assess the profound effects of empagliflozin on endothelial function in patients with type 2 diabetes and established cardiovascular diseases: The placebo-controlled double-blind randomized effect of empagliflozin on endothelial function in cardiovascular high risk diabetes mellitus: Multi-center placebo-controlled double-blind randomized trial. *J. Diabetes Investig.* **2020**, *11*, 1551–1563. [CrossRef]
29. Nowak, J.; Murray, J.J.; Oates, J.A.; Fitzgerald, G.A. Biochemical evidence of a chronic abnormality in platelet and vascular function in healthy individuals who smoke cigarettes. *Circulation* **1987**, *76*, 6–14. [CrossRef]
30. Raghuveer, G.; White, D.A.; Hayman, L.L.; Woo, J.G.; Villafane, J.; Celermajer, D.; Ward, K.D.; de Ferranti, S.D.; Zachariah, J.; American Heart Association Committee on Atherosclerosis; et al. Cardiovascular consequences of childhood secondhand tobacco smoke exposure: Prevailing evidence, burden, and racial and socioeconomic disparities: A scientific statement from the American Heart Association. *Circulation* **2016**, *134*, e336–e359. [CrossRef]
31. Sugiishi, M.; Takatsu, F. Cigarette smoking is a major risk factor for coronary spasm. *Circulation* **1993**, *87*, 76–79. [CrossRef]
32. Harle, T.; Luz, M.; Meyer, S.; Kronberg, K.; Nickau, B.; Escaned, J.; Davies, J.; Elsasser, A. Effect of coronary anatomy and hydrostatic pressure on intracoronary indices of stenosis severity. *JACC Cardiovasc. Interv.* **2017**, *10*, 764–773. [CrossRef]

33. Kawaguchi, Y.; Ito, K.; Kin, H.; Shirai, Y.; Okazaki, A.; Miyajima, K.; Watanabe, T.; Tatsuguchi, M.; Wakabayashi, Y.; Maekawa, Y. Impact of hydrostatic pressure variations caused by height differences in supine and prone positions on fractional flow reserve values in the coronary circulation. *J. Interv. Cardiol.* **2019**, *2019*, 4532862. [CrossRef]
34. Nagamatsu, S.; Sakamoto, K.; Yamashita, T.; Sato, R.; Tabata, N.; Motozato, K.; Yamanaga, K.; Ito, M.; Fujisue, K.; Kanazawa, H.; et al. Impact of hydrostatic pressure on fractional flow reserve: In vivo experimental study of anatomical height difference of coronary arteries. *J. Cardiol.* **2020**, *76*, 73–79. [CrossRef]
35. Pirozzolo, G.; Martinez Pereyra, V.; Hubert, A.; Guenther, F.; Sechtem, U.; Bekeredjian, R.; Mahrholdt, H.; Ong, P.; Seitz, A. Coronary artery spasm and impaired myocardial perfusion in patients with ANOCA: Predictors from a multimodality study using stress CMR and acetylcholine testing. *Int. J. Cardiol.* **2021**, *343*, 5–11. [CrossRef]
36. Sugisawa, J.; Matsumoto, Y.; Takeuchi, M.; Suda, A.; Tsuchiya, S.; Ohyama, K.; Nishimiya, K.; Akizuki, M.; Sato, K.; Ohura, S.; et al. Beneficial effects of exercise training on physical performance in patients with vasospastic angina. *Int. J. Cardiol.* **2021**, *328*, 14–21. [CrossRef]
37. Ohyama, K.; Matsumoto, Y.; Takanami, K.; Ota, H.; Nishimiya, K.; Sugisawa, J.; Tsuchiya, S.; Amamizu, H.; Uzuka, H.; Suda, A.; et al. Coronary adventitial and perivascular adipose tissue inflammation in patients with vasospastic angina. *J. Am. Coll. Cardiol.* **2018**, *71*, 414–425. [CrossRef]
38. Akasaka, T.; Yoshida, K.; Hozumi, T.; Takagi, T.; Kawamoto, T.; Kaji, S.; Morioka, S.; Yoshikawa, J. Comparison of coronary flow reserve between focal and diffuse vasoconstriction induced by ergonovine in patients with vasospastic angina. *Am. J. Cardiol.* **1997**, *80*, 705–710. [CrossRef]

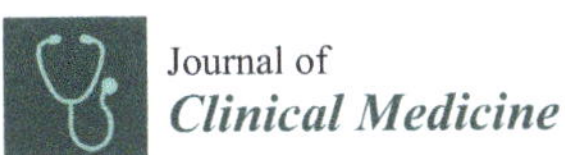
Journal of
Clinical Medicine

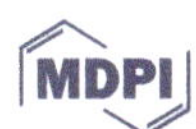

Article

Adjunctive Catheter-Directed Thrombolysis during Primary PCI for ST-Segment Elevation Myocardial Infarction with High Thrombus Burden

Satsuki Noma [1,2], Hideki Miyachi [1,2,*], Isamu Fukuizumi [1,2], Junya Matsuda [1,2], Hideto Sangen [1,2], Yoshiaki Kubota [2], Yoichi Imori [1,2], Yoshiyuki Saiki [1,2], Yusuke Hosokawa [1,2], Shuhei Tara [1,2], Yukichi Tokita [1,2], Koichi Akutsu [1,2], Wataru Shimizu [1,2], Takeshi Yamamoto [1] and Hitoshi Takano [2]

[1] Division of Cardiovascular Intensive Care, Nippon Medical School Hospital, Tokyo 113-8603, Japan; satsuki-n@nms.ac.jp (S.N.); isamu-f@nms.ac.jp (I.F.); jun1984087@nms.ac.jp (J.M.); sangen777@nms.ac.jp (H.S.); s9012@nms.ac.jp (Y.I.); s8043@nms.ac.jp (Y.S.); y-hosokawa@nms.ac.jp (Y.H.); s5062@nms.ac.jp (S.T.); yukichi@nms.ac.jp (Y.T.); koichi-a@nms.ac.jp (K.A.); wshimizu@nms.ac.jp (W.S.); yamamoto56@nms.ac.jp (T.Y.)

[2] Department of Cardiovascular Medicine, Nippon Medical School, Tokyo 113-8603, Japan; ykubota@nms.ac.jp (Y.K.); htakano@nms.ac.jp (H.T.)

* Correspondence: hidep-@nms.ac.jp; Tel.: +81-3-3822-2131

Citation: Noma, S.; Miyachi, H.; Fukuizumi, I.; Matsuda, J.; Sangen, H.; Kubota, Y.; Imori, Y.; Saiki, Y.; Hosokawa, Y.; Tara, S.; et al. Adjunctive Catheter-Directed Thrombolysis during Primary PCI for ST-Segment Elevation Myocardial Infarction with High Thrombus Burden. *J. Clin. Med.* **2022**, *11*, 262. https://doi.org/10.3390/jcm11010262

Academic Editors: Koichi Node

Received: 3 December 2021
Accepted: 31 December 2021
Published: 4 January 2022

Abstract: Background: High coronary thrombus burden has been associated with unfavorable outcomes in patients with ST-segment elevation myocardial infarction (STEMI), the optimal management of which has not yet been established. Methods: We assessed the adjunctive catheter-directed thrombolysis (CDT) during primary percutaneous coronary intervention (PCI) in patients with STEMI and high thrombus burden. CDT was defined as intracoronary infusion of tissue plasminogen activator (t-PA; monteplase). Results: Among the 1849 consecutive patients with STEMI, 263 had high thrombus burden. Moreover, 41 patients received t-PA (CDT group), whereas 222 did not receive it (non-CDT group). No significant differences in bleeding complications and in-hospital and long-term mortalities were observed (9.8% vs. 7.2%, $p = 0.53$; 7.3% vs. 2.3%, $p = 0.11$; and 12.6% vs. 17.5%, $p = 0.84$, CDT vs. non-CDT). In patients who underwent antecedent aspiration thrombectomy during PCI (75.6% CDT group and 87.4% non-CDT group), thrombolysis in myocardial infarction grade 2 or 3 flow rate after thrombectomy was significantly lower in the CDT group than in the non-CDT group (32.2% vs. 61.0%, $p < 0.01$). However, the final rates improved without significant difference (90.3% vs. 97.4%, $p = 0.14$). Conclusions: Adjunctive CDT appears to be tolerated and feasible for high thrombus burden. Particularly, it may be an option in cases with failed aspiration thrombectomy.

Keywords: high coronary thrombus burden; tissue plasminogen activator; catheter-directed thrombolysis

1. Introduction

In patients with ST-segment elevation myocardial infarction (STEMI), the preferred reperfusion regimen is primary percutaneous coronary intervention (PCI) [1,2]. However, even in cases where primary PCI is needed, high thrombus burden presents difficulties. High thrombus burden is associated with distal embolization, the slow-/no-reflow phenomenon, abrupt closure, stent thrombosis, and poor prognosis [3–6]. The therapeutic strategy for STEMI with high thrombus burden includes intracoronary thrombolysis, aspiration thrombectomy, distal embolic protection, excimer laser coronary angioplasty, balloon angioplasty, and stenting. However, interventional cardiologists find it challenging to establish an optimal treatment for high thrombus burden. It has been reported in small case series and studies that intracoronary administration of tissue plasminogen activator (t-PA) reduces coronary thrombus and improves thrombolysis in myocardial infarction (TIMI) flow grade [7,8].

Monteplase (Eisai Co. Ltd, Tokyo, Japan) is a mutant t-PA made by substituting only one amino acid in the epidermal growth factor domain and expressed in baby Syrian hamster kidney cells. It has a half-life of >20 min, which is long compared with the native t-PA half-life of four minutes [9], and it can be administered intravenously by a bolus injection. Kawai et al. reported that a single bolus injection of monteplase produces a higher rate of early recanalization of infarct-related coronary arteries than native t-PA [10]. Moreover, several studies have reported the usefulness of intravenous monteplase before PCI in the treatment of acute myocardial infarction [9,11]. Monteplase is classified as a third-generation thrombolytic drug and an intravenous bolus of 0.22 mg (27.500 IU)/kg of monteplase is equivalent to an intravenous infusion of 100 mg of alteplase and an intravenous bolus of 0.5 mg/kg of tenecteplase [12]. However, t-PA is known to cause paradoxical activation of thrombin, clot formation, and bleeding. Therefore, current guidelines recommend fibrinolytic therapy including t-PA within 12 h of symptom onset if primary PCI cannot be performed within 120 min after the diagnosis of STEMI. A T-time study showed that adjunctive low-dose intracoronary alteplase administered during primary PCI does not reduce microvascular obstruction in patients with STEMI within six hours of symptom onset [13]. However, it is unclear whether catheter-directed thrombolysis (CDT) using intracoronary monteplase during primary PCI constitutes effective treatment for patients with STEMI and high thrombus burden. Thus, the aim of this study was to evaluate the safety and feasibility of adjunctive CDT during primary PCI in patients with STEMI and high thrombus burden and to identify suitable candidates for this therapy.

2. Materials and Methods

2.1. Study Protocol

Between January 2005 and December 2017, 1849 consecutive patients with STEMI were transferred to Nippon Medical School Hospital, Tokyo, Japan. We found that 263 of these patients had high thrombus burden (i.e., an intracoronary thrombus of length >20 mm). Of the 263 patients, 41 were administered adjunctive CDT with intracoronary infusion of t-PA (monteplase) during primary PCI (CDT group) and 222 were not administered the adjunctive therapy during primary PCI (non-CDT group). The diagnosis of STEMI was based on findings of characteristic symptoms of myocardial ischemia, electrocardiographic change (ST-segment elevation in at least two contiguous leads and new-onset complete left bundle branch block), and subsequent release of biomarkers of myocardial necrosis [2]. Following STEMI diagnosis and provision of informed consent, all patients underwent primary PCI according to guideline-based practices with the early use of concomitant antiplatelet and anticoagulant medications. Antiplatelet therapy consisted of aspirin and a thienopyridine derivative (clopidogrel, prasugrel, or ticlopidine). With regard to anticoagulant therapy, intravenous unfractionated heparin (100 U/kg) was administered before primary PCI.

High thrombus burden was defined as the presence of an intracoronary thrombus of length >20 mm that is visible on angiography. If there was complete obstruction of an infarct-related artery by an angiographic thrombus, high thrombus burden was evaluated after minimal coronary flow was recovered after wire cross, aspiration thrombectomy, or balloon angioplasty. In our criteria, high thrombus burden corresponded to TIMI thrombus grades 4 (i.e., definite thrombus with the largest dimension $\geq$2 vessel diameters) and 5 (i.e., total occlusion) [14].

The PCI strategy depended on individual interventional cardiologists, and CDT was performed according to their judgements. However, in our hospital, the basic treatment protocol for STEMI patients with high thrombus burden is defined as follows (Figure 1). The final goal of the primary PCI is coronary reperfusion and not complete removal of the thrombus. First of all, aspiration thrombectomy is often performed for the reduction in thrombus volume in cases where coronary flow can be occluded even after wire crossing, when it is limited to STEMI patients with high thrombus burden. Balloon dilation may be preferred in cases where coronary flow can be resumed just by wire crossing. If successful distal flow is obtained, PCI may be completed without stent implantation. If distal flow is unsuccessful, thrombus aspiration and balloon dilation are repeatedly performed. If necessary, stents may also be implanted with distal embolic protection. If coronary flow is still inadequate even after repeated balloon dilatation and/or aspiration thrombectomy, intracoronary injection of nitroprusside/nicorandil and/or CDT are added, or intra-aortic balloon pump (IABP) is inserted. In this study, we focused the adjunctive CDT during primary PCI.

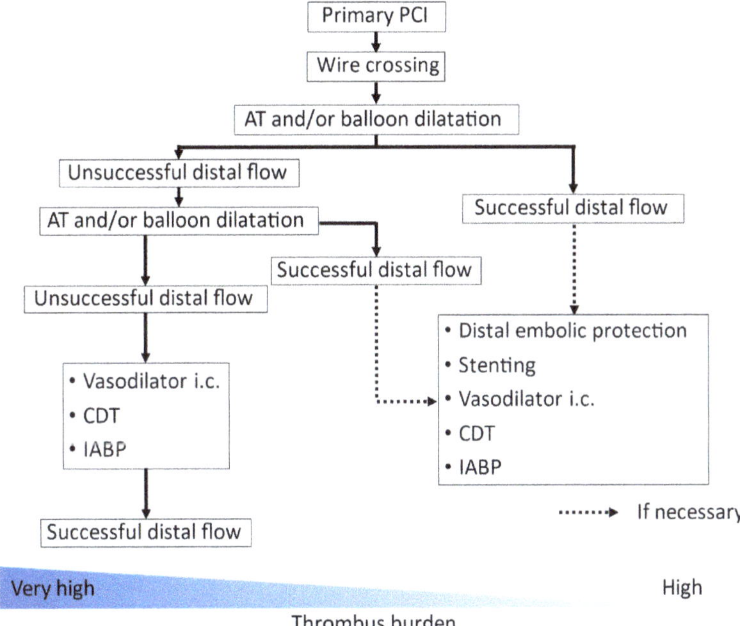

Figure 1. Basic protocol of primary PCI for STEMI patients with high thrombus burden. PCI, percutaneous coronary intervention; AT, aspiration thrombectomoy; CDT, catheter-directed thrombolysis; IABP, intra-aortic balloon pump.

The following data were collected and compared between the two groups: medical history, coronary risk factors, clinical characteristics, coronary angiographic findings, therapeutic strategies, PCI procedures, bleeding complications, in-hospital mortality, long-term mortality, major adverse cardiac events (MACEs), TIMI flow grades, myocardial blush grade, and corrected TIMI frame count. MACE was defined as all causes of death, reinfarction, and ischemia-driven target vessel revascularization. TIMI flow grade and corrected TIMI frame count (cTFC) were measured as the assessment of coronary flow [15,16]. Myocardial blush grade was measured as the parameter of myocardial reperfusion after PCI [17]. Data on bleeding complication as defined using TIMI bleeding criteria were collected [18]. TIMI major bleeding was defined as bleeding leading to death, intracranial bleeding, or a decrease in hemoglobin level greater than 5 g/dL from the baseline. TIMI minor bleeding was defined as spontaneous and observed blood loss with a decrease in hemoglobin level greater than 3 g/dL, but less than 5 g/dL from baseline or unobserved blood loss with a decrease in hemoglobin level greater than 4 g/dL but less than 5 g/dL from baseline [19]. We assessed TIMI bleeding criteria as the safety and in-hospital and long-term mortalities and long-term MACE as the feasibility of CDT. TIMI flow grade, cTFC, and myocardial blush grade were assessed as the efficacy of additional CDT.

2.2. Statistical Analysis

All continuous variables are presented as means and standard deviations. Categorical variables are presented as numbers or percentages. Categorical variables were tested using the Chi-square test or Fisher's exact test. Continuous variables were tested using Student's *t*-test or the Mann–Whitney U test. To evaluate MACE and long-term mortality, we compared the Kaplan–Meier curve using the log-rank test. Propensity score matching analysis was performed to assess the association between t-PA and outcomes to balance for risk factors. A propensity score for t-PA was generated based on a multivariable logistic regression model using the following variables: age, sex, body mass index, Killip class, hypertension, dyslipidemia, diabetes mellitus, and smoking. Propensity score matching was conducted using 4-digit nearest neighbor matching with a 0.20 caliper and a 1:1 match ratio. Values of $p < 0.05$ were considered to be statistically significant. All statistical analyses were performed using IBM SPSS statistics 26 (IBM Corporation, Armonk, NY, USA).

3. Results

3.1. Study Population

Data on the baseline characteristics of the CDT and non-CDT groups are shown in Table 1. The CDT group had a higher percentage of men and a lower mean age than the non-CDT group. There were no significant differences in blood pressure, heart rate, maximum creatine kinase level, and maximum creatine kinase-MB level between the two groups. The usage rates of aspirin, thienopyridine derivatives, and unfractionated heparin were similar between the two groups. A similarly high proportion of patients in both groups had coronary risk factors.

Table 1. Patients' clinical characteristics.

	CDT Group (*n* = 41)	**Non-CDT Group (*n* = 222)**	***p* Value**
Age (years)	59.4 ± 12.8	66.9 ± 13.0	<0.01
Male (%)	92.7	73.0	<0.01
BMI (kg/m^2)	25.1 ± 4.8	24.2 ± 3.8	0.20
Systolic BP (mmHg)	118.5 ± 32.9	120.3 ± 31.2	0.77
Diastolic BP (mmHg)	68.6 ± 20.4	68.9 ± 19.7	0.94
HR (beats/min)	76.1 ± 23.4	77.4 ± 20.5	0.77
EF (%)	57.6 ± 7.6	49.4 ± 12.6	0.06
Creatine kinase (CK)			
Max CK (IU/L)	3467 ± 2999	3314 ± 2649	0.74
Max CKMb (IU/L)	294 ± 308	311 ± 3250.72	
Cardiovascular history			
MI (%)	17.1	13.2	0.55
PCI (%)	8.6	14.7	0.42
CABG surgery (%)	2.9	1.5	0.50
Heart failure (%)	2.9	1.5	0.50
Cerebral infarction (%)	11.4	10.3	0.77
Hemodialysis (%)	0.0	1.5	1.00
PAD (%)	2.9	1.5	0.50

Table 1. *Cont.*

	CDT Group (*n* = 41)	Non-CDT Group (*n* = 222)	*p* Value
Coronary risk factor			
Hypertension (%)	58.5	74.8	0.03
Dyslipidemia (%)	53.7	56.8	0.71
Diabetes mellitus (%)	24.4	31.1	0.39
Smoking (%)	63.4	62.2	0.88
Hyperuricemia (%)	19.8	19.5	0.46
Killip classification			
Class 1 (%)	70.7	74.3	0.85
Class 2 (%)	14.6	10.8	
Class 3 (%)	4.9	6.8	
Class 4 (%)	9.8	8.1	
Medication before primary PCI			
Aspirin (%)	100	97.3	0.59
Thienopyridine (%)	97.6	97.3	1.00
Ticlopidine (%)	36.6	14.4	<0.01
Clopidogrel (%)	48.8	59.5	0.27
Prasugrel (%)	12.2	23.4	0.15
Unfractionated heparin	97.6	100	0.16

CDT, catheter-directed thrombolysis; BMI, body mass index; BP, blood pressure; HR, heart rate; EF, ejection fraction; CK, creatine kinase; MI, myocardial infarction; PCI, percutaneous coronary intervention; CABG, coronary artery bypass grafting; PAD, peripheral artery disease.

3.2. Angiographic Findings, Procedural Data, Outcomes, and Complications

Data on angiographic findings, PCI technical procedures, and TIMI flow grade before and after PCI are shown in Table 2. About 68% of culprit lesions in the CDT group and 57.2% of the culprit lesions in the non-CDT group were found in the right coronary artery (RCA). With regard to PCI procedures, a significantly higher contrast medium volume was used in the CDT group than in the non-CDT group (219.0 ± 56.9 mL vs. 182.1 ± 64.0 mL, $p = 0.02$). Radiation time was significantly longer in the CDT group than in the non-CDT group (45.0 ± 26.4 min vs. 35.3 ± 21.8 min, $p = 0.02$). As described in the Materials and Methods, PCI was performed according to each interventional cardiologist's judgement, however, PCI strategy was based on the basic protocol. Aspiration thrombectomy was performed in over 90% of patients in both groups. The majority of patients in both groups underwent balloon dilatation (80.5% vs. 73.9%, $p = 0.48$). There were no significant differences in the use of distal protection devices (19.5% vs. 21.6%, $p = 0.76$). Significantly fewer stents were used in the CDT group than in the non-CDT group (58.5% vs. 96.8%, $p < 0.01$). There were no significant differences on intracoronary administration of nitroprusside or nicorandil (24.4% vs. 15.8%, $p = 0.18$). The use frequency of IABP was significantly higher in the CDT group than in the non-CDT group (41.5% vs. 21.2%, $p < 0.01$). In this manner, patients in the CDT group tended to require more procedures than non-CDT group. However, in those patients, stent implantation was avoided because of the risk of distal embolization and in-stent thrombus protrusion due to residual thrombus.

Table 2. Angiographic findings, PCI procedures, and outcomes.

	CDT Group (n = 41)	Non-CDT Group (n = 222)	p Value
Culprit lesion			
RCA (%)	68.3	57.2	0.47
LAD (%)	24.4	35.1	
LCX (%)	7.3	6.3	
LMT (%)	0.0	1.3	
PCI procedure			
Onset-to-PCI time (min)	235 (IQR 138–698)	260 (IQR 137–575)	0.90
Devices			
Aspiration thrombectomy (%)	90.2	93.2	0.50
Balloon dilatation (%)	80.5	73.9	0.48
Distal protection (%)	19.5	21.6	0.76
Stent (%)	58.5	96.8	<0.01
Vasodilator i.c. (%)*	24.4	15.8	0.18
IABP (%)	41.5	21.2	<0.01
Contrast medium			
Dose (mL)	219.0 ± 56.9	182.1 ± 64.0	0.02
Radiation time (min)	45.0 ± 26.4	35.3 ± 21.8	0.02
TIMI flow grade before PCI			
0 (%)	92.7	89.6	0.68
1 (%)	4.9	5.4	
2 (%)	0.0	3.6	
3 (%)	2.4	1.4	
Final TIMI flow grade			
0 (%)	9.7	0.0	<0.01
1 (%)	7.3	1.8	
2 (%)	31.7	1.3	
3 (%)	51.2	96.9	
Final myocardial blush grade			
0 (%)	19.5	10.4	<0.01
1 (%)	17.1	8.6	
2 (%)	36.6	26.1	
3 (%)	26.8	55.0	
cTFC before PCI	96.7 ± 15.0	97.5 ± 11.7	0.74
cTFC after PCI	53.7 ± 29.4	33.4 ± 18.2	<0.01
Outcomes			
In-hospital mortality (%)	7.3	2.3	0.11
Long-term mortality (%)	12.6	17.5	0.84

Table 2. *Cont.*

	CDT Group (n = 41)	Non-CDT Group (n = 222)	p Value
Bleeding complications			
TIMI major bleeding (%)	4.9	0.9	0.11
TIMI minor bleeding (%)	9.8	7.2	0.53

PCI, percutaneous coronary intervention; IQR, interquartile range; RCA, right coronary artery; LAD, left anterior descending artery; LCX, left circumflex; LMT, left main trunk; IABP, intra-aortic balloon pump; Vasodilator*, Nitroprusside or Nicorandil; i.c., intra-coronary; TIMI, thrombolysis in myocardial infarction.

Regarding the invasive therapeutic strategy, when coronary flow did not improve sufficiently after various invasive procedures, adjunctive CDT was performed. To definitely inject monteplase into the coronary artery, intracoronary monteplase was administered using a guiding catheter (n = 24) and other catheters such as microcatheters and aspiration catheters (Lumine infusion catheter: n = 11; Thrombuster II or III: n = 5; Rebirth: n = 2; Eliminate: n = 1; Pronto V3: n = 1; ST01: n = 1) (Table 3). The mean dose was 702,439 ± 519,850 U. Each dose is shown in Figure 2, which was used within the insurance coverage. Monteplase was initially injected as a single bolus (400,000 IU) and added with each additional bolus.

Table 3. t-PA intracoronary administration catheter.

Catheter	n
Guiding catheter	24
Lumine infusion catheter®, Gadelius Medical K.K., Tokyo, Japan	11
Thrombuster II or III®, Kaneka Medix Co., Tokyo, Japan	5
Rebirth®, Nipro Co., Osaka, Japan	2
Eliminate®, Terumo Co., Tokyo, Japan	1
Pronto V3®, Teleflex, Wayne, PA, USA	1
ST01®, Terumo Co., Tokyo, Japan	1

t-PA, tissue plasminogen activator.

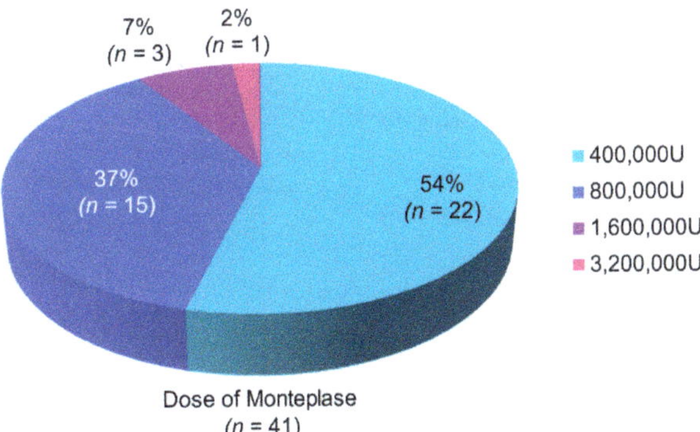

Figure 2. Dose of monteplase administered and proportion of patients.

The TIMI major and minor bleeding rates were not significantly different between the two groups (Table 2). In-hospital mortality was also similar between the two groups (7.3% versus 2.3%, p = 0.11) (Table 2), and there was no significant difference in the cumulative mortality rate between both groups (12.6% versus 17.5%, log-rank p = 0.84) (Figure 3A).

Furthermore, there was no significant difference in MACEs between the two groups (19.9% versus 20.5%, log-rank $p = 0.55$) (Figure 3B).

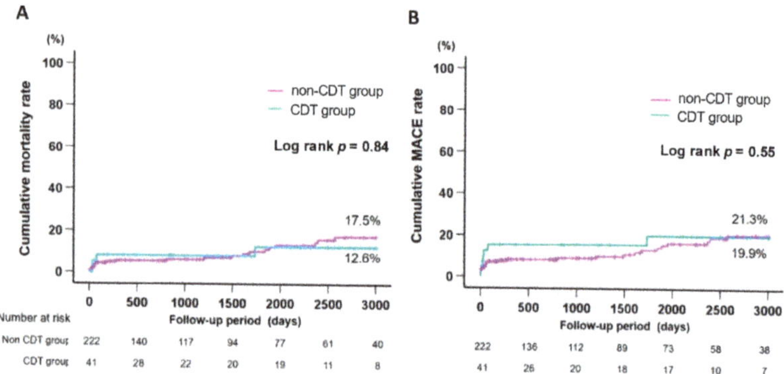

Figure 3. Cumulative mortality rates (**A**) and MACE rates (**B**) in the CDT and non-CDT groups. Kaplan–Meier curves for cumulative mortality rate and MACE (death, reinfarction, or ischemia-driven target vessel revascularization) rate are shown in Figure 3A and 3B, respectively. CDT, catheter-directed thrombolysis; MACE, major adverse cardiac event.

As shown in Table 2, approximately 90% of patients in both groups had TIMI grade 0 flow before PCI. After PCI, the proportion of patients with TIMI grade ≥2 flow increased from 5.0% to 98.2% in the non-CDT group and from 2.4% to 82.9% in the CDT group. Moreover, there was a significant difference in the distribution of TIMI flow grade after PCI between the two groups ($p < 0.01$). Myocardial blush grade distribution also differed significantly between both groups. Final myocardial blush grade 3 accounted for 55.0% and 26.8% in the non-CDT and CDT groups, respectively. The mean value of cTFC before PCI was high and not different significantly between both groups. The mean value of cTFC decreased after PCI, however, it was higher in the CDT group than in the non-CDT group. Despite adjunctive CDT, coronary flow did not recover as well as those in the non-CDT group.

3.3. *Propensity Score Matching Analysis*

Propensity score matching analysis was conducted in selected patients with similar characteristics and comorbidities within each group. After propensity score matching, 74 patients (37 in each group) were included. Baseline patient characteristics and medications of the matched groups are shown in Table 4. Both groups matched well for clinical variables. Even after propensity score matching analysis, in-hospital mortality, major bleeding, and minor bleeding did not differ significantly between both groups (8.1% vs. 5.4%, $p = 1.00$; 5.4% vs. 5.4%, $p = 1.00$; and 10.8% vs. 8.1%, $p = 1.00$, respectively). The Kaplan–Meier curves for cumulative mortality rates and MACEs revealed no differences between the CDT and non-CDT group (13.7% vs. 27.5%, log-rank $p = 0.58$, 21.7% vs. 30.9%, log-rank $p = 0.90$, respectively) (Figure 4).

Table 4. Patients' clinical characteristics and outcomes after propensity score matching.

	CDT Group ($n = 37$)	Non-CDT Group ($n = 37$)	p Value
Age (years)	61.0 ± 12.2	63.2 ± 12.0	0.45
Male (%)	94.6	91.9	1.00
BMI (kg/m^2)	24.6 ± 4.8	24.4 ± 3.7	0.83
Systolic BP (mmHg)	124.6 ± 23.7	127.1 ± 28.0	0.68

Table 4. *Cont.*

	CDT Group (n = 37)	Non-CDT Group (n = 37)	p Value
Diastolic BP (mmHg)	73.4 ± 15.4	72.4 ± 18.6	0.81
HR (beats/min)	77.8 ± 19.4	81.7 ± 19.6	0.40
EF (%)	51.9 ± 12.2	49.9 ± 13.0	0.52
Creatine kinase (CK)			
Max CK (IU/L)	3271 ± 2840	3307 ± 2259	0.95
Max CKMb (IU/L)	295 ± 217	285 ± 181	0.82
Cardiovascular history			
MI (%)	13.5	13.5	1.00
PCI (%)	2.7	18.9	0.06
CABG surgery (%)	5.4	0.0	0.49
Heart failure (%)	2.7	5.4	1.00
Cerebral infarction (%)	10.8	10.8	1.00
Hemodialysis (%)	0.0	0.0	
PAD (%)	2.7	0.0	1.00
Coronary risk factor			
Hypertension (%)	64.9	67.6	1.00
Dyslipidemia (%)	54.1	45.9	0.64
Diabetes mellitus (%)	27.0	35.1	0.62
Smoking (%)	70.3	64.9	0.80
Killip classification			
Class 1 (%)	73.0	70.3	0.49
Class 2 (%)	13.5	5.4	
Class 3 (%)	5.4	18.9	
Class 4 (%)	8.1	5.4	
Final TIMI flow grade			
0 (%)	10.8	0.0	<0.01
1 (%)	8.1	5.4	
2 (%)	27.0	13.5	
3 (%)	54.1	81.1	
Final Myocardial blush grade			
0 (%)	18.9	24.3	0.08
1 (%)	13.5	8.1	
2 (%)	37.8	16.2	
3 (%)	29.7	51.4	
cTFC before PCI	96.3 ± 15.8	96.5 ± 12.7	0.96
cTFC after PCI	53.4 ± 30.6	37.3 ± 21.2	0.01
Outcomes			
In-hospital mortality (%)	8.1	5.4	1.00

Table 4. *Cont.*

	CDT Group (*n* = 37)	Non-CDT Group (*n* = 37)	*p* Value
Bleeding complications			
TIMI major bleeding (%)	5.4	5.4	1.00
TIMI minor bleeding (%)	10.8	8.1	1.00

CDT, catheter-directed thrombolysis; BMI, body mass index; BP, blood pressure; HR, heart rate; EF, ejection fraction; CK, creatine kinase; MI, myocardial infarction; PCI, percutaneous coronary intervention; CABG, coronary artery bypass grafting; PAD, peripheral artery disease; TIMI, thrombolysis in myocardial infarction; cTFC, corrected TIMI frame count.

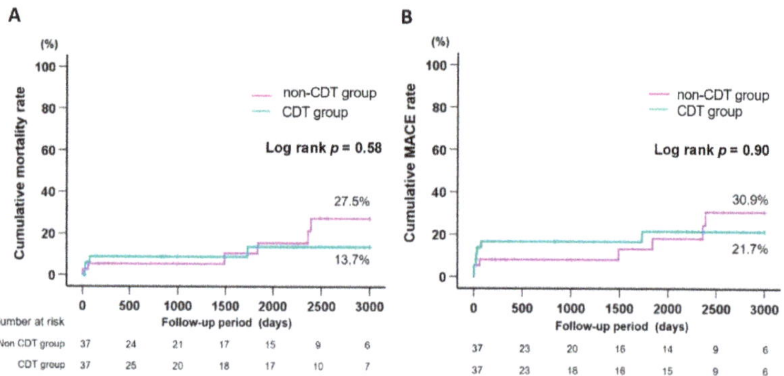

Figure 4. Cumulative mortality rates (**A**) and MACE rates (**B**) after propensity score matching. After propensity score matching, Kaplan–Meier curves for cumulative mortality rate and MACE (death, reinfarction, or ischemia-driven target vessel revascularization) rate are shown in Figure 4A and 4B, respectively. CDT, catheter-directed thrombolysis; MACE, major adverse cardiac event.

3.4. Antecedent Aspiration Thrombectomy Cases

As described before, aspiration thrombectomy was initially performed to remove high thrombus burden in a number of patients (CDT group: n = 31 (75.6%); non-CDT group: n = 194 (87.4%)). Subsequently, several therapeutic procedures such as balloon dilatation, distal embolic protection, stenting, intracoronary vasodilator infusion, IABP, and CDT were performed, if necessary. Therefore, we also analyzed antecedent aspiration thrombectomy cases. In most patients in the CDT group, TIMI flow grade did not improve substantially after aspiration thrombectomy. TIMI flow increased to grades 2 or 3 after aspiration thrombectomy in only 32.2% of patients in the CDT group (Figure 5). Thereafter, intracoronary t-PA administration and other procedures were added. As a result, most patients (90.3%) finally had TIMI grade 2 or 3 flow. In contrast, in the non-CDT group, initial aspiration thrombectomy drastically improved TIMI flow grade (TIMI grade 2 or 3 flow: from 4.6% to 60.8%). Finally, TIMI grade 2 or 3 flow was achieved in 96.9% of patients in the non-CDT group, and this was not significantly different compared with that in the CDT group (p = 0.14).

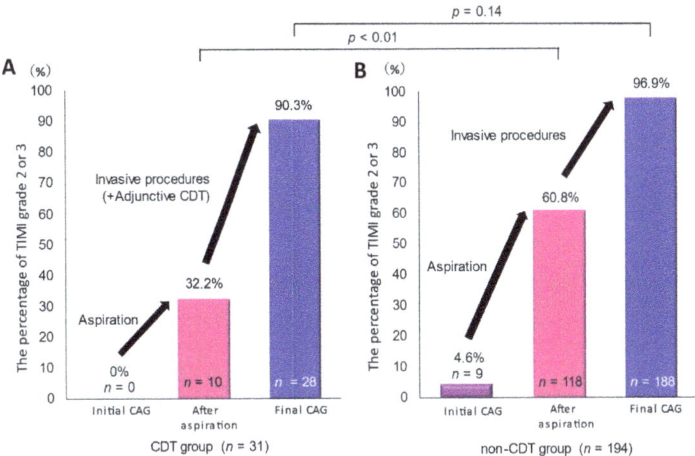

Figure 5. Change of TIMI grade 2 or 3 flow in antecedent aspiration thrombectomy cases. We performed subgroup analysis of antecedent aspiration thrombectomy cases (CDT group: $n = 31$; non-CDT group: $n = 194$). (**A**,**B**) show the rate of TIMI grade 2 or 3 flow during PCI in the CDT group and the non-CDT group, respectively. TIMI, thrombolysis in myocardial infarction; CDT, catheter-directed thrombolysis; IABP, intra-aortic balloon pump.

On the other hand, cTFC distributions were quite different between both groups (Figure 6). At the initial CAG, cTFCs were 100 in most cases within both groups, and no significant differences between both groups were observed ($p = 0.70$). After aspiration thrombectomy, mean cTFC in the non-CDT group drastically decreased and was significantly lower than that in the CDT group ($p < 0.01$). The final median cTFC in the CDT group also decreased, although it remained higher than that in the non-CDT group ($p < 0.01$). Additionally, the final cTFC in the CDT group was more widely distributed than that in the non-CDT group.

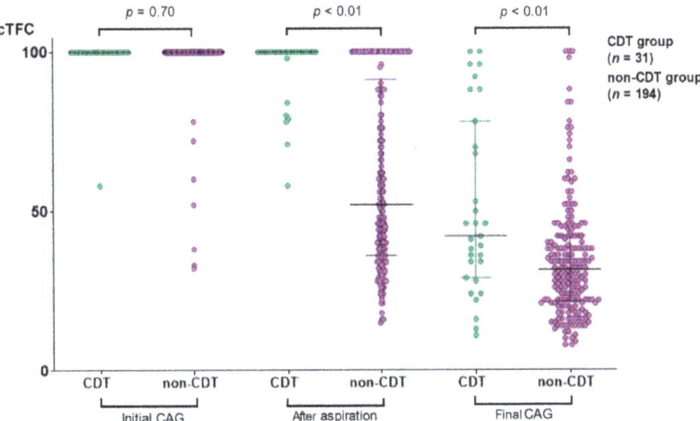

Figure 6. Change in corrected TIMI frame count in antecedent aspiration thrombectomy cases. In antecedent aspiration thrombectomy cases (CDT group: $n = 31$; non-CDT group: $n = 194$), Figure 6 shows the distribution of cTFC at the initial CAG, after aspiration, and final CAG. TIMI, thrombolysis in myocardial infarction; CDT, catheter-directed thrombolysis; CTFC, corrected TIMI frame count; CAG, coronary arteriography; IQR, interquartile range.

3.5. Clinical Characteristics of Patients in the CDT Group with Final TIMI Flow Grade 0 or 1

Despite intracoronary t-PA administration, the final TIMI flow grade of six patients with STEMI and high thrombus burden did not improve but remained at grade 0 or 1. The clinical characteristics of these six patients are shown in Table 5. All patients were men, and half of the infarct-related lesions were distal branch lesions (#4AV lesions in two patients and a #14 lesion in one patient). Four patients had plaque rupture lesions, and two patients had embolism. One patient died due to ventricular septal perforation (patient 5). An RCA #3 lesion with TIMI flow grade 0 was the culprit lesion. Due to the severely tortuous nature of the RCA, devices could not be passed across the lesion. Therefore, the interventional cardiologist administered an intracoronary t-PA injection.

Table 5. Clinical characteristics in STEMI patients with final TIMI 0 or 1 in the CDT group.

Case	Age (y.o)	Sex	IRL	Prior MI	Killip	Lesion Characteristics	The Reason of t-PA Administration	Other Therapeutic Strategies	Initial TIMI Grade	Death
1	71	M	LAD (#7)	-	3	Embolism	Unsuccessful thrombectomy	Thrombectomy IABP	1	-
2	70	M	RCA (4AV)	-	1	Embolism	Peripheral lesion unsuitable for PCI	-	0	-
3	67	M	LCX (#14)	-	1	Plaque rupture	Acute stent thrombosis	Thrombectomy stenting	0	-
4	58	M	RCA (4AV)	+	2	Plaque rupture	Guide-wire induced coronary dissection	Thrombectomy	1	-
5	70	M	RCA (#3)	-	3	Plaque rupture	Devices were undelivered. (severe tortuous)	IABP	0	+ (VSR)
6	59	M	RCA (#2)	-	1	Plaque rupture	Unsuccessful thrombectomy	Thrombectomy IABP stenting Nitroprusside i.c.	0	-

STEMI, ST-elevation myocardial infarction; t-PA, tissue plasminogen activator; TIMI, thrombolysis in myocardial infarction; IRL, infarct-related lesion; LAD, left anterior descending; RCA, right coronary artery; PCI, percuraneous coronary intervention; LCX, left circumflex; IABP, intra-aortic balloon pump; VSR, Ventricular septal rupture; i.c., Intra-coronary.

4. Discussion

This study revealed several important findings. First, adjunctive CDT during primary PCI for patients with STEMI and high thrombus burden resulted in favorable outcomes. Although the outcomes including in-hospital and long-term mortalities and long-term MACE were not superior to those of patients who did not require adjunctive CDT, it should be considered that adjunctive CDT was performed in refractory patients that coronary flow did not improve even after various invasive procedures. Next, adjunctive CDT improved coronary flow, however, the final coronary flow after adjunctive CDT evaluated by TIMI flow grade and cTFC were inferior to those of patients who did not require adjunctive CDT. Third, limited to patients who underwent antecedent aspiration thrombectomy according to our therapeutic strategy, those in the CDT group had poorer coronary flow after thrombectomy compared to those in the non-CDT group. However, the final coronary flow dramatically improved, and the TIMI flow grade 2 or 3 rate was similar between both groups. This study showed that adjunctive CDT may be an option in selected cases such as patients with failed aspiration thrombectomy.

Historically, urokinase, streptokinase, and t-PA have been used as thrombolysis options. In a previous study in which intracoronary urokinase was administered after thrombus development during PCI, there was no reported in-hospital death, but 10% of the patients required blood transfusions [20]. The results of the Thrombolysis and Angioplasty in Unstable Angina study and those of several other studies show that the effectiveness of intracoronary urokinase in the treatment of stable and unstable anginas is largely discouraging [21–23]. In the Intracoronary t-PA Registry, the bleeding complication rate of thrombolysis was shown to be high (9.2%) [24]. As a result, intracoronary thrombolysis is rarely used in clinical practice. Furthermore, there have been advancements in device technologies and pharmacology such as aspiration thrombectomy, distal protection devices, dual antiplatelet therapy, and glycoprotein IIb/IIIa inhibitors [25,26].

Conversely, several other studies support the usefulness of intracoronary thrombolysis in select cases [7,24,27,28]. It was reported in some case reports that adjunctive CDT during PCI is useful as a therapeutic strategy for high thrombus burden [29–32]. In particular, two case reports showed that post-intracoronary thrombolytic therapy is a good option for patients who previously underwent failed thrombectomy during primary PCI [30,31]. These case findings are consistent with the results of our study. In our study, adjunctive CDT was administered to patients whose coronary flow could not be improved using aspiration thrombectomy. Post-procedurally, the adjunctive CDT strategy led to favorable outcomes, and final coronary flow was almost similar to those of the non-CDT strategy. Therefore, adjunctive CDT may be an option for cases of high thrombus burden in which coronary flow does not improve after aspiration thrombectomy.

Recent studies have revealed the unusefulness of intracoronary thrombolysis in microvascular obstruction due to distal embolization of the thrombus [13,33,34]. Although the current study showed that intracoronary thrombolysis improved the coronary flow, a few cases still had slow flow or no reflow. In such cases, poor coronary flow may be attributed to microvascular obstruction due to distal embolism from proximal high thrombus burden. Moreover, adjunctive CDT has some safety concerns such as bleeding complications. However, previous studies have shown that low-dose intracoronary t-PA administration did not increase the bleeding risk [13,33]. The current study also found no significant difference in bleeding complication between both groups, and mean dose of monteplase in this study corresponded to the low dose in previous studies. However, the rates of bleeding complications were higher in the CDT group than in the non-CDT group, and the number of patients was so small in this study. Thus, further research is required to address concerns over bleeding complications.

The clinical characteristics of patients in the CDT group with final TIMI grade 0 or 1 flow are shown in Table 4. RCA and/or distal lesions accounted for four of six (66%) cases of infarct-related lesions. Thus, even with adjunctive CDT, it may be difficult to obtain good TIMI flow in the case of an RCA lesion with high thrombus burden at the distal branch. To prevent the no-reflow phenomenon, it is important to reduce thrombus burden using thrombectomy devices or other means. However, recent large-scale studies and meta-analyses indicated that routine thrombus aspiration during PCI for STEMI increases the risk of stroke and/or transient ischemic attack and does not improve clinical outcomes [35–38]. Therefore, routine thrombus aspiration is not recommended in recent guidelines [2]. However, in a previous study, the subgroup analysis of patients with high thrombus burden (i.e., TIMI thrombus grade $\geq$3) suggested that thrombus aspiration improves cardiovascular mortality [39]. Thus, it seems reasonable that many patients with high thrombus burden initially underwent aspiration thrombectomy in this study. In addition, it was reported in the ASSENT-4 PCI trial that compared with primary PCI, full-dose tenecteplase combined with PCI is associated with an increase in the primary end point of death, congestive heart failure, or shock within 90 days [40]. Thus, adjunctive CDT during PCI should not be routinely recommended but should be limited to patients with STEMI and high thrombus burden, as shown in this study.

Several important limitations of our study should be noted. First, because this study was a retrospective nonrandomized trial with a small sample size that was performed at a single institute, there may be selection bias. In particular, it is noteworthy as a selection bias that additional CDT was performed in selected patients with poor coronary flow after invasive procedures. Additionally, other treatment options such as aspiration thrombectomy, distal embolic protection, IABP, and intracoronary nitroprusside or nicorandil may have contributed to the final patient outcomes. The administration technique for CDT was different and t-PA was performed using a guiding catheter, microcatheter, or aspiration catheter. It was evaluated whether t-PA was effectively delivered to coronary thrombus using any catheter. Second, thrombus burden was higher in this study than in other studies. Previous studies defined high thrombus burden as the presence of accumulated thrombus >3 times the luminal diameter of the infarct-related artery or TIMI thrombus grade >3 [6,41]. In contrast, we defined high thrombus burden as the presence of an intracoronary thrombus of length >20 mm that is visible in the angiography and corresponds to TIMI thrombus grade >4. This difference may underestimate the effectiveness of adjunctive CDT. In contrast, detailed quantitative evaluation of thrombus burden was not performed in this study. Thus, thrombus burden size may be associated with efficacy of adjunctive CDT strategy. Third, because the efficacy of an intravenous bolus injection of abciximab in the prevention of post-PCI coronary events in Japanese patients has not been confirmed [42], the glycoprotein IIb/IIIa receptor antagonist is not available in Japan and was not used in this study. Additionally, the usage rate of the anticoagulation drug was not analyzed in this study; therefore, its effect may be underestimated. Finally, the pathophysiology of STEMI such as plaque rupture, plaque erosion, or calcified nodules was not considered in this study, which may have had an effect on the results. These limitations deserve confirmation in a large randomized controlled trial.

5. Conclusions

Adjunctive CDT during primary PCI is tolerated and feasible for STEMI patients with high thrombus burden. Particularly, it may be a useful therapeutic option in cases of high thrombus burden in which coronary flow cannot be significantly improved using aspiration thrombectomy.

Author Contributions: H.M. and T.Y. designed this study. S.N., I.F., J.M., H.S., Y.K., Y.I., Y.S., Y.H., S.T., Y.T. and K.A. performed the data acquisition. S.N., H.M. and T.Y. analyzed and interpretated the data. S.N. and H.M. performed the statistical analysis. T.Y. was involved in the critical revision of the manuscript. W.S. and H.T. approved the final version prior to submission. All authors have read and agreed to the published version of the manuscript.

Funding: This research received no grant from any funding agency in the public, commercial, or not-for-profit sector.

Institutional Review Board Statement: This study was approved by the Nippon Medical School Hospital Ethics Committee (Reference no. B-2020-242).

Informed Consent Statement: The requirement for informed consent was waived because all data were anonymized.

Data Availability Statement: The data presented in this study are available on request from the corresponding author.

Acknowledgments: The authors thank all those who have been involved with patient care including emergency medical services, technicians, medical engineers, nurses, pharmacists, and physicians at the Nippon Medical School Hospital.

Conflicts of Interest: The authors declare no conflict of interest.

References

1. Steg, P.G.; James, S.K.; Atar, D.; Badano, L.P.; Blomstrom-Lundqvist, C.; Borger, M.A.; Di Mario, C.; Dickstein, K.; Ducrocq, G.; Fernandez-Aviles, F.; et al. ESC Guidelines for the management of acute myocardial infarction in patients presenting with ST-segment elevation. *Eur. Heart J.* **2012**, *33*, 2569–2619. [CrossRef]
2. Ibanez, B.; James, S.; Agewall, S.; Antunes, M.J.; Bucciarelli-Ducci, C.; Bueno, H.; Caforio, A.L.P.; Crea, F.; Goudevenos, J.A.; Halvorsen, S.; et al. 2017 ESC Guidelines for the management of acute myocardial infarction in patients presenting with ST-segment elevation. *Rev. Esp. Cardiol. (Engl. Ed.)* **2017**, *70*, 1082. [CrossRef]
3. Falk, E. Unstable angina with fatal outcome: Dynamic coronary thrombosis leading to infarction and/or sudden death. Autopsy evidence of recurrent mural thrombosis with peripheral embolization culminating in total vascular occlusion. *Circulation* **1985**, *71*, 699–708. [CrossRef]
4. Singh, M.; Reeder, G.S.; Ohman, E.M.; Mathew, V.; Hillegass, W.B.; Anderson, R.D.; Gallup, D.S.; Garratt, K.N.; Holmes, D.R., Jr. Does the presence of thrombus seen on a coronary angiogram affect the outcome after percutaneous coronary angioplasty? An Angiographic Trials Pool data experience. *J. Am. Coll. Cardiol.* **2001**, *38*, 624–630. [CrossRef]
5. Sianos, G.; Papafaklis, M.I.; Daemen, J.; Vaina, S.; van Mieghem, C.A.; van Domburg, R.T.; Michalis, L.K.; Serruys, P.W. Angiographic stent thrombosis after routine use of drug-eluting stents in ST-segment elevation myocardial infarction: The importance of thrombus burden. *J. Am. Coll. Cardiol.* **2007**, *50*, 573–583. [CrossRef]
6. Jolly, S.S.; Cairns, J.A.; Lavi, S.; Cantor, W.J.; Bernat, I.; Cheema, A.N.; Moreno, R.; Kedev, S.; Stankovic, G.; Rao, S.V.; et al. Thrombus Aspiration in Patients with High Thrombus Burden in the TOTAL Trial. *J. Am. Coll. Cardiol.* **2018**, *72*, 1589–1596. [CrossRef]
7. Kelly, R.V.; Crouch, E.; Krumnacher, H.; Cohen, M.G.; Stouffer, G.A. Safety of adjunctive intracoronary thrombolytic therapy during complex percutaneous coronary intervention: Initial experience with intracoronary tenecteplase. *Catheter. Cardiovasc. Interv. Off. J. Soc. Card. Angiogr. Interv.* **2005**, *66*, 327–332. [CrossRef]
8. Saito, T.; Taniguchi, I.; Nakamura, S.; Oka, H.; Mizuno, Y.; Noda, K.; Yamashita, S.; Oshima, S. Pulse-spray thrombolysis in acutely obstructed coronary artery in critical situations. *Catheter. Cardiovasc. Diagn.* **1997**, *40*, 101–108. [CrossRef]
9. Inoue, T.; Yaguchi, I.; Takayanagi, K.; Hayashi, T.; Morooka, S.; Eguchi, Y. A new thrombolytic agent, monteplase, is independent of the plasminogen activator inhibitor in patients with acute myocardial infarction: Initial results of the COmbining Monteplase with Angioplasty (COMA) trial. *Am. Heart J.* **2002**, *144*, E5. [CrossRef]
10. Kawai, C.; Yui, Y.; Hosoda, S.; Nobuyoshi, M.; Suzuki, S.; Sato, H.; Takatsu, F.; Motomiya, T.; Kanmatsuse, K.; Kodama, K.; et al. A Prospective, Randomized, Double-Blind Multicenter Trial of a Single Bolus Injection of the Novel Modified t-PA E6010 in the Treatment of Acute Myocardial Infarction: Comparison with Native t-PA. *J. Am. Coll. Cardiol.* **1997**, *29*, 1447–1453. [CrossRef]
11. Kurihara, H.; Matsumoto, S.; Tamura, R.; Yachiku, K.; Nakata, A.; Nakagawa, T.; Yoshino, T.; Matsuyama, T. Clinical outcome of percutaneous coronary intervention with antecedent mutant t-PA administration for acute myocardial infarction. *Am. Heart J.* **2004**, *147*, E14. [CrossRef]
12. Verstraete, M. Third-generation thrombolytic drugs. *Am. J. Med.* **2000**, *109*, 52–58. [CrossRef]
13. McCartney, P.J.; Eteiba, H.; Maznyczka, A.M.; McEntegart, M.; Greenwood, J.P.; Muir, D.F.; Chowdhary, S.; Gershlick, A.H.; Appleby, C.; Cotton, J.M.; et al. Effect of Low-Dose Intracoronary Alteplase during Primary Percutaneous Coronary Intervention on Microvascular Obstruction in Patients with Acute Myocardial Infarction: A Randomized Clinical Trial. *JAMA* **2019**, *321*, 56–68. [CrossRef]
14. Gibson, C.M.; de Lemos, J.A.; Murphy, S.A.; Marble, S.J.; McCabe, C.H.; Cannon, C.P.; Antman, E.M.; Braunwald, E. Combination therapy with abciximab reduces angiographically evident thrombus in acute myocardial infarction: A TIMI 14 substudy. *Circulation* **2001**, *103*, 2550–2554. [CrossRef]
15. Group, T.S. Comparison of invasive and conservative strategies after treatment with intravenous tissue plasminogen activator in acute myocardial infarction. Results of the thrombolysis in myocardial infarction (TIMI) phase II trial. *N. Engl. J. Med.* **1989**, *320*, 618–627.
16. Gibson, C.M.; Cannon, C.P.; Daley, W.L.; Dodge, J.T., Jr.; Alexander, B., Jr.; Marble, S.J.; McCabe, C.H.; Raymond, L.; Fortin, T.; Poole, W.K.; et al. TIMI frame count: A quantitative method of assessing coronary artery flow. *Circulation* **1996**, *93*, 879–888. [CrossRef]
17. van 't Hof, A.W.; Liem, A.; Suryapranata, H.; Hoorntje, J.C.; de Boer, M.J.; Zijlstra, F. Angiographic assessment of myocardial reperfusion in patients treated with primary angioplasty for acute myocardial infarction: Myocardial blush grade. Zwolle Myocardial Infarction Study Group. *Circulation* **1998**, *97*, 2302–2306. [CrossRef]
18. Chesebro, J.H.; Knatterud, G.; Roberts, R.; Borer, J.; Cohen, L.S.; Dalen, J.; Dodge, H.T.; Francis, C.K.; Hillis, D.; Ludbrook, P.; et al. Thrombolysis in Myocardial Infarction (TIMI) Trial, Phase I: A comparison between intravenous tissue plasminogen activator and intravenous streptokinase. Clinical findings through hospital discharge. *Circulation* **1987**, *76*, 142–154. [CrossRef]
19. Rao, A.K.; Pratt, C.; Berke, A.; Jaffe, A.; Ockene, I.; Schreiber, T.L.; Bell, W.R.; Knatterud, G.; Robertson, T.L.; Terrin, M.L. Thrombolysis in Myocardial Infarction (TIMI) Trial–phase I: Hemorrhagic manifestations and changes in plasma fibrinogen and the fibrinolytic system in patients treated with recombinant tissue plasminogen activator and streptokinase. *J. Am. Coll. Cardiol.* **1988**, *11*, 1–11. [CrossRef]

20. Schieman, G.; Cohen, B.M.; Kozina, J.; Erickson, J.S.; Podolin, R.A.; Peterson, K.L.; Ross, J., Jr.; Buchbinder, M. Intracoronary urokinase for intracoronary thrombus accumulation complicating percutaneous transluminal coronary angioplasty in acute ischemic syndromes. *Circulation* **1990**, *82*, 2052–2060. [CrossRef]
21. Ambrose, J.A.; Almeida, O.D.; Sharma, S.K.; Torre, S.R.; Marmur, J.D.; Israel, D.H.; Ratner, D.E.; Weiss, M.B.; Hjemdahl-Monsen, C.E.; Myler, R.K.; et al. Adjunctive thrombolytic therapy during angioplasty for ischemic rest angina. Results of the TAUSA Trial. TAUSA Investigators. Thrombolysis and Angioplasty in Unstable Angina trial. *Circulation* **1994**, *90*, 69–77. [CrossRef]
22. DiSciascio, G.; Kohli, R.S.; Goudreau, E.; Sabri, N.; Vetrovec, G.W. Intracoronary recombinant tissue-type plasminogen activator in unstable angina: A pilot angiographic study. *Am. Heart J.* **1991**, *122 Pt 1*, 1–6. [CrossRef]
23. Goudreau, E.; DiSciascio, G.; Vetrovec, G.W.; Chami, Y.; Kohli, R.; Warner, M.; Sabri, N.; Cowley, M.J. Intracoronary urokinase as an adjunct to percutaneous transluminal coronary angioplasty in patients with complex coronary narrowings or angioplasty-induced complications. *Am. J. Cardiol.* **1992**, *69*, 57–62. [CrossRef]
24. Ferguson, J.J. Clinical experience with intracoronary tissue plasminogen activator: Results of a multicenter registry. Intracoronary t-PA Registry Investigators. *Catheter. Cardiovasc. Diagn.* **1995**, *34*, 196–201. [CrossRef]
25. Svilaas, T.; Vlaar, P.J.; van der Horst, I.C.; Diercks, G.F.; de Smet, B.J.; van den Heuvel, A.F.; Anthonio, R.L.; Jessurun, G.A.; Tan, E.S.; Suurmeijer, A.J.; et al. Thrombus aspiration during primary percutaneous coronary intervention. *N. Engl. J. Med.* **2008**, *358*, 557–567. [CrossRef]
26. Dangas, G.; Stone, G.W.; Weinberg, M.D.; Webb, J.; Cox, D.A.; Brodie, B.R.; Krucoff, M.W.; Gibbons, R.J.; Lansky, A.J.; Mehran, R. Contemporary outcomes of rescue percutaneous coronary intervention for acute myocardial infarction: Comparison with primary angioplasty and the role of distal protection devices (EMERALD trial). *Am. Heart J.* **2008**, *155*, 1090–1096. [CrossRef]
27. Gurbel, P.A.; Navetta, F.I.; Bates, E.R.; Muller, D.W.; Tenaglia, A.N.; Miller, M.J.; Muhlstein, B.; Hermiller, J.B.; Davidson, C.J.; Aguirre, F.V.; et al. Lesion-directed administration of alteplase with intracoronary heparin in patients with unstable angina and coronary thrombus undergoing angioplasty. *Catheter. Cardiovasc. Diagn.* **1996**, *37*, 382–391. [CrossRef]
28. Barua, S.; Geenty, P.; Deshmukh, T.; Ada, C.; Tanous, D.; Cooper, M.; Fahmy, P.; Denniss, A.R. The role of intracoronary thrombolysis in selected patients presenting with ST-elevation myocardial infarction: A case series. *Eur. Heart J. Case Rep.* **2020**, *4*, 1–10. [CrossRef]
29. Agarwal, S.K. Pharmacoinvasive therapy for acute myocardial infarction. *Catheter. Cardiovasc. Interv. Off. J. Soc. Card. Angiogr. Interv.* **2011**, *78*, 72–75. [CrossRef]
30. Gallagher, S.; Jain, A.K.; Archbold, R.A. Intracoronary thrombolytic therapy: A treatment option for failed mechanical thrombectomy. *Catheter. Cardiovasc. Interv. Off. J. Soc. Card. Angiogr. Interv.* **2012**, *80*, 835–837. [CrossRef]
31. Higashi, H.; Inaba, S.; Nishimura, K.; Hamagami, T.; Fujita, Y.; Ogimoto, A.; Okayama, H.; Higaki, J. Usefulness of adjunctive pulse infusion thrombolysis after failed aspiration for massive intracoronary thrombus. *Can. J. Cardiol.* **2011**, *27*, 869.e1–869.e2. [CrossRef]
32. Kim, J.S.; Kim, J.H.; Jang, H.H.; Lee, Y.W.; Song, S.G.; Park, J.H.; Chun, K.J. Successful revascularization of coronary artery occluded by massive intracoronary thrombi with alteplase and percutaneous coronary intervention. *J. Atheroscler. Thromb.* **2010**, *17*, 768–770. [CrossRef]
33. Gibson, C.M.; Kumar, V.; Gopalakrishnan, L.; Singh, P.; Guo, J.; Kazziha, S.; Devireddy, C.; Pinto, D.; Marshall, J.J.; Stouffer, G.A.; et al. Feasibility and Safety of Low-Dose Intra-Coronary Tenecteplase during Primary Percutaneous Coronary Intervention for ST-Elevation Myocardial Infarction (ICE T-TIMI 49). *Am. J. Cardiol.* **2020**, *125*, 485–490. [CrossRef]
34. Alyamani, M.; Campbell, S.; Navarese, E.; Welsh, R.C.; Bainey, K.R. Safety and Efficacy of Intracoronary Thrombolysis as Adjunctive Therapy to Primary PCI in STEMI: A Systematic Review and Meta-Analysis. *Can. J. Cardiol.* **2021**, *37*, 339–346. [CrossRef]
35. Frobert, O.; Lagerqvist, B.; Olivecrona, G.K.; Omerovic, E.; Gudnason, T.; Maeng, M.; Aasa, M.; Angeras, O.; Calais, F.; Danielewicz, M.; et al. Thrombus aspiration during ST-segment elevation myocardial infarction. *N. Engl. J. Med.* **2013**, *369*, 1587–1597. [CrossRef]
36. Jolly, S.S.; Cairns, J.A.; Yusuf, S.; Meeks, B.; Pogue, J.; Rokoss, M.J.; Kedev, S.; Thabane, L.; Stankovic, G.; Moreno, R.; et al. Randomized trial of primary PCI with or without routine manual thrombectomy. *N. Engl. J. Med.* **2015**, *372*, 1389–1398. [CrossRef]
37. Mastoris, I.; Giustino, G.; Sartori, S.; Baber, U.; Mehran, R.; Kini, A.S.; Sharma, S.K.; Dangas, G.D. Efficacy and safety of routine thrombus aspiration in patients with ST-segment elevation myocardial infarction undergoing primary percutaneous coronary intervention: An updated systematic review and meta-analysis of randomized controlled trials. *Catheter. Cardiovasc. Interv. Off. J. Soc. Card. Angiogr. Interv.* **2016**, *87*, 650–660. [CrossRef]
38. Meneguz-Moreno, R.A.; Costa, J.R., Jr.; Oki, F.H.; Costa, R.A.; Abizaid, A. Thrombus aspiration in STEMI patients: An updated systematic review and meta-analysis. *Minerva Cardioangiol.* **2017**, *65*, 648–658. [CrossRef]
39. Jolly, S.S.; James, S.; Dzavik, V.; Cairns, J.A.; Mahmoud, K.D.; Zijlstra, F.; Yusuf, S.; Olivecrona, G.K.; Renlund, H.; Gao, P.; et al. Thrombus Aspiration in ST-Segment-Elevation Myocardial Infarction: An Individual Patient Meta-Analysis: Thrombectomy Trialists Collaboration. *Circulation* **2017**, *135*, 143–152. [CrossRef]
40. Assessment of the Safety and Efficacy of a New Treatment Strategy with Percutaneous Coronary Intervention (ASSENT-4 PCI) Investigators. Primary versus tenecteplase-facilitated percutaneous coronary intervention in patients with ST-segment elevation acute myocardial infarction (ASSENT-4 PCI): Randomised trial. *Lancet* **2006**, *367*, 569–578. [CrossRef]

41. Echavarria-Pinto, M.; Lopes, R.; Gorgadze, T.; Gonzalo, N.; Hernandez, R.; Jimenez-Quevedo, P.; Alfonso, F.; Banuelos, C.; Nunez-Gil, I.J.; Ibanez, B.; et al. Safety and efficacy of intense antithrombotic treatment and percutaneous coronary intervention deferral in patients with large intracoronary thrombus. *Am. J. Cardiol.* **2013**, *111*, 1745–1750. [CrossRef]
42. Nakagawa, Y.; Nobuyoshi, M.; Yamaguchi, T.; Meguro, T.; Yokoi, H.; Kimura, T.; Hosoda, S.; Kanmatsuse, K.; Matsumori, A.; Sasayama, S. Efficacy of abciximab for patients undergoing balloon angioplasty: Data from Japanese evaluation of c7E3 Fab for elective and primary PCI organization in randomized trial (JEPPORT). *Circ. J.* **2009**, *73*, 145–151. [CrossRef]

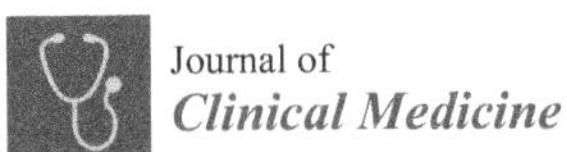
Journal of
Clinical Medicine
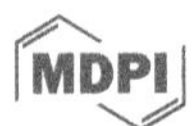

Article

A Prospective Randomized, Double-Blind, Multi-Center, Phase III Clinical Trial Evaluating the Efficacy and Safety of Olmesartan/Amlodipine plus Rosuvastatin Combination Treatment in Patients with Concomitant Hypertension and Dyslipidemia: A LEISURE Study

Sang-Ho Jo [1], Seok Min Kang [2], Byung Su Yoo [3], Young Soo Lee [4], Ho Joong Youn [5], Kyungwan Min [6], Jae Myung Yu [7], Hyun Ju Yoon [8], Woo Shik Kim [9], Gee Hee Kim [10], Jae Hyoung Park [11], Seok Yeon Kim [12] and Cheol Ho Kim [13,*]

1 Department of Internal Medicine, Division of Cardiology, Hallym University Sacred Heart Hospital, Anyang 14068, Korea; sophi5neo@gmail.com
2 Department of Internal Medicine, Yonsei University College of Medicine, Seoul 03722, Korea; SMKANG@yuhs.ac
3 Department of Internal Medicine, Division of Cardiology, Wonju College of Medicine, Yonsei University, Wonju 26426, Korea; yubs@yonsei.ac.kr
4 Department of Internal Medicine, Division of Cardiology, Daegu Catholic University Medical Center, Daegu 42472, Korea; mdleeys@cu.ac.kr
5 Department of Internal Medicine, Division of Cardiology, Seoul St. Mary's Hospital, The Catholic University of Korea, Seoul 06591, Korea; hjy@catholic.ac.kr
6 Nowon Eulji Medical Center, Department of Internal Medicine, Division of Endocrinology, Eulji University, Seoul 01830, Korea; minyungwa@gmail.com
7 Department of Internal Medicine, Division of Endocrinology, Hallym University Kangnam Sacred Heart Hospital, Seoul 07441, Korea; jaemyungyu@hotmail.com
8 Department of Internal Medicine, Division of Cardiology, Chonnam National University Hospital, Gwangju KS018, Korea; ann426@hanmail.net
9 Department of Cardiology, Kyunghee Medical Center, Seoul 02447, Korea; wskim1125@khu.ac.kr
10 Department of Internal Medicine, Division of Cardiology, St. Vincent's Hospital, College of Medicine, The Catholic University of Korea, Seoul 06591, Korea; jiheekim@catolic.ac.kr
11 Department of Internal Medicine, Division of Cardiology, Korea University Anam Hospital, Seoul 02841, Korea; jhpark3992@naver.com
12 Department of Internal Medicine, Division of Cardiology, Seoul Medical Center, Seoul 02053, Korea; ks7688@hanmail.net
13 Department of Internal Medicine, Division of Cardiology, Seoul National University Bundang Hospital, Seongnam 13620, Korea
* Correspondence: cheolkim@snubh.org; Tel.: +82-31-380-3722; Fax: +82-31-386-2269

Citation: Jo, S.-H.; Kang, S.M.; Yoo, B.S.; Lee, Y.S.; Youn, H.J.; Min, K.; Yu, J.M.; Yoon, H.J.; Kim, W.S.; Kim, G.H.; et al. A Prospective Randomized, Double-Blind, Multi-Center, Phase III Clinical Trial Evaluating the Efficacy and Safety of Olmesartan/Amlodipine plus Rosuvastatin Combination Treatment in Patients with Concomitant Hypertension and Dyslipidemia: A LEISURE Study. *J. Clin. Med.* **2022**, *11*, 350. https://doi.org/10.3390/jcm11020350

Academic Editors: Koichi Node, Atsushi Tanaka and Arrigo Cicero

Received: 1 December 2021
Accepted: 8 January 2022
Published: 11 January 2022

Abstract: Background: This study was a multicenter, randomized, double-blinded, placebo-controlled phase III clinical trial to investigate the efficacy and safety of an olmesartan/amlodipine single pill plus rosuvastatin combination treatment for patients with concomitant hypertension and dyslipidemia. Methods: Patients with both hypertension and dyslipidemia aged 20–80 were enrolled from 36 tertiary hospitals in Korea from January 2017 to April 2018. Patients were randomized to three groups in a 1:1:0.5 ratio, olmesartan/amlodipine single pill plus rosuvastatin (olme/amlo/rosu) or olmesartan plus rosuvastatin (olme/rosu) or olmesartan/amlodipine single pill (olme/amlo) combination. The primary endpoints were change of sitting systolic blood pressure (sitSBP) from baseline in the olme/amlo/rosu vs. olme/rosu groups and the percentage change of low-density lipoprotein cholesterol (LDL-C) from baseline in the olme/amlo/rosu vs. olme/amlo groups after 8 weeks of treatment. Results: A total of 265 patients were randomized, 106 to olme/amlo/rosu, 106 to olme/rosu and 53 to olme/amlo groups. Baseline characteristics among the three groups did not differ. The mean sitSBP change was significantly larger in the olme/amlo/rosu group with −24.30 ± 12.62 mmHg (from 153.58 ± 10.90 to 129.28 ± 13.58) as compared to the olme/rosu group, −9.72 ± 16.27 mmHg (from 153.71 ± 11.10 to 144.00 ± 18.44 mmHg). The difference in change of sitSBP between the two groups was −14.62± 1.98 mmHg with significance (95% CI −18.51 to −10.73, $p < 0.0001$). The mean LDL-C reduced significantly in the olme/amlo/rosu group, −52.31 ± 16.63% (from 154.52 ± 30.84 to 72.72 ± 26.08 mg/dL) as compared to the olme/amlo group with no change, −2.98 ± 16.16% (from 160.42 ± 32.05 to 153.81 ± 31.57 mg/dL). Significant difference in change was found in LDL-C between the two groups with −50.10 ± 2.73% (95% CI −55.49 to −44.71, $p < 0.0001$). Total adverse drug reaction rates were 10.48%, 5.66% and 3.7% in the olme/amlo/rosu, olme/rosu and olme/amlo groups, respectively with no statistical significance among the three groups. Serious adverse drug reactions did not occur. Conclusions: Olmesartan/amlodipine single pill plus rosuvastatin combination treatment for patients with both hypertension and dyslipidemia is effective and safe as compared to either olmesartan plus rosuvastatin or olmesartan plus amlodipine treatment.

Keywords: olmesartan; amlodipine; rosuvastatin; single pill combination; phase III clinical trial

1. Introduction

Single pill combination (SPC) of two or more antihypertensive drugs has shown promising results in improving drug compliance, lowering blood pressure and potentially providing better clinical outcomes [1–4].

There have been many clinical trials to evaluate the efficacy and safety of the SPC of 2–3 classes of antihypertensive or dyslipidemia drug [5–7]. Moreover, SPCs with both antihypertensive and anti-dyslipidemia drugs have been developed and tested [4,8–11]. Most of these studies showed promising efficacy and safety data as compared to monotherapy or equivalent doses of separate pill combinations. Reflecting these results, recent guidelines regarding hypertension management specifically indicated the use of single-pill combinations for the simple purpose of improving drug adherence [12]. The concept of single pill, or fixed dose combination, or poly-pill has broadened its scope beyond hypertension or dyslipidemia treatment. A recent clinical trial assessing the separate small dose combination of four classes of cardiovascular drugs suggests promising use of the poly-pill in reducing cardiovascular disease [10,13]. The performance of this kind of clinical trial suggests the popularity and promising future directions for the poly=pill or SPC in treating hypertension and cardiovascular disease. Patients with hypertension had high probability of dyslipidemia and vice versa. Therefore, concomitant prescription of antihypertensive and anti-dyslipidemia drugs is not rare and this will increase in the future as the elderly and co-morbid population grows. Accordingly, the SPC of different kinds of antihypertensive and anti-dyslipidemia drugs is needed in the context of compliance improvement and for better clinical outcome. Moreover, reflecting the recommendation of recent hypertension treatment guidelines regarding the initial two-drug combination for blood pressure management, even in stage I hypertensive patients, a three-drug combination with two antihypertensive drugs and one anti-dyslipidemia drug for patients with combined risk of hypertension and dyslipidemia is a reasonable strategy and needs to be tested [12]. We tested a well-known drugs combination, olmesartan and amlodipine as antihypertensive medication, and rosuvastatin as an anti-dyslipidemia drug. Olmesartan showed signs of harm by a greater occurrence rate of fatal cardiovascular events in a large scale prospective clinical, even if it showed promising results in reducing microalbuminuria [14]. However, other clinical trials showed safety and benefits in preventing cardiovascular events [15,16]. Furthermore, olmesartan is one of the most widely used antihypertensive drugs in Korea and globally [17].

We performed a prospective multi-center randomized double blinded placebo-controlled phase III clinical trial to assess an SPC drug composed of olmesartan/amlodipine plus a separate dose of rosuvastatin to examine its efficacy and safety in controlling blood pressure and serum lipid level. The final study purpose was to develop a triple SPC with these three drugs.

2. Methods

2.1. Purpose

This multicenter double blind phase III clinical trial was performed from January 2017 to April 2018 in 36 tertiary hospitals in Korea. The study purpose was to test the blood pressure (BP) lowering and low-density lipoprotein cholesterol (LDL-C) reducing effect of olmesartan/amlodipine plus a separate dose of rosuvastatin as compared to olmesartan plus rosuvastatin or olmesartan plus amlodipine.

The trial protocol was approved by the institutional review board at Seoul National University Bundang Hospital (IRB No. B-1610-368-002) and Hallym University Sacred Heart Hospital (IRB No. 2016-S072). All patients provided written informed consent at the time of enrolment and randomization. This study was performed under the standards specified in the International Council for Harmonization Guidelines for Good Clinical Practice and the principles of the Declaration of Helsinki. This trial was registered at ClinicalTrials.gov, with Identifier NCT03009487.

2.2. Patients

Patients aged 20–80 who had concomitant hypertension and dyslipidemia participated in this study. The patients had to have been prescribed both anti-hypertensive and anti-dyslipidemic drugs or meet the diagnosis criteria for hypertension and dyslipidemia (Supplementary Tables S1 and S2).

Exclusion criteria were (1) mean sitting systolic BP (sitSBP) difference of 20 mmHg or over among three readings or sitDBP 10 mmHg or over, (2) mean sitting diastolic BP (sitDBP) $\geq$ 110 mmHg in three readings at randomization visit (visit 2), (3) compliance to olmesartan 40 mg was under 70% or over 130%, (4) those with symptomatic orthostatic hypotension, (5) likely to have secondary hypertension, (6) severe heart failure with NYHA class III-IV symptom, severe aortic or mitral stenosis, those with obstructive hypertrophic cardiomyopathy or severe coronary obstructive disease, (7) critical arrhythmia, (8) those with stroke or transient ischemic attack, acute coronary syndrome, peripheral arterial disease or coronary revascularization within 6 months, (9) uncontrolled diabetes (HbA1c $\geq$ 9.0% or fasting blood glucose $\geq$ 160 mg/dL), (10) uncontrolled thyroid abnormalities, (11) chronic kidney disease (serum creatinine $\geq$ 2 mg/dL or renal replacement therapy or hepatic failure patients and with AST or ALT over 2 times of upper normal limit, (12) Crohn's disease, active hemorrhagic ulcer and acute and chronic pancreatitis, (13) chronic inflammation status requiring anti-inflammatory drugs, (14) myopathy or history of rhabdomyolysis, (15) critical hyperuricemia (uric acid > 10 mg/dL) or hyperkalemia (K > 5.5 mmol/L), (16) clinically meaningful hyponatremia (Na < 130 mmol/L) or volume depletion status, (17) malignancy within 5 years, (18) alcohol or drug abuser within 1 year, (19) pregnancy or breast feeding.

2.3. Study Drugs

The study drug was olmesartan 40 mg/amlodipine 10 mg (SPC) plus rosuvastatin 20 mg, olme/rosu group drug was olmesartan 40 mg plus rosuvastatin 20 mg (separate drug), and olme/amlo group drug was olmesartan 40 mg/amlodipine 10 mg (single pill combination). Study drug group received olmesartan 40 mg/amlodipine 10 mg (2 drug single-pill) plus rosuvastatin 20 mg plus placebo of olmesartan 40 mg. Olme/rosu group received olmesartan 40 mg plus rosuvastatin 20 mg plus placebo of olmesartan 40 mg/amlodipine 10 mg and olme/amlo group patients received olmesartan 40 mg/amlodipine 10 mg plus placebo of olmesartan 40 mg plus placebo of rosuvastatin 20 mg.

2.4. Study Procedures

After screening for eligibility (visit 1) and before randomization (visit 2), if subjects already took these medications, they stopped both antihypertensive and anti-dyslipidemia medications including fenofibrate, and took only olmesartan at 40 mg per day combined with therapeutic life style changes after patients agreed and provided informed consent at study entrance for 6 weeks of washout period (Figure 1).

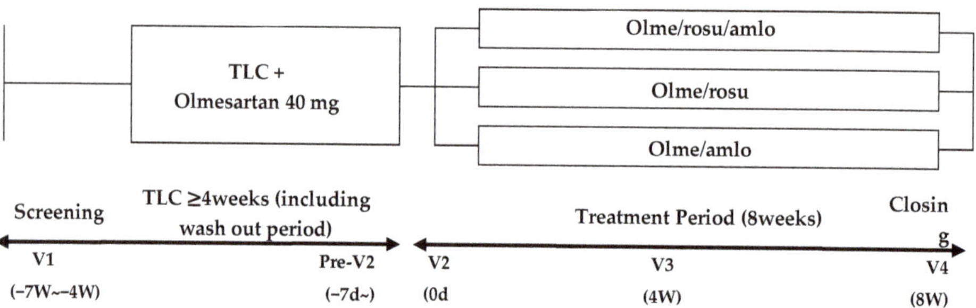

Figure 1. Study scheme. TLC, therapeutic life style change; olme, olmesartan; rosu, rosuvastatin; amlo, amlodipine; v, visit.

Their sitSBP ought to have been within 140 to 180 mmHg at randomization time point (visit 2) and their lipid profile ought to have met the criteria (visit 2) (Figure 1, Supplementary Tables S1 and S2). The BP was measured at the arm, with higher BP taken. After checking the BP and lipid profile at visit 2, patients were randomly assigned to three groups consecutively, study drug group (olme/amlo/rosu), olme/rosu and olme/amlo groups, with 1:1:0.5 ratio and with PROC plan in SAS system V9.3. by an independent statistician who do not know the study performance. We allocated half the number of patients to the/amlo group as compared to the other groups because of an ethical issue; those in the olme/amlo group did not receive anti-dyslipidemia drugs.

After being randomized to each group, patient received investigational drugs for 8 weeks and were followed up for safety and efficacy at 4 and 8 weeks of treatment (Figure 2).

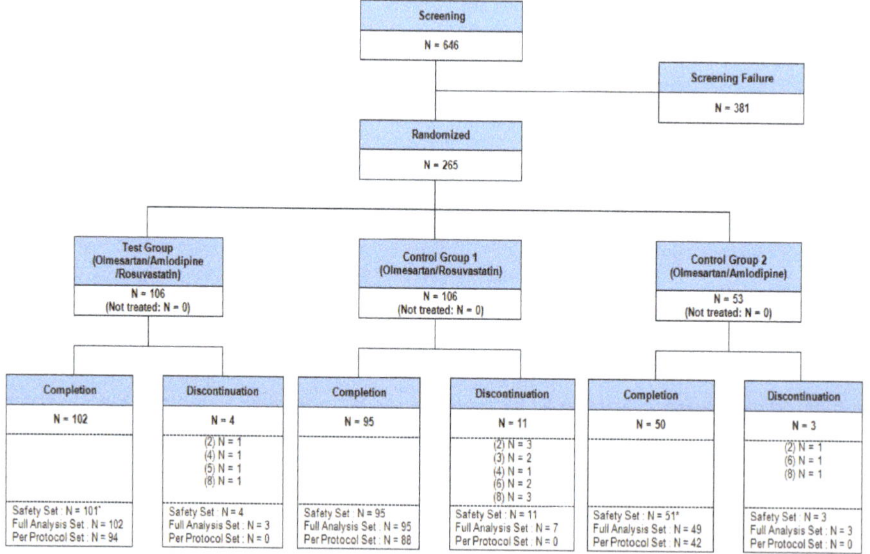

Figure 2. Study patients flow. * = 1 person was classified into olme/amlo group instead of olme/amlo/rosu group in safety analysis due to study investigational product was falsely distributed.

Drug compliance was estimated by checking the remaining drugs at visit 2 and calculating real intake dose/planned dose.

2.4.1. Sample Size Estimation and Statistical Analysis

For sample size estimation in the aspect of sitSBP change, the sitSBP change was −21.53 mmHg in amlo group and −13.30 in non-amlo group, with maximal standard deviation of 16.58 mmHg.

Thus, null hypothesis was $H_0 = \mu_t - \mu_c \geq 0$

μ_t: Mean sitSBP change in Olmesartan/Amlodipine/Rosuvastatin group.

μ_c: Mean sitSBP change in Olmesartan/Rosuvastatin group.

$$n = \frac{2(Z_\alpha+Z_\beta)^2\sigma^2}{(\mu_t-\mu_c)^2} = \frac{2\times(1.96+1.282)^2\times 16.58^2}{(-8.23)^2} = 85.32 \approx 86$$

Thus, 86 patients in each group were required to allow for 2.5% alpha and 10% beta error.

For samples size estimation in the aspect of LDL-C change, we referred to relevant references and found minimal −48.0% LDL-C difference between rosuvastatin and no-rosuvastatin groups. We assumed maximal standard deviation as 11.1% and we hypothesized as follows;

Thus, null hypothesis was $H_0 = \mu_t - \mu_c \geq 0$

μ_t: LDL-C change in Olmesartan/Amlodipine/Rosuvastatin group

μ_c: LDL-C change in Olmesartan/Amlodipine group

$$n = \frac{2(Z_\alpha+Z_\beta)^2\sigma^2}{(\mu_t-\mu_c)^2} = \frac{2\times(1.96+1.282)^2\times(0.111)^2}{(-0.48)^2} = 1.12 \approx 2$$

Thus, two patients in each group were required to allow for 2.5% alpha and 10% beta error.

Combining the above two calculations, final study population was 86 in each group. Considering 15% lost to follow-up, 102 patients in the olme/amlo/rosu and olme/rosu groups and 51 in the olme/amlo group were required with 1:1:0.5 ratio.

The efficacy was evaluated mainly with a full analysis set (FAS) along with a Per-protocol Set (PPS) and safety was tested with a safety set (SS). In dealing with the missing values for the efficacy analysis, we used Last Observation Carried Forward (LOCF) methods for adjustment, and for safety analysis we used original data, with missing for without LOCF. Categorical variables were presented with numbers and percentages and compared using the Pearson's chi-square test or Fisher's exact test. Continuous variables with normal distribution were presented as the mean ± standard deviation and compared using the paired sample *t*-test, or one sample *t*-test or Wilcoxon singed rank test for intra-group comparison. To test the inter-group differences for continuous variables, ANCOVA test was performed. *p* value of <0.05 was considered to be significant. Statistical analysis was carried out using SAS version 9.4.

2.4.2. Endpoints

Primary endpoints were sitSBP change from baseline at 8 week treatment in olme/amlo/rosu vs. olme/rosu group and percentage change of LDL-C from baseline in olme/amlo/rosu vs. olme/amlo group. The differences from baseline between two groups in sitSBP and LDL-C were also compared (study drug group vs. each of two comparator groups).

Secondary endpoint was (1) sitSBP change from baseline in olme/amlo/rosu and olme/amlo, (2) LDL-C change from baseline in olme/amlo/rosu and olme/rosu, (3) sitDBP change from baseline in olme/amlo/rosu, olme/rosu and olme/amlo, (4) target BP and LDL-C attainment rate in olme/amlo/rosu vs. olme/rosu vs. olme/amlo.

(5) Total cholesterol, triglyceride (TG), HDL-C, APO-A1 and AP-B change.

3. Results

A total of 646 patients participated in the study from 29 tertiary hospitals in Korea. After 381 patients dropped out in screening, 265 patients were randomized. FAS (patients taking drug at least once and having efficacy evaluation at least once) included

259 (olme/amlo/rosu group 105, olme/rosu group 102, olme/amlo group 52), and per-protocol set (completing the study) included 224 patients (olme/amlo/rosu group 94, olme/rosu group 88, olm/amlo group 42) and safety set (patients taking drug at least once and followed-up at least once) included 265 patients (olme/amlo/rosu group 105, olme/rosu group 106, olm/amlo group 54) (Table 1, Figure 2, Supplementary Table S3). The overall drug adherence rate was 97.42 ± 4.73%. In the individual group, the rates were 97.01 ± 5.29% in olme/amlo/rosu, 98.24 ± 2.75% in olme/rosu and 96.65 ± 6.24% in olme/amlo group, with no statistical difference among the three groups ($p = 0.9706$).

Table 1. Baseline characteristics.

	Olme/Amlo/Rosu (n = 105)	Olme/Rosu (n = 102)	Olme/Amlo (n = 52)	p-Value
Age (years), Mean (SD)	65.18 (9.34)	63.49 (9.76)	64.06 (8.94)	0.3817
Sex, n (%)				
Male	59 (56.19)	58 (56.86)	31 (59.62)	0.9176
Height (cm)				
Mean (SD)	162.64 (9.58)	161.31 (8.52)	162.21 (8.64)	0.5609
Weight (kg)				
Mean (SD)	70.96 (11.92)	69.48 (11.34)	70.50 (12.50)	0.6018
Body Mass Index (kg/m^2)				
Mean (SD)	26.75 (3.28)	26.60 (3.01)	26.67 (3.26)	0.9949
Smoking Status, n (%)				0.7611
Never	57 (54.29)	56 (54.90)	30 (57.69)	
Current	21 (20.00)	26 (25.49)	10 (19.23)	
Former	27 (25.71)	20 (19.61)	12 (23.08)	
Drinking Status, n (%)				0.1590
Never	57 (54.29)	48 (47.06)	20 (38.46)	
Current	41 (39.05)	51 (50.00)	27 (51.92)	
Former	7 (6.67)	3 (2.94)	5 (9.62)	
Total Cholesterol (mg/dL)				0.6331
Mean (SD)	216.98 (34.82)	220.63 (35.24)	223.48 (37.24)	
HDL-C (mg/dL)				0.3811
Mean (SD)	49.23 (11.95)	46.87 (11.45)	48.65 (10.74)	
SBP (mmHg)				0.6207
Mean (SD)	153.58 (10.90)	153.71 (11.10)	151.30 (8.87)	
10-year risk assessment (score)				0.6538
Mean (SD)	16.38 (8.19)	17.22 (7.48)	16.25 (7.87)	
Risk Factor, n (%)				
hypertension	105 (100.00)	102 (100.00)	52 (100.00)	1
HDL-C < 40 mg/dL	25 (23.81)	24 (23.53)	13 (25.00)	0.7561
Age ≥45 in male, ≥55 in female	95 (90.48)	94 (92.16)	47 (90.38)	0.8543
Coronary heart disease	1 (0.95)	1 (0.95)	0	0.9978
Family history of premature CAD	8 (7.62)	9 (8.82)	4 (7.69)	0.3195

HDL, high density lipoprotein; CAD, coronary artery disease.

3.1. *Efficacy Outcomes*

3.1.1. Primary Endpoint

The primary outcome was comparison of sitSBP change after 8 weeks of treatment between olme/amlo/rosu ($n = 105$) vs. olme/rosu groups ($n = 102$) and comparison of LDL-C change between olme/amlo/rosu vs. olme/ amlo groups (FAS analysis). The mean sitSBP change was significantly larger in olme/amlo/rosu group with −24.30 ± 12.62mmHg (from 153.58 ± 10.90 to 129.28 ± 13.58) as compared to olme/rosu group, −9.72 ± 16.27 mmHg (from 153.71 ± 11.10 to 144.00 ± 18.44 mmHg) (Table 2 and Figure 2). The change of sitSBP from baseline at 8 weeks was more pronounced in olme/amlo/rosu group as compared to olme/rosu group, and the difference of change between 2 groups was −14.62 ± 1.98 mmHg with significance (95% CI −18.51 to −10.73, $p < 0.0001$). (Table 2 and Figure 2).

The mean LDL-C percentage reduction was significantly more in the olme/amlo/rosu group, −52.41 ± 16.63% (from 154.52 ± 30.84 to 72.72 ± 26.08 mg/dL) compared to that of the olme/amlo group, −2.98 ± 16.16% (from 160.42 ± 32.05 to 153.81 ± 31.57 mg/dL) with $p < 0.0001$. More LDL-C reduction was found in the olme/amlo/rosu group compared to the olme/amlo group, with a significant difference of change between the two groups with −50.10 ± 2.73% (95% CI −55.49 to −44.71, $p < 0.0001$) (Table 3 and Figure 3).

Table 2. Change of sitSBP at 8 weeks comparing olme/amlo/rosu and olme/rosu group.

SBP, mmHg	Olme/Amlo/Rosu (n = 105)	Olme/Rosu (n = 102)	p-Value
At Baseline, Mean(SD)	153.58 (10.90)	153.71 (11.10)	0.9639
At Week 8, Mean(SD)	129.28 (13.58)	144.00 (18.44)	<0.0001
Change form baseline at 8 week, Mean(SD)	−24.30 (12.62)	−9.72 (16.27)	<0.0001

Table 3. Change of LDL-C at 8 weeks comparing olme/amlo/rosu and olme/amlo group.

LDL-C, mg/dL	Olme/Amlo/Rosu (n = 105)	Olme/Rosu (n = 52)	p-Value
At Baseline, Mean(SD)	154.52 (30.84)	160.42 (32.05)	0.2672
At Week 8, Mean(SD)	72.72 (26.08)	153.81 (31.57)	<0.0001
Percent Change form baseline at 8 week, Mean(SD)%	−52.31 (16.63)	−2.98 (16.16)	<0.0001

By per-protocol set analysis, sitSBP significantly reduced by −24.60 ± 12.0 mmHg in the olme/amlo/rosu group (n = 94) and −9.93 ± 14.90 mmHg in the olme/rosu groups (n = 88) at 8 weeks with statistical significance (both $p < 0.0001$). Inter-group difference in sitSBP change from baseline was −14.57 ±1.95 mmHg with significance ($p < 0.0001$). With per-protocol set analysis by ANCOVA, LDL-C was significantly reduced by −52.92 ± 15.23% in the olme/amlo/rosu group ($p < 0.0001$) and but not reduced in the olme/amlo group, 3.10 ± 17.27% (p = 0.2513) The change of LDL-C from baseline is significantly higher in the olme/amlo/rosu group; inter-group difference of LDL-C change was −50.06 ± 2.9%.

3.1.2. Secondary Endpoints

The sitSBP change from baseline between olme/amlo/rosu vs. olme/amlo were −24.30 ± 12.62 mmHg and −22.89 ± 11.74 mmHg, respectively, with no difference (LS mean difference (SE), −0.63 ± 2.02 mmHg, p = 0.7555) despite that intra-group BP reduction in each group was significant (both $p < 0.0001$). The LDL-C change in olme/amlo/rosu was −52.31 ± 16.63% and −51.38 ± 17.46% in olme/rosu group at 8-week with statistic significance in each intra-group, but inter-group difference of change between 2 groups was −1.34 ± 2.33% with no difference (p = 0.5667).

The change of sitDBP in olme/amlo/rosu vs. olme/rosu vs. olme/amlo at 4- and 8-week were −11.83 ± 7.52 mmHg, −4.23 ± 8.52 mmHg, −10.21 ± 7.50 mmHg and −12.06 ± 7.81 mmHg, −4.72 ± 9.01 mmHg, −12.46 ± 7.01 mmHg, respectively, with statistical significance in each group (all $p < 0.0001$ as compared to baseline in each group at 4 and 8 weeks). The change of sitDBP in olme/amlo/rosu at 4 and 8 weeks was significantly greater as compared to that of olme/rosu with group difference of −8.53 ± 1.07 mmHg (LS mean difference (SE), $p < 0.0001$) at 4 weeks and −8.33 ± 1.11mmHg (LS mean difference [SE], $p < 0.0001$) at 8 weeks, but the difference of sitDBP change from baseline at 4 and 8 weeks between olme/amlo/rosu vs. olme/amlo were not different with LS mean difference (SE), −1.51 ± 1.12 mmHg, (p = 0.1806) and 0.57 ± 1.14 mmHg, (p = 0.6160), respectively.

The rate of target BP attainment at 8 weeks, defined as sitSBP < 140 and/or sitDBP < 90 mmHg (for those with ≥60 years, sitSBP < 150 and/or sitDBP < 90 mmHg) was 84.76% (89/105) in olme/amlo/rosu group, 47.06% (48/102) in olme/rosu, and 76.92% (40/52) in olme/amlo group. This rate was significantly higher in the olme/amlo/rosu group as compared to the olme/rosu group ($p < 0.0001$) but did not differ between olme/amlo/rosu vs. olme/amlo group (p = 0.2272).

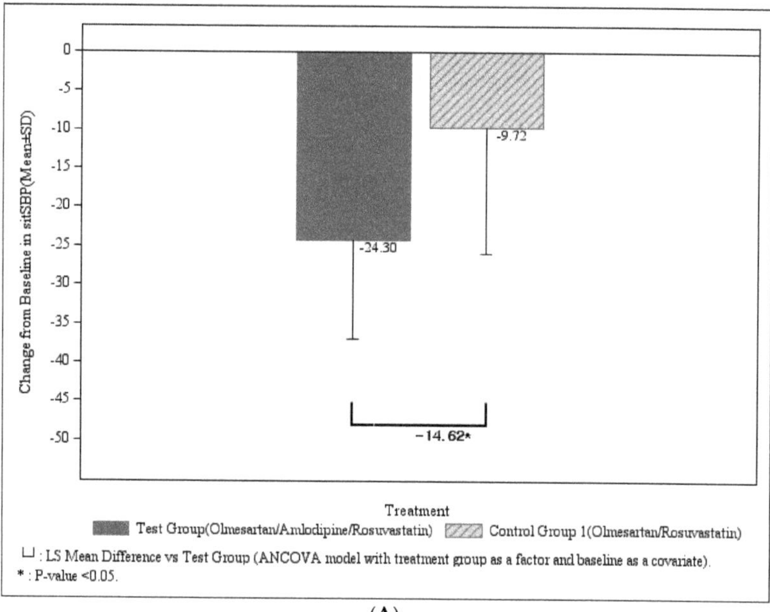

(A)

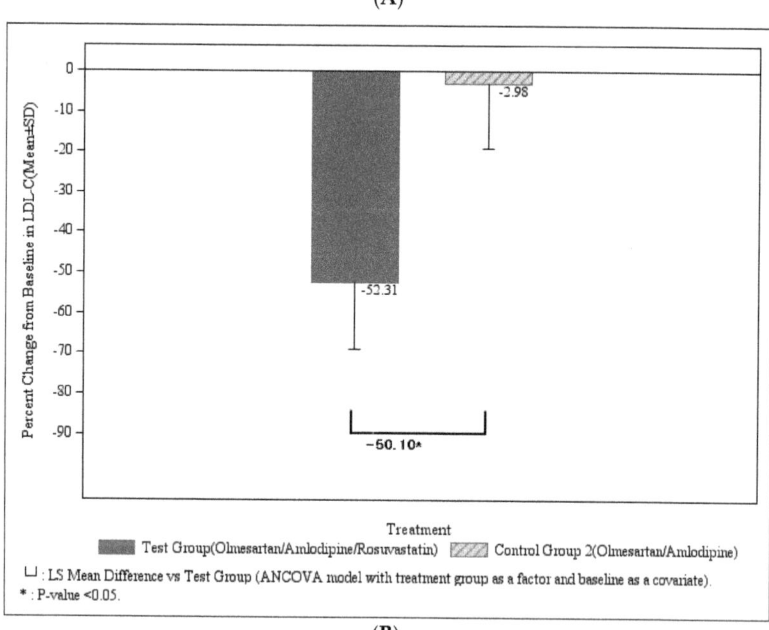

(B)

Figure 3. (**A**) Change of sitSBP in olme/amlo/rosu vs. olme/rosu after 8 week treatment (**B**) Change of LDL-C in olme/amlo/rosu vs. olme/amlo after 8 week treatment.

The rate of target LDL-C attainment according to the risk category of the NCEP ATP III guideline (for example, if risk factor 0–1, responder had LDL-C < 160 mg/dL, if risk factor ≥ 2 and 10 year risk ≤ 20%, responder had LDL-C < 130 mg/dL, and if coronary heart disease (CHD) or CHD risk equivalents or 10 year risk > 20%, responder had LDL-C < 100 mg/dL) was 84.76% (89/105) in olme/amlo/rosu, 83.33% (85/102) in olme/rosu and 15.38% (8/52) in olme/amlo groups, with no difference between 1st and 2nd groups, and significantly higher in 1st group as compared to 3rd group ($p < 0.0001$). Total cholesterol, TG and APO-B reduced significantly and HDL-C and APO-A1 increased significantly both in olme/amlo/rosu group and olme/rosu groups. However no change was found in olme/amlo group (Supplementary Table S4).

3.2. Subgroup Analysis

We stratified the patients according to age (65 years old over or not), sex and chronic kidney disease. Same findings were detected in all subgroups, more reduced sitSBP in olme/amlo/rosu group as compared to olme/rosu group and more lowered LDL-C in olme/amlo/rosu group as compared to olme/amlo group (Supplementary Table S5).

3.3. Safety Outcomes

Total adverse drug events rate was 7.1% (19/265) in all population. 10.48% (11/105), and 5.66% (6/106) and 3.7% (2/54) in the olme/amlo/rosu, olme/rosu and olme/amlo groups, respectively; no serious adverse drug event occurred in all groups. No significant differences among the three groups were detected ($p = 0.2163$). Regarding the severity, mild drug reaction was most common (Table 4).

Table 4. Adverse drug reactions.

Patients Number (%) (Event No)	Olme/Amlo/Rosu ($n = 105$)	Olme/Rosu) ($n = 106$)	Olme/Amlo ($n = 54$)	Total ($n = 265$)
Subjects with ADRs	11 (10.48)	6 (5.66)	2 (3.70)	19 (7.17)
95% Confidence Interval	(4.62, 16.33)	(1.26, 10.06)	(0.00, 8.74)	(4.06, 10.28)
p-value *				0.2163 (c)
Severity				
Mild	14	6	2	22
Moderate	0	2	0	2
Severe	0	0	0	0
Relationship with drugs				
Certain	0	0	0	0
Probable/Likely	0	2	1	3
Possible	7	3	0	10
Unlikely	7	3	1	11
Not related	0	0	0	0
Unassessable/Unclassifiable	0	0	0	0
Subjects with Serious ADRs	0	0	0	0
Exact 95% Confidence Interval	(0.00, 3.45)	(0.00, 3.42)	(0.00, 6.60)	(0.00, 1.38)
p-value *				NC
Subjects with ADRs Leading to drug Discontinuation	1 (0.95) (2)	0	0	1 (0.38) (2)
Exact 95% Confidence Interval	(0.02, 5.19)	(0.00, 3.42)	(0.00, 6.60)	(0.01, 2.08)
p-value *				0.6000 (f)
Subjects with ADRs Leading to Fatal circumstances	0	0	0	0
Exact 95% Confidence Interval	(0.00, 3.45)	(0.00, 3.42)	(0.00, 6.60)	(0.00, 1.38)
p-value *				NC

Olme, Olmesartan; Amlo, Amlodipine; Rosu, Rosuvastatin; ADR, adverse drug reaction; NC, not calculated. * Testing for difference among treatment groups, chi-square test (c) or Fisher's exact test (f). Note: Denominator of percentage is the number of subjects in each group. Severity and relationship are displayed as 'number of events' and others are displayed as 'number of subjects (percentage of subjects) (number of events)'. ADR is the adverse event whose relationship to the study drug is 'Certain', 'Probable/Likely', 'Possible', 'Unlikely', 'Unassessable/Unclassifiable'.

4. Discussion

Our study demonstrated the efficacy of the triple combination of olm/amlo/rosu on BP and LDL-C lowering, as well as safety, compared to olme/rosu or olme/amlo dual combination. Treatment with olme/amlo/rosu significantly reduced SBP by 24 mmHg and LDL-C by 52% compared to olme/rosu or olme/amlo. The attainment rates of target BP and LDL-C at 8 weeks were both 85%. Our data confirmed the efficacy of the triple combination of antihypertensive and anti-dyslipidemia drugs. In the safety profile, the olme/amlo/rosu combination shows similar results with the other two groups.

As the co-morbid and elderly population is growing more and more, the need for medication tends to increase. As such, drug compliance is likely to getting poorer as the number of pills increases. Recent studies have repeatedly provided evidence of the relationship of poor compliance and poor control of BP and LDL-C [18,19]. Poor compliance could be associated finally with poor clinical outcomes [20]. Therefore recent guidelines on hypertension management suggested single pill combination drugs to enhance drug compliance [12,21].

Our study had value in reflecting current the prevailing metabolic syndrome and testing the potential of a combination of different classes of drug, anti-hypertension and anti-dyslipidemia. These two diseases are frequently encountered in daily practice and are major components of metabolic syndrome. The drugs used in our study for BP lowering were olmesartan and amlodipine. Amlodipine is widely used in Korea as well as globally with myriad clinical data on improving clinical outcomes, as well as BP lowering, from large scale randomized clinical trials [17,21].

On the other hand, olmesartan is controversial regarding cardiovascular safety, because a ROADMAP trial showed more frequent development of fatal cardiovascular event in olmesartan users, 0.7% (15/2232) vs. 0.1% (3/2215), despite it improved primary endpoint of microalbuminuria. However, in that study, cardiovascular event was the secondary endpoint and the events rate was very small, 0.7% (15/2232) vs. 0.1% (3/2215) [14]. Moreover, the event was attributed to cardiovascular death among patients with preexisting coronary heart disease (2% [11/564] vs. 0.2% [1/540]). Considering our study population had simple hypertension and dyslipidemia (Table 1, only two patients have coronary heart disease) and the target patient group for this triple combination treatment was those with combined risks of simple hypertension and dyslipidemia rather than those with established coronary artery disease, olmesartan can be a good option for controlling hypertension. Other clinical studies performed after the ROADMAP trial and retrospective studies argue that the harm caused by olmesartan was not so robust and reported data for better cardiovascular outcome with that drug [15,16,22]. Noticeably, in a recent trial comparing BP target in elderly patients, one of the study drugs was olmesartan and this study showed reduced cardiovascular events in olmesartan users, so the previous concern can be diminished [16]. This drug also has potential for reducing albuminuria, improving renal function, improving left ventricular hypertrophy and halting coronary plaque progression [14,23,24].

The statin used in our study was rosuvastatin, and this also is associated with numerous data on improving hard clinical endpoints, especially in primary prevention of cardiovascular disease, as well as efficacy in lowering LDL-C [25,26]. Because rosuvastatin also has the property of delaying plaque regression, the combination of rosuvastatin with olmesartan could have potential in reducing or at least halting coronary plaque progression [27].

This combination of angiotensin receptor blockers (ARBs), angiotensin-converting enzyme inhibitors (ACEIs) and calcium channel blockers (CCBs) is first recommended as combination in major guidelines and is the most widely used combination in Korea and globally [17,21]. Thus there is a rationale for the two antihypertensive drugs with olmesartan and amlodipine in our trial. The combination of olmesartan/amlodipine was reported to be superior to perindopril/amlodipine in central BP reduction in a randomized, double blind trial [28]. When we consider that central BP lowering could play a role in improving outcomes, this result also supports the combination of olmesartan and amlodipine. In addition to this combination, we added rosuvastatin as a separate pill. This triple combination as SPC provided good safety and efficacy data and pharmacokinetic profile [29].

When we compare our results with other similar studies, the efficacy in attaining the BP target in our study was 85% which is equivalent to the olmesartan plus amlodipine plus hydrochlorothiazide triple combination of antihypertensive drugs, for which control rate was 83% from a large scale retrospective observational study [30]. In the safety profile, all adverse events occurred at 8.46% in that study, which was similar to our 7.17% [30].

The magnitude of reduction of LDL-C in olme/amlo/rosu arm (−52.41%) in our study, was very similar to that of the previous study (−52.3%) assessing the efficacy of olmesartan/rosuvastatin SPC reduction [11]. These results coincide well with previous studies, similar to ours in study design and drug used. Our results clearly demonstrated efficacy and safety and provide the rationale for developing a triple combination of olmesartan/amlodipine/rosuvastatin for treatment of hypertension and dyslipidemia.

Although this phase III trial was performed to develop the triple SPC drug for ease of drug compliance, the result is meaningful because it can provide physicians with efficacy and safety data for this SPC of antihypertensive and anti-dyslipidemia drugs and can help to treat patients with combined risks.

Limitations

Our study has limitations. Firstly, a larger study population would be better to assess the primary end-point of sitSBP and LDL-C reduction and target level attainment after 8 weeks with three subset groups. Secondly, a larger population in olme/amlo could balance each group's population and can give more concrete data, despite the ethical issue that the olme/amlo group do not receive anti-dyslipidemia drugs.

5. Conclusions

A triple combination of olmesartan/amlodipine/rosuvastatin treatment is safe and effective in reducing blood pressure and LDL-C. This combination will help to improve drug compliance in patients with co-morbidity. Future studies investigating whether this combination could increase the adherence rate and improve clinical outcomes are warranted.

Supplementary Materials: The following supporting information can be downloaded at: https://www.mdpi.com/xxx/s1, Table S1. Inclusion criteria. Table S2. Pre-visit 2 inclusion criteria for dyslipidemia according to cardiovascular risk. Table S3. Final patients included. Table S4. Lipid levels other than LDL-C in 3 groups after 8week treatment. Table S5. Subgroup analysis.

Author Contributions: Conceptualization, C.H.K.; formal analysis, S.-H.J.; funding acquisition, S.-H.J. and C.H.K.; investigation, S.-H.J., S.M.K., B.S.Y., Y.S.L., H.J.Y. (Ho Joong Youn), K.M., J.M.Y., H.J.Y. (Hyun Ju Yoon), W.S.K., G.H.K., J.H.P., S.Y.K. and C.H.K.; methodology, C.H.K.; project administration, C.H.K.; writing—original draft, S.-H.J.; writing—review & editing, S.-H.J. and C.H.K. All authors have read and agreed to the published version of the manuscript.

Funding: This work was supported by Daewoong Pharmaceutical Co., Ltd.

Institutional Review Board Statement: The trial protocol was approved by the institutional review board at Seoul National University Bundang Hospital (IRB No. B-1610-368-002) and Hallym University Sacred Heart Hospital (IRB No. 2016-S072). This study was performed under the standards specified in the International Council for Harmonization Guidelines for Good Clinical Practice and the principles of the Declaration of Helsinki. This trial was registered at ClinicalTrials.gov, with ClinicalTrials.gov Identifier NCT03009487.

Informed Consent Statement: Informed consent was obtained from all subjects involved in the study.

Data Availability Statement: Not applicable.

Conflicts of Interest: The authors declare no conflict of interest.

References

1. Bangalore, S.; Kamalakkannan, G.; Parkar, S.; Messerli, F.H. Fixed-dose combinations improve medication compliance: A meta-analysis. *Am. J. Med.* **2007**, *120*, 713–719. [CrossRef] [PubMed]
2. Wald, D.S.; Law, M.; Morris, J.K.; Bestwick, J.P.; Wald, N.J. Combination therapy versus monotherapy in reducing blood pressure: Meta-analysis on 11,000 participants from 42 trials. *Am. J. Med.* **2009**, *122*, 290–300. [CrossRef]
3. Parati, G.; Kjeldsen, S.; Coca, A.; Cushman, W.C.; Wang, J. Adherence to Single-Pill versus Free-Equivalent Combination Therapy in Hypertension: A Systematic Review and Meta-Analysis. *Hypertension* **2021**, *77*, 692–705. [CrossRef]

4. Weisser, B.; Predel, H.G.; Gillessen, A.; Hacke, C.; Vor dem Esche, J.; Rippin, G.; Noetel, A.; Randerath, O. Single Pill Regimen Leads to Better Adherence and Clinical Outcome in Daily Practice in Patients Suffering from Hypertension and/or Dyslipidemia: Results of a Meta-Analysis. *High Blood Press. Cardiovasc. Prev.* **2020**, *27*, 157–164. [CrossRef]
5. Gupta, A.K.; Arshad, S.; Poulter, N.R. Compliance, safety, and effectiveness of fixed-dose combinations of antihypertensive agents: A meta-analysis. *Hypertension* **2010**, *55*, 399–407. [CrossRef] [PubMed]
6. Chow, C.K.; Atkins, E.R.; Hillis, G.S.; Nelson, M.R.; Reid, C.M.; Schlaich, M.P.; Hay, P.; Rogers, K.; Billot, L.; Burke, M.; et al. Initial treatment with a single pill containing quadruple combination of quarter doses of blood pressure medicines versus standard dose monotherapy in patients with hypertension (QUARTET): A phase 3, randomised, double-blind, active-controlled trial. *Lancet* **2021**, *398*, 1043–1052. [CrossRef]
7. Vattimo, A.C.A.; Fonseca, F.A.H.; Morais, D.C.; Generoso, L.F.; Herrera, R.; Barbosa, C.M.; de Oliveira Izar, M.C.; Cardoso, R.A.; Zung, S. Efficacy and Tolerability of a Fixed-Dose Combination of Rosuvastatin and Ezetimibe Compared with a Fixed-Dose Combination of Simvastatin and Ezetimibe in Brazilian Patients with Primary Hypercholesterolemia or Mixed Dyslipidemia: A Multicenter, Randomized Trial. *Curr. Ther. Res. Clin. Exp.* **2020**, *93*, 100595. [PubMed]
8. Kim, W.; Chang, K.; Cho, E.J.; Ahn, J.C.; Yu, C.W.; Cho, K.I.; Kim, Y.J.; Kang, D.H.; Kim, S.Y.; Lee, S.H.; et al. A randomized, double-blind clinical trial to evaluate the efficacy and safety of a fixed-dose combination of amlodipine/rosuvastatin in patients with dyslipidemia and hypertension. *J. Clin. Hypertens.* **2020**, *22*, 261–269. [CrossRef]
9. Chung, S.; Ko, Y.G.; Kim, J.S.; Kim, B.K.; Ahn, C.M.; Park, S.; Hong, S.J.; Lee, S.H.; Choi, D. Effect of FIXed-dose combination of ARb and statin on adherence and risk factor control: The randomized FIXAR study. *Cardiol. J.* **2020**. [CrossRef]
10. Joseph, P.; Roshandel, G.; Gao, P.; Pais, P.; Lonn, E.; Xavier, D.; Avezum, A.; Zhu, J.; Liu, L.; Sliwa, K.; et al. Fixed-dose combination therapies with and without aspirin for primary prevention of cardiovascular disease: An individual participant data meta-analysis. *Lancet* **2021**, *398*, 1133–1146. [CrossRef]
11. Park, J.S.; Shin, J.H.; Hong, T.J.; Seo, H.S.; Shim, W.J.; Baek, S.H.; Jeong, J.O.; Ahn, Y.; Kang, W.C.; Kim, Y.H.; et al. Efficacy and safety of fixed-dose combination therapy with olmesartan medoxomil and rosuvastatin in Korean patients with mild to moderate hypertension and dyslipidemia: An 8-week, multicenter, randomized, double-blind, factorial-design study (OLSTA-D RCT: OLmesartan rosuvaSTAtin from Daewoong). *Drug Des. Devel. Ther.* **2016**, *10*, 2599–2609.
12. Williams, B.; Mancia, G.; Spiering, W.; Agabiti Rosei, E.; Azizi, M.; Burnier, M.; Clement, D.L.; Coca, A.; de Simone, G.; Dominiczak, A.; et al. 2018 ESC/ESH Guidelines for the management of arterial hypertension. *Eur. Heart J.* **2018**, *39*, 3021–3104. [CrossRef] [PubMed]
13. Roshandel, G.; Khoshnia, M.; Poustchi, H.; Hemming, K.; Kamangar, F.; Gharavi, A.; Ostovaneh, M.R.; Nateghi, A.; Majed, M.; Navabakhsh, B.; et al. Effectiveness of polypill for primary and secondary prevention of cardiovascular diseases (PolyIran): A pragmatic, cluster-randomised trial. *Lancet* **2019**, *394*, 672–683. [CrossRef]
14. Haller, H.; Ito, S.; Izzo, J.L.; Jr Januszewicz, A.; Katayama, S.; Menne, J.; Mimran, A.; Rabelink, T.J.; Ritz, E.; Ruilope, L.M.; et al. Olmesartan for the delay or prevention of microalbuminuria in type 2 diabetes. *N. Engl. J. Med.* **2011**, *364*, 907–917. [CrossRef]
15. Hirohata, A.; Yamamoto, K.; Miyoshi, T.; Hatanaka, K.; Hirohata, S.; Yamawaki, H.; Komatsubara, I.; Hirose, E.; Kobayashi, Y.; Ohkawa, K.; et al. Four-year clinical outcomes of the OLIVUS-Ex (impact of Olmesartan on progression of coronary atherosclerosis: Evaluation by intravascular ultrasound) extension trial. *Atherosclerosis* **2012**, *220*, 134–138. [CrossRef]
16. Zhang, W.; Zhang, S.; Deng, Y.; Wu, S.; Ren, J.; Sun, G.; Yang, J.; Jiang, Y.; Xu, X.; Wang, T.D.; et al. Trial of Intensive Blood-Pressure Control in Older Patients with Hypertension. *N. Engl. J. Med.* **2021**, *385*, 1268–1279. [CrossRef] [PubMed]
17. Kim, H.C.; Cho, S.M.J.; Lee, H.; Lee, H.H.; Baek, J.; Heo, J.E. Korea hypertension fact sheet 2020: Analysis of nationwide population-based data. *Clin. Hypertens.* **2021**, *27*, 8. [CrossRef]
18. Osterberg, L.; Blaschke, T. Adherence to medication. *N. Engl. J. Med.* **2005**, *353*, 487–497. [CrossRef] [PubMed]
19. Burnier, M.; Egan, B.M. Adherence in Hypertension. *Circ. Res.* **2019**, *124*, 1124–1140. [CrossRef]
20. Verma, A.A.; Khuu, W.; Tadrous, M.; Gomes, T.; Mamdani, M.M. Fixed-dose combination antihypertensive medications, adherence, and clinical outcomes: A population-based retrospective cohort study. *PLoS Med.* **2018**, *15*, e1002584. [CrossRef] [PubMed]
21. Whelton, P.K.; Carey, R.M.; Aronow, W.S.; Casey, D.E., Jr.; Collins, K.J.; Dennison Himmelfarb, C.; DePalma, S.M.; Gidding, S.; Jamerson, K.A.; Jones, D.W.; et al. 2017 ACC/AHA/AAPA/ABC/ACPM/AGS/APhA/ASH/ASPC/NMA/PCNA Guideline for the Prevention, Detection, Evaluation, and Management of High Blood Pressure in Adults: Executive Summary: A Report of the American College of Cardiology/American Heart Association Task Force on Clinical Practice Guidelines. *Hypertension* **2018**, *71*, 1269–1324.
22. You, S.C.; Park, H.; Yoon, D.; Park, S.; Joung, B.; Park, R.W. Olmesartan is not associated with the risk of enteropathy: A Korean nationwide observational cohort study. *Korean J. Intern. Med.* **2019**, *34*, 90–98. [CrossRef]
23. Hirohata, A.; Yamamoto, K.; Miyoshi, T.; Hatanaka, K.; Hirohata, S.; Yamawaki, H.; Komatsubara, I.; Murakami, M.; Hirose, E.; Sato, S.; et al. Impact of olmesartan on progression of coronary atherosclerosis a serial volumetric intravascular ultrasound analysis from the OLIVUS (impact of OLmesarten on progression of coronary atherosclerosis: Evaluation by intravascular ultrasound) trial. *J. Am. Coll. Cardiol.* **2010**, *55*, 976–982. [CrossRef]
24. Swindle, J.P.; Buzinec, P.; Iorga, S.R.; Ramaswamy, K.; Panjabi, S. Long-term clinical and economic outcomes associated with angiotensin II receptor blocker use in hypertensive patients. *Curr. Med. Res. Opin.* **2011**, *27*, 1719–1731. [CrossRef]

25. Ridker, P.M.; Danielson, E.; Fonseca, F.A.; Genest, J.; Gotto, A.M., Jr.; Kastelein, J.J.; Koenig, W.; Libby, P.; Lorenzatti, A.J.; MacFadyen, J.G.; et al. Rosuvastatin to prevent vascular events in men and women with elevated C-reactive protein. *N. Engl. J. Med.* **2008**, *359*, 2195–2207. [CrossRef] [PubMed]
26. Yusuf, S.; Lonn, E.; Pais, P.; Bosch, J.; López-Jaramillo, P.; Zhu, J.; Xavier, D.; Avezum, A.; Leiter, L.A.; Piegas, L.S.; et al. Blood-Pressure and Cholesterol Lowering in Persons without Cardiovascular Disease. *N. Engl. J. Med.* **2016**, *374*, 2032–2043. [CrossRef] [PubMed]
27. Lee, C.W.; Kang, S.J.; Ahn, J.M.; Song, H.G.; Lee, J.Y.; Kim, W.J.; Park, D.W.; Lee, S.W.; Kim, Y.H.; Park, S.W.; et al. Comparison of effects of atorvastatin (20 mg) versus rosuvastatin (10 mg) therapy on mild coronary atherosclerotic plaques (from the ARTMAP trial). *Am. J. Cardiol.* **2012**, *109*, 1700–1704. [CrossRef] [PubMed]
28. Ruilope, L.; Schaefer, A. The fixed-dose combination of olmesartan/amlodipine was superior in central aortic blood pressure reduction compared with perindopril/amlodipine: A randomized, double-blind trial in patients with hypertension. *Adv. Ther.* **2013**, *30*, 1086–1099. [CrossRef]
29. Oh, M.; Shin, J.G.; Ahn, S.; Kim, B.H.; Kim, J.Y.; Shin, H.J.; Shin, H.J.; Ghim, J.L. Pharmacokinetic comparison of a fixed-dose combination versus concomitant administration of amlodipine, olmesartan, and rosuvastatin in healthy adult subjects. *Drug Des. Devel. Ther.* **2019**, *13*, 991–997. [CrossRef]
30. Park, S.J.; Rhee, S.J. Real-World Effectiveness and Safety of a Single-Pill Combination of Olmesartan/Amlodipine/Hydrochlorothiazide in Korean Patients with Essential Hypertension (RESOLVE): A Large, Observational, Retrospective, Cohort Study. *Adv. Ther.* **2020**, *37*, 3500–3514. [CrossRef]

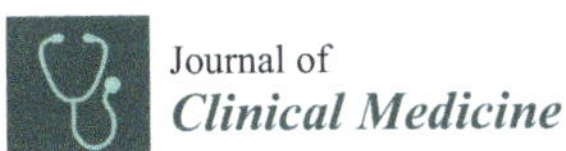
Journal of
Clinical Medicine

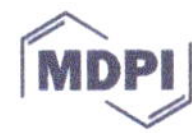

Article

A Novel Quantitative Parameter for Static Myocardial Computed Tomography: Myocardial Perfusion Ratio to the Aorta

Takanori Kouchi [1], Yuki Tanabe [1,*], Takumasa Takemoto [1], Kazuki Yoshida [1], Yuta Yamamoto [1], Shigehiro Miyazaki [2], Naoki Fukuyama [1], Hikaru Nishiyama [1], Shinji Inaba [2], Naoto Kawaguchi [1], Tomoyuki Kido [1], Osamu Yamaguchi [2] and Teruhito Kido [1]

1 Department of Radiology, Graduate School of Medicine, Ehime University, Shitsukawa, Toon 791-0295, Japan; taka.xlay56@gmail.com (T.K.); take10toku6@gmail.com (T.T.); kn0wn951753@gmail.com (K.Y.); please_zantetsu@yahoo.co.jp (Y.Y.); n.fukuyama68@gmail.com (N.F.); nishiyama.hikaru.mj@ehime-u.ac.jp (H.N.); n.kawa1113@gmail.com (N.K.); tomozo0421@gmail.com (T.K.); terukido@m.ehime-u.ac.jp (T.K.)
2 Department of Cardiology, Pulmonology, Hypertension and Nephrology, Graduate School of Medicine, Ehime University, Shitsukawa, Toon 791-0295, Japan; shigehiro.miyazaki.0123@gmail.com (S.M.); inaba226@gmail.com (S.I.); yamaguti@m.ehime-u.ac.jp (O.Y.)
* Correspondence: yuki.tanabe.0225@gmail.com

Abstract: We evaluated the feasibility of myocardial perfusion ratio to the aorta (MPR) in static computed tomography perfusion (CTP) for detecting myocardial perfusion abnormalities assessed by single-photon emission computed tomography (SPECT). Twenty-five patients with suspected coronary artery disease who underwent dynamic CTP and SPECT were retrospectively evaluated. CTP images scanned at a sub-optimal phase for detecting myocardial perfusion abnormalities were selected from dynamic CTP images and used as static CTP images in the present study. The diagnostic accuracy of MPR derived from static CTP was compared to those of visual assessment and conventional quantitative parameters such as myocardial CT attenuation (HU) and transmural perfusion ratio (TPR). The area under the curve of MPR (0.84; 95% confidence interval [CI], 0.76–0.90) was significantly higher than those of myocardial CT attenuation (0.73; 95% CI, 0.65–0.79) and TPR (0.76; 95% CI, 0.67–0.83) ($p < 0.05$). Sensitivity and specificity were 67% (95% CI, 54–77%) and 90% (95% CI, 86–92%) for visual assessment, 51% (95% CI, 39–63%) and 86% (95% CI, 82–89%) for myocardial CT attenuation, 63% (95% CI, 51–74%) and 84% (95% CI, 80–88%) for TPR, and 78% (95% CI, 66–86%) and 84% (95% CI, 80–88%) for MPR, respectively. MPR showed higher diagnostic accuracy for detecting myocardial perfusion abnormality compared with myocardial CT attenuation and TPR.

Keywords: computed tomography; computed tomography perfusion; myocardial perfusion abnormality

Citation: Kouchi, T.; Tanabe, Y.; Takemoto, T.; Yoshida, K.; Yamamoto, Y.; Miyazaki, S.; Fukuyama, N.; Nishiyama, H.; Inaba, S.; Kawaguchi, N.; et al. A Novel Quantitative Parameter for Static Myocardial Computed Tomography: Myocardial Perfusion Ratio to the Aorta. *J. Clin. Med.* **2022**, *11*, 1816. https://doi.org/10.3390/jcm11071816

Academic Editors: Koichi Node and Atsushi Tanaka

Received: 17 December 2021
Accepted: 22 March 2022
Published: 25 March 2022

1. Introduction

In coronary artery disease (CAD), it is important to assess the significance of myocardial ischemia to determine the optimal treatment strategy before revascularization [1,2]. In current practice, various myocardial perfusion imaging (MPI) techniques such as single-photon emission computed tomography (SPECT), magnetic resonance (MR) imaging, or positron emission tomography (PET) have been widely used [3–6]. Recently, developments in computed tomography (CT) technology have fulfilled the technical prerequisites for the application of stress myocardial CT perfusion (CTP) for the evaluation of CAD [7]. Two main techniques have been applied for myocardial CTP imaging: static CTP and dynamic CTP [8]. Static CTP is mainly evaluated by visual assessment, while dynamic CTP is assessed using several quantitative parameters derived from the time attenuation curve, which is advantageous for adapting to varying ischemic severities and for assessing the therapeutic effect of revascularization therapy with high objectivity and reproducibility [9,10]. However, dynamic CTP has a disadvantage; its radiation exposure is relatively high compared with that for static CTP (9.23 mSv vs. 5.93 mSv) [11]. Moreover, dynamic CTP requires wide detector coverage and high temporal resolution to obtain the data of the whole heart without temporal and spatial gaps [12]. Hence, a robust quantitative evaluation of static CTP imaging is required. Semi-quantitative parameters for static CTP imaging have been proposed, such as myocardial CT attenuation and transmural perfusion ratio (TPR), but the diagnostic accuracy of these parameters has been reported to be inferior to that of visual assessment for the detection of myocardial ischemia [13]. We introduced the myocardial perfusion ratio to the aorta (MPR) as a new quantitative parameter for static CTP and evaluated its feasibility for identifying myocardial perfusion abnormalities.

2. Materials and Methods

2.1. Study Population

This retrospective study was approved by our institution's human research committee (registration number: 1810021). The need for informed consent was waived due to the retrospective nature of the study. Thirty patients from our cardiac database who underwent stress dynamic myocardial CTP and SPECT-MPI between February 2013 and March 2015 were enrolled in this study. In the present study, static myocardial CTP images were retrospectively extracted from dynamic myocardial CTP imaging data. The attending physician determined the indications for myocardial CTP and SPECT for the assessment of CAD due to effort angina via ST-T changes on electrocardiography, reduction in angina symptoms after administration of nitroglycerin, or multiple coronary risk factors. The exclusion criteria were as follows: (1) cardiomyopathy; (2) left ventricular ejection fraction <20%; (3) greater than first-degree atrioventricular block; (4) left complete bundle branch block; (5) valvular heart disease; (6) history of coronary artery bypass grafting; and (7) poor image quality of stress dynamic CTP and SPECT. The radiation exposure was calculated using the dose-length product with a conversion factor of 0.014, as described previously [14].

2.2. Dynamic Myocardial CTP Scan Protocol

An established dynamic myocardial CTP scan protocol was performed for this study [15]. All stress dynamic myocardial CTP scans were performed using a 256-slice multidetector row CT scanner (Brilliance iCT; Philips Healthcare, Cleveland, OH, USA) and an automatic dual injector (Stellant DualFlow; Nihon Medrad KK, Osaka, Japan). A timing bolus scan was performed to estimate the scan timing and contrast medium (CM) concentration for coronary CT angiography (CTA) using a 20% solution of the CM (iopamidol 370 mg iodine/mL; Bayer Yakuhin, Ltd., Osaka, Japan) diluted with saline (5.0 mL/s for 10 s), followed by a saline chaser (5.0 mL/s for 4 s) [16]. The timing bolus scan was performed with axial data acquisition at the level of the ascending aorta. Three minutes after stress loading via intravenous infusion of adenosine triphosphate (Adetphos-L KOWA injection 20 mg; Kowa Company Ltd., Tokyo, Japan; 0.16 mg/kg/min, for 5 min), a stress dynamic CTP scan was performed for 30 consecutive cardiac cycles with the prospective electrocardiography-gated dynamic mode, which targets a phase of 40% RR interval using a bolus of CM (50 mL, 5.0 mL/s for 10 s) followed by a saline chaser (5.0 mL/s for 4 s). The scan parameters for the timing bolus scan were as follows: tube current of 50 mA; tube voltage of 120 kVp; and collimation at 2 × 16 × 0.625 mm. The scan parameters of the dynamic CTP scan were as follows: tube current of 80 mAs; tube voltage of 100 kVp; and collimation at 64 × 1.25 mm. Subsequently, CTA was performed using a diluted CM followed by a saline chaser, as previously described [16].

2.3. Analysis of Aortic Peak Enhancement in Timing Bolus and Dynamic CTP Scans

The timing bolus scan and dynamic CTP scan data sets were transferred to a dedicated software (Synapse Vincent ver.5; Fujifilm Medical Systems, Tokyo, Japan). A radiological technologist (9 years of experience in cardiac imaging) independently set the regions of interest (ROI) within the ascending aorta and measured aortic peak enhancement (PE) for each timing bolus scan and dynamic CTP scan data.

2.4. Post-Processing and Image Analysis of Myocardial CTP Imaging

A series of dynamic CTP images were reconstructed using a 360° reconstruction algorithm. Elastic registration and a spatiotemporal filter were used to reduce the image noise spatially and temporally through a dedicated workstation (IntelliSpace Portal; Philips Healthcare, Amsterdam, The Netherlands). For all cases, one radiological technologist (9 years of experience in cardiac CT imaging) selected a sub-optimal phase from dynamic CTP images as static CTP images according to the results of a previous study [17]. A short-axis view from the base to the apex of the left ventricle with 5 mm thickness without overlap was obtained using multi-planar reformation.

For qualitative assessment, one radiologist and cardiologist (6 years of experience in cardiac CT imaging each), both of whom were blinded to all other data, visually assessed all static CTP images to identify myocardial perfusion abnormalities as low-attenuation areas according to the 16-segment model [18]. The window width and level were arbitrarily adjusted to the optimal settings in each case. The final assessment was obtained through consensus. For quantitative assessment, another radiologist (7 years of experience in cardiac CT imaging) analyzed endocardial CT attenuation, TPR, and MPR using commercially available software (Synapse Vincent ver.5; Fujifilm Medical Systems, Tokyo, Japan) according to the 16-segment model [18]. The ROIs were set within both the endocardial and epicardial myocardium in each segment to calculate myocardial CT attenuation. MPR was defined as the endocardial CT enhancement of a specific segment divided by the PE of the ascending aorta in the timing bolus scan (Figure 1). TPR was defined as the endocardial CT attenuation of a specific segment divided by the mean of the epicardial CT attenuation of all segments [19]. To determine the inter-observer agreement of quantitative parameters, ten randomly selected patients were analyzed by a radiologist blinded to all other data (8 years of experience in cardiac CT imaging).

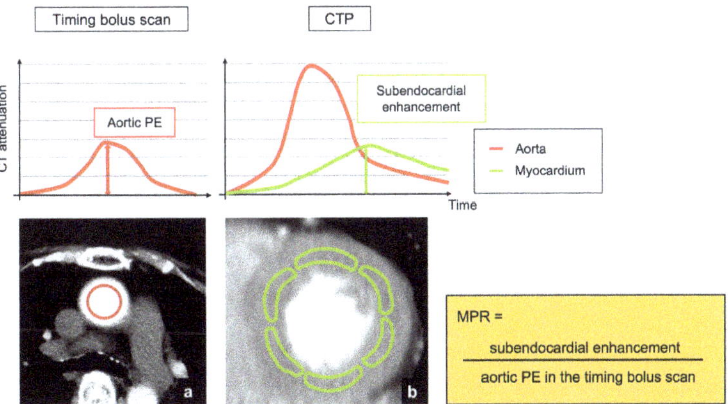

Figure 1. Analysis of MPR derived from myocardial CTP and timing bolus scan. (**a**) An axial image at the level of the ascending aorta in the timing bolus scan. (**b**) A short-axis view of left ventricle which was obtained from the static CTP image. PE was defined as the difference between baseline and peak CT attenuation of the aorta. A sub-optimal phase of dynamic CTP series was selected as static CTP image. MPR was calculated as follows: MPR = subendocardial enhancement/aortic PE in the timing bolus scan. CTP, computed tomography perfusion; PE, peak enhancement; MPR, myocardial perfusion ratio.

2.5. SPECT-MPI Scan Protocol and Image Analysis

A stress/rest SPECT-MPI was performed using a cadmium zinc telluride camera (Discovery NM 530c, GE Healthcare, Princeton, NJ, USA), as previously described [20]. Stress SPECT scans were performed 60 min after an injection of 99mTc-tetrofosmin (Myoview; Nihon Medi-Physics Co., Ltd., Tokyo, Japan) or 99mTc-sestamibi (Cardiolite; FUJIFILM RI Pharma Co., Ltd., Tokyo, Japan) at a dose range of 296–370 MBq. Four hours later, a rest SPECT scan was performed with 740 MBq of 99mTc myocardial perfusion agent. Cardiac long- and short-axis views were obtained using acquired perfusion data of the patients in the supine position.

Two radiologists (7 and 12 years of experience in SPECT-MPI), who were blinded to all other data, semi-quantitatively assessed stress and rest SPECT images using a 5-point scale (0 = normal, 1 = mildly reduced; 2 = moderately reduced; 3 = severely reduced, and 4 = absent). Discrepancies were resolved by consensus. A myocardial segment with a score ≥2 in the stress image was defined as an abnormal perfusion segment [21]. Reversible perfusion abnormality that was present in the stress state and resolved at rest state indicated ischemia. Fixed perfusion abnormality, which was present in both stress and rest states in the same segment, indicated infarction.

2.6. Statistical Analysis

Continuous variable data were expressed as mean (standard deviation) or median (25th–75th percentiles) based on the Shapiro–Wilk test results. The scan heart rates were compared during stress and resting CT using a paired *t*-test. The correlation in the aortic peak enhancement between the timing bolus and dynamic CTP scans was evaluated using Pearson's correlation coefficient. The inter-observer agreements for visual assessment of static myocardial CTP and SPECT-MPI were assessed using the Cohen κ value. The inter-observer agreement for endocardial CT attenuation, TPR, and MPR was assessed using the interclass correlation coefficient (ICC). The endocardial CT attenuation, TPR, and MPR were compared between normal and abnormal perfusion segments using the Mann–Whitney U test. The diagnostic accuracy of visual assessment, endocardial CT attenuation, TPR, and MPR for detecting myocardial perfusion abnormality assessed by SPECT-MPI were analyzed by receiver operating characteristic curve analysis (ROC) and compared using Delong's test [22]. The cut-off values of endocardial CT attenuation, TPR, and MPR for identifying myocardial perfusion abnormality were determined using Youden's index. The sensitivity, specificity, positive predictive value, negative predictive value, and area under the receiver operating characteristic curve (AUC) with 95% confidence intervals were also analyzed for visual assessment, endocardial CT attenuation, TPR, and MPR. Statistical significance was set at $p < 0.05$. Statistical analyses were performed using JMP software (version 13.0; SAS Institute, Cary, NC, USA).

3. Results

3.1. Study Population

Of the 30 patients, 5 were excluded because of a history of coronary artery bypass grafting ($n = 1$), cardiomyopathy ($n = 1$), and poor image quality in dynamic CTP due to insufficient breath-hold ($n = 3$), with 25 patients finally enrolled. Table 1 shows patient characteristics. No patient experienced any cardiac events during their imaging session. The scan heart rate increased significantly from 65.4 (10.2) beats/min at rest to 80.0 (8.0) beats/min at stress CTP scans ($p < 0.0001$). The mean effective radiation doses for timing bolus scan and dynamic CTP were 75.1 (8.4) and 754.4 (0.7) (DLP), respectively. The total amount of CM used in the timing bolus scan and dynamic CTP was 59.1 (2.6) mL.

Table 1. Patient characteristics.

Age (Years)	70.5 (9.5)
Men (%)	19 (76%)
Body mass index (kg/m^2)	24.1 (3.1)
Coronary risk factors (number [%])	
Hypertension	18 (72%)
Dyslipidemia	12 (48%)
Diabetes mellitus	8 (32%)
Positive smoking history	16 (64%)
Family history of coronary artery disease	10 (40%)
HR (bpm)	
Baseline	65.4 (10.2)
Stress	80.0 (8.0)
Time periods between CT and SPECT (days)	27 (13–43)

Data are expressed as mean (standard deviation), median (interquartile range), or N (%). HR, heart rate; CT, computed tomography; SPECT, single-photon emission computed tomography.

3.2. Characteristics of Myocardial Segments Assessed by SPECT-MPI

The interobserver agreement for perfusion abnormality on SPECT-MPI assessment was 0.83, and we concluded that the reliability was satisfactory (>0.70). Of the 400 segments, 63 were diagnosed as abnormal perfusion segments. Of the abnormal perfusion segments, 14 were diagnosed as ischemic segments and 49 were diagnosed as infarcted segments.

3.3. Aortic Peak Enhancement in Timing Bolus Scan and Dynamic CTP Scan

The aortic peak enhancements were 80.8 (18.1) HU in the timing bolus scan and 393.8 (91.7) HU in the dynamic CTP scan. There was a significant correlation between the aortic peak enhancement of the timing bolus and dynamic CTP scans ($r = 0.84$, $p < 0.0001$).

3.4. Comparisons in Endocardial CT Attenuation, TPR, and MPR between Normal and Abnormal Perfusion Segments

The interobserver agreement of the endocardial CT attenuation, TPR, and MPR were 0.96 (0.95–0.97), 0.84 (0.79–0.88), and 0.95 (0.94–0.97), respectively. The endocardial CT attenuations in normal and abnormal perfusion segments were 128 (112–144) and 106 (95–124) HU; TPR in normal and abnormal perfusion segments were 1.0 (0.9–1.0) and 0.9 (0.8–1.0); and MPR in normal and abnormal perfusion segments were 1.0 (0.9–1.1) and 0.7 (0.5–0.8). There were significant differences in endocardial CT attenuation, TPR, and MPR between the normal and abnormal perfusion segments ($p < 0.0001$).

3.5. Diagnostic Accuracy of Visual Assessment, Endocardial CT Attenuation, TPR, and MPR

The interobserver agreement for perfusion abnormality on visual CTP assessment was 0.74, and we concluded that the reliability was satisfactory (>0.70). The cut-off values of endocardial CT attenuation, TPR, and MPR were 106 HU, 0.92, and 0.81, respectively. The diagnostic accuracy for identifying myocardial perfusion abnormalities is summarized in Table 2. The sensitivity and specificity levels for detecting myocardial perfusion abnormalities were 67% (54–77%) and 90% (86–92%) for visual assessment, 51% (39–63%) and 86% (82–89%) for endocardial CT attenuation, 63% (51–74%) and 84% (80–88%) for TPR, and 78% (66–86%) and 84% (80–88%) for MPR, respectively. The AUC for identifying myocardial perfusion abnormality was 0.78 (0.71–0.84) for visual assessment, 0.73 (0.65–0.79) for endocardial CT attenuation, 0.76 (0.67–0.83) for TPR, and 0.84 (0.76–0.9) for MPR (Figure 2). The AUC of MPR was significantly higher than that of endocardial CT attenuation and TPR ($p = 0.0013$ for endocardial CT attenuation; $p = 0.044$ for TPR), while there was no significant difference in the AUC between MPR and visual assessment ($p = 0.103$). Representative clinical cases are shown in Figures 3–5.

Table 2. Diagnostic accuracy of MPR, TPR, endocardial CT attenuation, and visual assessment for detection of myocardial perfusion abnormality.

	Sensitivity (%)	Specificity (%)	PPV (%)	NPV (%)
MPR	78 (66–86)	84 (80–88)	48 (39–58)	95 (92–97)
TPR	63 (51–74)	84 (80–88)	43 (33–53)	92 (89–95)
CT attenuation (HU)	51 (39–63)	86 (82–89)	41 (30–52)	90 (87–93)
Visual assessment	67 (54–77)	90 (86–92)	55 (43–65)	93 (90–96)

Data are expressed as percentage (95% confidence interval). MPR, myocardial perfusion ratio; TPR, transmural perfusion ratio; CT, computed tomography; PPV, positive predictive value; NPV, negative predictive value.

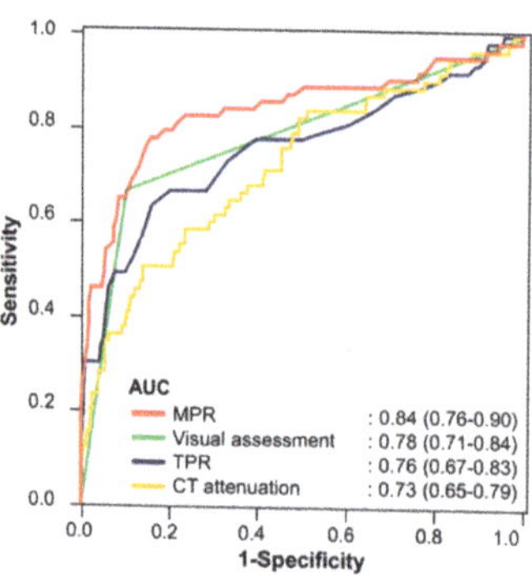

Figure 2. ROC curves of MPR, TPR, endocardial CT attenuation, and visual assessment for the detection of myocardial perfusion abnormality. The AUCs of MPR and visual assessment are comparable, and the AUC of MPR is significantly higher than those of TPR and endocardial CT attenuation. The 95% confidence intervals of the AUCs are shown in parentheses. ROC, receiver operating characteristic; MPR, myocardial perfusion ratio; TPR, transmural perfusion ratio; CT, computed tomography; AUC, area under the curve.

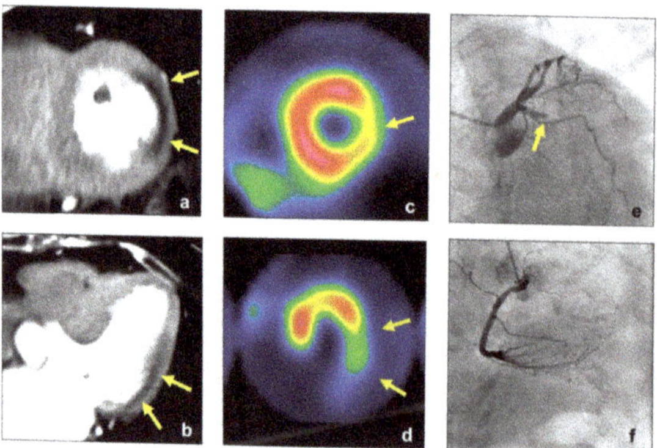

Figure 3. A 75-year-old woman with effort angina. Stress CTP image of the left ventricle showed a perfusion abnormality in the lateral wall (yellow arrow, (**a**,**b**)), and MPR in this lesion was lower than the cut-off value of MPR in this study (0.60 < cut-off value: 0.81). SPECT ((**c**,**d**), stress) showed a perfusion abnormality in the lateral wall (yellow arrow). ICA ((**e**), LCA, (**f**), RCA) revealed chronic total occlusion within the LCX. CTP, computed tomography perfusion; MPR, myocardial perfusion ratio; SPECT, single-photon emission computed tomography; ICA, invasive coronary angiography; LCA, left coronary artery; RCA, right coronary artery; LCX, left circumflex coronary artery.

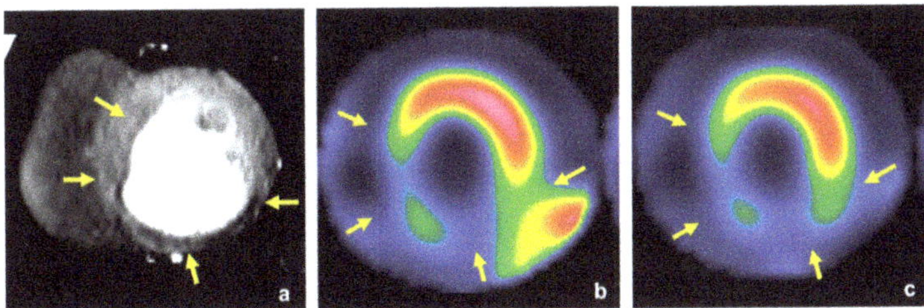

Figure 4. A 58-year-old man with effort angina. Stress CTP image of the left ventricle showed extensive myocardial perfusion abnormalities in the inferior, septal, and lateral inferior wall (yellow arrow, (**a**)). The perfusion abnormalities were detected with MPR (0.50 < cut-off value: 0.81), but not detected with TPR (0.96 > cut-off value: 0.92). SPECT ((**b**), stress; (**c**), rest) showed fixed perfusion abnormalities in these lesions, which indicated extensive old myocardial infarction (yellow arrow). CTP, computed tomography perfusion; MPR, myocardial perfusion ratio; TPR, transmural perfusion ratio; SPECT, single-photon emission computed tomography.

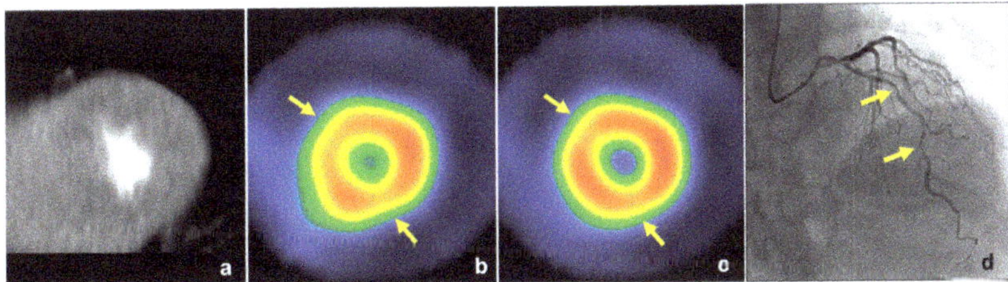

Figure 5. A 64-year-old man with effort angina. No obvious low-attenuation area was observed in the stress CTP image for the visual assessment (**a**), but the perfusion abnormalities were detected with MPR in the anterior and inferior myocardium of the apex (MPR: 0.69 and 0.71 < cut-off value: 0.81, respectively). SPECT ((**b**), stress; (**c**), rest) showed reversible perfusion abnormalities in the anterior and inferior myocardium in the apex (yellow arrow). ICA revealed tandem lesions with moderate and severe stenosis in the LAD (yellow arrow, (**d**)). The FFR of LAD was 0.68. CTP, computed tomography perfusion; MPR, myocardial perfusion ratio; SPECT, single-photon emission computed tomography; ICA, invasive coronary angiography; LAD, left anterior descending artery; FFR, fractional flow reserve.

4. Discussion

The main findings of this study were as follows: (1) there were significant differences in MPR, myocardial CT attenuation, and TPR when comparing a myocardium with normal and abnormal perfusion; (2) the MPR had significantly higher diagnostic accuracy for detecting myocardial perfusion abnormality than myocardial CT attenuation and TPR; and (3) the MPR had higher sensitivity for detecting myocardial perfusion abnormality in comparison with visual assessment.

For static CTP imaging, myocardial CT attenuation is a simple quantitative parameter, but it is affected by various pathophysiological differences, such as the patient's body weight and cardiac function [15]. Indeed, myocardial blood flow assessed by [^{15}O] H_2O PET was variable even in healthy people [23]. Tanabe et al. reported that these variations could be corrected by calculating the PE ratio of the myocardium to the aorta [24]. However, this correction method is not available for static CTP because it is impossible to accurately measure aortic PE. In this study, we corrected for myocardial CT enhancement with aortic PE obtained in a timing bolus scan with diluted CM, which was scanned for coronary CTA. Kawaguchi et al. reported that observed enhancement within coronary CTA was made uniform by adjusting the amount of CM based on the results of the timing bolus scan, despite individual differences regarding clinical background [15]. The aortic PE in dynamic CTP scan can be predicted using timing bolus scan data, and there was a good correlation in the aortic PE between the timing bolus and dynamic CTP scans in our results. Therefore, MPR could correct the variability of myocardial CT attenuation and showed higher diagnostic accuracy for detecting myocardial perfusion abnormalities than myocardial CT attenuation.

TPR is another quantitative parameter proposed in static CTP scans. TPR is a stable parameter that can be used to calculate the ratio of subendocardial CT attenuation to subepicardial CT attenuation [19]. Yang et al. reported that TPR had higher diagnostic accuracy for the detection of myocardial ischemia than myocardial CT attenuation, as replicated in the present results [13]. Furthermore, the MPR had a significantly higher diagnostic accuracy than TPR in our study. The reason for this was that TPR showed higher false-negative results compared with MPR. Ko et al. reported that TPR was falsely normalized in the presence of balanced transmural ischemia because both subendocardial and subepicardial CT attenuation were decreased [25]. In the present study, most of the false-negative results were observed in patients with extensive perfusion abnormalities. That being said, MPR is an enhancement ratio of the subendocardial myocardium to the ascending aorta; thus, it has a robust capability for detecting myocardial abnormalities even in cases with extensive perfusion abnormality.

Visual assessment is a standard method for the assessment of static myocardial CTP imaging. According to our results, the visual assessment had higher specificity and lower sensitivity than the MPR. Yuehua et al. also reported a low sensitivity and high specificity of visual assessment (62.7% and 97.7%, respectively) for detecting myocardial ischemia [26]. The reason for the high specificity in visual assessment is that it has the advantage of clarifying false perfusion abnormalities, such as beam hardening artifacts and motion artifacts. Visual assessment can identify these artifacts, which usually have a triangular shape, originate from the region of high attenuation next to it, and do not conform to vascular territories [27]. The reason for the low sensitivity in visual assessment is that it might miss mild perfusion abnormality due to the small difference in CT attenuation between normal and ischemic myocardium [26]. A previous animal study showed that the difference in myocardial CT attenuation between normal and ischemic myocardium was small in mild CAD [28]. Therefore, visual assessment requires an optimal adjustment of window width/level and substantial experience in myocardial CTP imaging. MPR allows for the quantitative assessment of myocardial perfusion using the cut-off value, which leads to lower dependence on the experience of observers than with visual assessment. Indeed, the MPR showed higher sensitivity for detecting myocardial perfusion abnormality than the visual assessment in the present study.

In the present study, we suggested the MPR as a novel quantitative parameter for static myocardial CTP imaging. MPR has the potential to reveal myocardial perfusion abnormalities that may be difficult for conventional quantitative parameters (e.g., myocardial CT attenuation, TPR) to detect. Then, MPR could be complementarily useful by utilizing the higher sensitivity for the cases in which myocardial perfusion abnormalities are not clearly detected by the visual assessment such as mild CAD in clinical practice. In a meta-analysis, myocardial CTP imaging had comparable diagnostic accuracy with conventional MPI (SPECT, MR, and PET) for detecting hemodynamically significant CAD [29]. Additionally, myocardial CTP imaging had some clinical advantages in comparison with these conventional MPI, such as higher accessibility, lower cost, and integration with coronary CTA [30,31]. Recently, new CT technologies such as ultra-high spatial resolution CT and photon-counting CT have been developed, which will lead to the further evolution of myocardial CTP imaging [32,33]. Myocardial CTP imaging has the potential to be widespread in future, and MPR will be one of the quantitative parameters for myocardial CTP imaging.

This study had several limitations. First, it was a retrospective, single-center study with a small sample size. Second, we did not evaluate coronary CTA because we focused on the feasibility of MPR for detecting myocardial perfusion abnormalities in static myocardial CTP imaging. Third, patients with myocardial infarction were not excluded from the present study population, which might have led to the lower diagnostic accuracy of TPR. However, myocardial CTP imaging will be performed in patients with myocardial infarction in the real world, especially in patients with unrecognized myocardial infarction. Finally, the static CTP images were derived from the dynamic CTP data in the present study, and the scan parameters might not be optimal for static CTP imaging. Further studies are required to evaluate the feasibility of MPR in the optimal setting for static CTP imaging.

In conclusion, MPR of the myocardium to the aorta using a timing bolus scan is a feasible quantitative parameter for assessing myocardial perfusion in static CTP imaging. MPR has a high diagnostic accuracy for detecting myocardial perfusion abnormalities, independent of substantial individual variations.

Author Contributions: Conceptualization, T.K. (Takanori Kouchi), and Y.T.; methodology, T.K. (Takanori Kouchi), and Y.T.; validation, all authors; formal analysis, T.K. (Takanori Kouchi), and Y.T.; investigation, T.K. (Takanori Kouchi), Y.T., T.T., K.Y., Y.Y., S.M., N.F., and H.N.; resources, S.M., S.I., and O.Y.; data curation, T.K. (Takanori Kouchi); writing—original draft preparation, T.K. (Takanori Kouchi), and Y.T.; writing—review and editing, N.K. and T.K. (Tomoyuki Kido); visualization, T.K. (Takanori Kouchi); supervision, O.Y. and T.K. (Teruhito Kido); project administration, T.K. (Teruhito Kido) All authors have read and agreed to the published version of the manuscript.

Funding: This work was supported by JSPS KAKENHI Grant Number JP20K16760.

Institutional Review Board Statement: This retrospective study was approved by the Institution's Human Research Committee (registration number: 1810021).

Informed Consent Statement: The need for patient consent was waived by the institutional ethics committee.

Data Availability Statement: Data can be obtained from the corresponding author upon reasonable request.

Conflicts of Interest: The authors declare no conflict of interest.

References

1. Moroi, M.; Yamashina, A.; Tsukamoto, K.; Nishimura, T. The J-ACCESS Investigators. Coronary revascularization does not decrease cardiac events in patients with stable ischemic heart disease but might do in those who showed moderate to severe ischemia. *Int. J. Cardiol.* **2012**, *158*, 246–252. [CrossRef] [PubMed]
2. Nudi, F.; Neri, G.; Schillaci, O.; Pinto, A.; Procaccini, E.; Vetere, M.; Tomai, F.; Frati, G.; Biondi-Zoccai, G. Time to and risk of cardiac events after myocardial perfusion scintigraphy. *J. Cardiol.* **2015**, *66*, 125–129. [CrossRef] [PubMed]
3. Hachamovitch, R.; Hayes, S.W.; Friedman, J.D.; Cohen, I.; Berman, D.S. Comparison of the Short-Term Survival Benefit Associated With Revascularization Compared With Medical Therapy in Patients with No Prior Coronary Artery Disease Undergoing Stress Myocardial Perfusion Single Photon Emission Computed Tomography. *Circulation* **2003**, *107*, 2900–2907. [CrossRef] [PubMed]
4. Shaw, L.J.; Berman, D.S.; Maron, D.J.; Mancini, G.B.J.; Hayes, S.W.; Hartigan, P.M.; Weintraub, W.S.; O'Rourke, R.A.; Dada, M.; Spertus, J.A.; et al. Optimal medical therapy with or without percutaneous coronary intervention to re- duce ischemic burden: Results from the Clinical Outcomes Utilizing Revascularization and Aggressive Drug Evaluation (COURAGE) trial nuclear substudy. *Circulation* **2008**, *117*, 1283–1291. [CrossRef]
5. Greenwood, J.P.; Maredia, N.; Younger, J.; Brown, J.M.; Nixon, J.; Everett, C.C.; Bijsterveld, P.; Ridgway, J.P.; Radjenovic, A.; Dickinson, C.J.; et al. Cardiovascular magnetic resonance and single-photon emission computed tomography for diagnosis of coronary heart disease (CE-MARC): A prospective trial. *Lancet* **2012**, *379*, 453–460. [CrossRef]
6. Jaarsma, C.; Leiner, T.; Bekkers, S.C.; Crijns, H.J.; Wildberger, J.E.; Nagel, E.; Nelemans, P.J.; Schalla, S. Diagnostic performance of noninvasive myocardial perfusion imaging using single-photon emission computed tomography, cardiac magnetic resonance, and positron emission tomography imaging for the detection of obstructive coronary artery disease: A meta-analysis. *J. Am. Coll. Cardiol.* **2012**, *59*, 1719–1728. [CrossRef]
7. Techasith, T.; Cury, R.C. Stress Myocardial CT Perfusion: An Update and Future Perspective. *JACC Cardiovasc. Imaging* **2011**, *4*, 905–916. [CrossRef]
8. Rossi, A.; Merkus, D.; Klotz, E.; Mollet, N.; De Feyter, P.; Krestin, G. Stress Myocardial Perfusion: Imaging with Multidetector CT. *Radiology* **2014**, *270*, 25–46. [CrossRef]
9. Bamberg, F.; Becker, A.; Schwarz, F.; Marcus, R.P.; Greif, M.; Von Ziegler, F.; Blankstein, R.; Hoffmann, U.; Sommer, W.H.; Hoffmann, V.S.; et al. Detection of Hemodynamically Significant Coronary Artery Stenosis: Incremental Diagnostic Value of Dynamic CT-based Myocardial Perfusion Imaging. *Radiology* **2011**, *260*, 689–698. [CrossRef]

10. Huber, A.M.; Leber, V.; Gramer, B.M.; Muenzel, D.; Leber, A.; Rieber, J.; Schmidt, M.; Vembar, M.; Hoffmann, E.; Rummeny, E. Myocardium: Dynamic versus Single-Shot CT Perfusion Imaging. *Radiology* **2013**, *269*, 378–386. [CrossRef]
11. Danad, I.; Szymonifka, J.; Schulman-Marcus, J.; Min, J.K. Static and dynamic assessment of myocardial perfusion by computed tomography. *Eur. Hear. J.-Cardiovasc. Imaging* **2016**, *17*, 836–844. [CrossRef]
12. Kurata, A.; Kawaguchi, N.; Kido, T.; Inoue, K.; Suzuki, J.; Ogimoto, A.; Funada, J.-I.; Higaki, J.; Miyagawa, M.; Vembar, M.; et al. Qualitative and Quantitative Assessment of Adenosine Triphosphate Stress Whole-Heart Dynamic Myocardial Perfusion Imaging Using 256-Slice Computed Tomography. *PLoS ONE* **2013**, *8*, e83950. [CrossRef] [PubMed]
13. Yang, D.H.; Kim, Y.-H.; Roh, J.-H.; Kang, J.-W.; Han, D.; Jung, J.; Kim, N.; Lee, J.B.; Ahn, J.-M.; Lee, J.-Y.; et al. Stress Myocardial Perfusion CT in Patients Suspected of Having Coronary Artery Disease: Visual and Quantitative Analysis—Validation by Using Fractional Flow Reserve. *Radiology* **2015**, *276*, 715–723. [CrossRef]
14. Shrimpton, P.C.; Hillier, M.C.; A Lewis, M.; Dunn, M. National survey of doses from CT in the UK: 2003. *Br. J. Radiol.* **2006**, *79*, 968–980. [CrossRef] [PubMed]
15. Kawaguchi, N.; Kurata, A.; Kido, T.; Nishiyama, Y.; Kido, T.; Miyagawa, M.; Ogimoto, A.; Mochizuki, T. Optimization of Coronary Attenuation in Coronary Computed Tomography Angiography Using Diluted Contrast Material. *Circ. J.* **2014**, *78*, 662–670. [CrossRef] [PubMed]
16. Tanabe, Y.; Kido, T.; Uetani, T.; Kurata, A.; Kono, T.; Ogimoto, A.; Miyagawa, M.; Soma, T.; Murase, K.; Iwaki, H.; et al. Differentiation of myocardial ischemia and infarction assessed by dynamic computed tomography perfusion imaging and comparison with cardiac magnetic resonance and single-photon emission computed tomography. *Eur. Radiol.* **2016**, *26*, 3790–3801. [CrossRef] [PubMed]
17. Tanabe, Y.; Kido, T.; Kurata, A.; Uetani, T.; Fukuyama, N.; Yokoi, T.; Nishiyama, H.; Kido, T.; Miyagawa, M.; Mochizuki, T. Optimal Scan Time for Single-Phase Myocardial Computed Tomography Perfusion to Detect Myocardial Ischemia—Derivation Cohort From Dynamic Myocardial Computed Tomography Perfusion–. *Circ. J.* **2016**, *80*, 2506–2512. [CrossRef]
18. Cerqueira, M.D.; Weissman, N.J.; Dilsizian, V.; Jacobs, A.K.; Kaul, S.; Laskey, W.K.; Pennell, D.J.; Rumberger, J.A.; Ryan, T.; Verani, M.S.; et al. Standardized myocardial segmentation and nomenclature for tomographic imaging of the heart. A statement for healthcare professionals from the Cardiac Imaging Committee of the Council on Clinical Cardiology of the American Heart Association. *Circulation* **2002**, *105*, 539–542. [CrossRef]
19. George, R.T.; Arbab-Zadeh, A.; Miller, J.M.; Kitagawa, K.; Chang, H.-J.; Bluemke, D.A.; Becker, L.; Yousuf, O.; Texter, J.; Lardo, A.C.; et al. Adenosine stress 64- and 256-row detector computed tomography angiography and perfusion imaging: A pilot study evaluating the transmural extent of perfusion abnormalities to predict atherosclerosis causing myocardial ischemia. *Circ. Cardiovasc. Imaging* **2009**, *2*, 174–182. [CrossRef]
20. Nishiyama, Y.; Miyagawa, M.; Kawaguchi, N.; Nakamura, M.; Kido, T.; Kurata, A.; Kido, T.; Ogimoto, A.; Higaki, J.; Mochizuki, T. Combined Supine and Prone Myocardial Perfusion Single-Photon Emission Computed Tomography With a Cadmium Zinc Telluride Camera for Detection of Coronary Artery Disease. *Circ. J.* **2014**, *78*, 1169–1175. [CrossRef]
21. Wang, Y.; Qin, L.; Shi, X.; Zeng, Y.; Jing, H.; Schoepf, U.J.; Jin, Z. Adenosine-Stress Dynamic Myocardial Perfusion Imaging With Second-Generation Dual-Source CT: Comparison With Conventional Catheter Coronary Angiography and SPECT Nuclear Myocardial Perfusion Imaging. *Am. J. Roentgenol.* **2012**, *198*, 521–529. [CrossRef] [PubMed]
22. Delong, E.R.; Delong, D.M.; Clarke-Pearson, D.L. Comparing the Areas under Two or More Correlated Receiver Operating Characteristic Curves: A Nonparametric Approach. *Biometrics* **1988**, *44*, 837–845. [CrossRef] [PubMed]
23. Danad, I.; Raijmakers, P.G.; Appelman, Y.E.; Harms, H.J.; de Haan, S.; Oever, M.L.P.V.D.; van Kuijk, C.; Allaart, C.P.; Hoekstra, O.S.; Lammertsma, A.A.; et al. Coronary risk factors and myocardial blood flow in patients evaluated for coronary artery disease: A quantitative [15O]H_2O PET/CT study. *Eur. J. Nucl. Med. Mol. Imaging* **2011**, *39*, 102–112. [CrossRef] [PubMed]
24. Tanabe, Y.; Kido, T.; Kurata, A.; Yokoi, T.; Fukuyama, N.; Uetani, T.; Nishiyama, H.; Kawaguchi, N.; Tahir, E.; Miyagawa, M.; et al. Peak enhancement ratio of myocardium to aorta for identification of myocardial ischemia using dynamic myocardial computed tomography perfusion imaging. *J. Cardiol.* **2017**, *70*, 565–570. [CrossRef] [PubMed]
25. Ko, B.S.; Cameron, J.D.; Leung, M.; Meredith, I.T.; Leong, D.P.; Antonis, P.R.; Crossett, M.; Troupis, J.; Harper, R.; Malaiapan, Y.; et al. Combined CT coronary angiography and stress myocardial perfusion imaging for hemodynamically significant stenoses in patients with suspected coronary artery disease: A comparison with fractional flow reserve. *JACC Cardiovasc. Imaging* **2012**, *5*, 1097–1111. [CrossRef] [PubMed]
26. Li, Y.; Dai, X.; Lu, Z.; Shen, C.; Zhang, J. Diagnostic performance of quantitative, semi-quantitative, and visual analysis of dynamic CT myocardial perfusion imaging: A validation study with invasive fractional flow reserve. *Eur. Radiol.* **2021**, *31*, 525–534. [CrossRef] [PubMed]
27. Pontone, G.; Andreini, D.; I Guaricci, A.; Guglielmo, M.; Baggiano, A.; Muscogiuri, G.; Fusini, L.; Soldi, M.; Fazzari, F.; Berzovini, C.; et al. Quantitative vs. qualitative evaluation of static stress computed tomography perfusion to detect haemodynamically significant coronary artery disease. *Eur. Hear. J.-Cardiovasc. Imaging* **2018**, *19*, 1244–1252. [CrossRef]
28. Schwarz, F.; Hinkel, R.; Baloch, E.; Marcus, R.P.; Hildebrandt, K.; Sandner, T.A.; Kupatt, C.; Hoffmann, V.; Wintersperger, B.J.; Reiser, M.F.; et al. Myocardial CT perfusion imaging in a large animal model: Comparison of dynamic versus single-phase acquisitions. *JACC Cardiovasc. Imaging* **2013**, *6*, 1229–1238. [CrossRef]

29. Takx, R.A.; Blomberg, B.A.; El Aidi, H.; Habets, J.; de Jong, P.A.; Nagel, E.; Hoffmann, U.; Leiner, T. Diagnostic Accuracy of Stress Myocardial Perfusion Imaging Compared to Invasive Coronary Angiography With Fractional Flow Reserve Meta-Analysis. *Circ. Cardiovasc. Imaging* **2015**, *8*, 1. [CrossRef]
30. Rochitte, C.E.; George, R.T.; Chen, M.Y.; Arbab-Zadeh, A.; Dewey, M.; Miller, J.M.; Niinuma, H.; Yoshioka, K.; Kitagawa, K.; Nakamori, S.; et al. Computed tomography angiography and perfusion to assess coronary artery stenosis causing perfusion defects by single photon emission computed tomography: The CORE320 study. *Eur. Hear. J.* **2014**, *35*, 1120–1130. [CrossRef]
31. Meyer, M.; Nance, J.W.; Schoepf, U.J.; Moscariello, A.; Weininger, M.; Rowe, G.W.; Ruzsics, B.; Kang, D.K.; Chiaramida, S.A.; Schoenberg, S.O.; et al. Cost-effectiveness of substituting dual-energy CT for SPECT in the assessment of myocardial perfusion for the workup of coronary artery disease. *Eur. J. Radiol.* **2012**, *81*, 3719–3725. [CrossRef] [PubMed]
32. Papazoglou, A.S.; Karagiannidis, E.; Moysidis, D.V.; Sofidis, G.; Bompoti, A.; Stalikas, N.; Panteris, E.; Arvanitidis, C.; Herrmann, M.D.; Michaelson, J.S.; et al. Current clinical applications and potential perspective of micro-computed tomography in cardiovascular imaging: A systematic scoping review. *Hell. J. Cardiol.* **2021**, *62*, 399–407. [CrossRef] [PubMed]
33. Si-Mohamed, S.A.; Boccalini, S.; Lacombe, H.; Diaw, A.; Varasteh, M.; Rodesch, P.-A.; Dessouky, R.; Villien, M.; Tatard-Leitman, V.; Bochaton, T.; et al. Coronary CT Angiography with Photon-counting CT: First-In-Human Results. *Radiology* **2022**, *15*, 211780. [CrossRef] [PubMed]

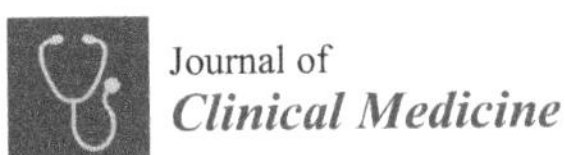

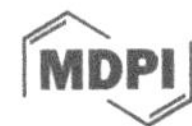

Article

A Japanese Dose of Prasugrel versus a Standard Dose of Clopidogrel in Patients with Acute Myocardial Infarction from the K-ACTIVE Registry

Hiroyoshi Mori [1,*], Takuya Mizukami [1], Atsuo Maeda [1], Kazuki Fukui [2], Yoshihiro Akashi [3], Junya Ako [4], Yuji Ikari [5], Toshiaki Ebina [6], Kouichi Tamura [7], Atsuo Namiki [8], Ichiro Michishita [9], Kazuo Kimura [10] and Hiroshi Suzuki [1]

1 Department of Cardiology, Showa University Fujigaoka Hospital, Yokohama 227-8501, Japan; mizukamit@med.showa-u.ac.jp (T.M.); atsuo@kt.rim.or.jp (A.M.); hrsuzuki@med.showa-u.ac.jp (H.S.)
2 Kanagawa Cardiovascular and Respiratory Center, Department of Cardiology, Yokohama 236-0051, Japan; fukui@kanagawa-junko.jp
3 Department of Cardiology, St. Marianna University School of Medicine, Kawasaki 216-8511, Japan; yoakashi-circ@umin.ac.jp
4 Department of Cardiology, Kitasato University School of Medicine, Sagamihiara 252-0375, Japan; jako@kitasato-u.ac.jp
5 Department of Cardiology, Tokai University School of Medicine, Isehara 259-1193, Japan; ikari@is.icc.u-tokai.ac.jp
6 Department of Laboratory Medicine, Yokohama City University Medical Center, Yokohama 232-0024, Japan; tebina@yokohama-cu.ac.jp
7 Department of Cardiology, Yokohama City University Graduate School of Medicine, Yokohama 236-0004, Japan; tamukou@med.yokohama-cu.ac.jp
8 Department of Cardiology, Kanto Rosai Hospital, Kawasaki 211-8510, Japan; namikiatsuo@kantoh.johas.go.jp
9 Department of Cardiology, Yokohama Sakae Kyosai Hospital, Yokohama 247-8581, Japan; i-michishita@yokohamasakae.jp
10 Department of Cardiology, Yokohama City University Medical Center, Yokohama 232-0024, Japan; c_kimura@yokohama-cu.ac.jp
* Correspondence: hymori@med.showa-u.ac.jp; Tel.: +81-459711151

Abstract: Background: Dual antiplatelet therapy (DAPT) with aspirin plus P2Y12 inhibitor is used as a standard therapy for patients with acute myocardial infarction (AMI) treated with drug-eluting stents (DESs). In Japan, clopidogrel was the major P2Y12 inhibitor used for a decade until the new P2Y12 inhibitor, prasugrel, was introduced. Based on clinical studies considering Japanese features, the set dose for prasugrel was reduced to 20 mg as a loading dose (LD) and 3.75 mg as a maintenance dose (MD); these values are 60 and 10 mg, respectively, globally. Despite this dose discrepancy, little real-world clinical data regarding its efficacy and safety exist. Methods: From the K-ACTIVE registry, based on the DAPT regimen, patients were divided into a prasugrel group and a clopidogrel group. The ischemic event was a composite of cardiovascular death, non-fatal MI, and non-fatal stroke. The bleeding event was type 3 or 5 bleeding based on the Bleeding Academic Research Consortium (BARC) criteria. Results: Substantially more patients were prescribed prasugrel ($n = 2786$) than clopidogrel ($n = 890$). Clopidogrel tended to be selected over prasugrel in older patients with numerous comorbidities. Before adjustments were made, the cumulative incidence of ischemic events at 1 year was significantly greater in the clopidogrel group than in the prasugrel group ($p = 0.007$), while the cumulative incidence of bleeding events at 1 year was comparable between the groups ($p = 0.131$). After adjustments were made for the age, sex, body weight, creatine level, type of AMI, history of MI, approach site, oral anticoagulation therapy, presence of multivessel disease, Killip classification, and presence of intra-aortic balloon pumping, both ischemic and bleeding events became comparable between the groups. Conclusion: A Japanese dose of prasugrel was commonly used in AMI patients in the real-world database. Both the prasugrel and clopidogrel groups showed comparable rates of 1 year ischemic and bleeding events.

Citation: Mori, H.; Mizukami, T.; Maeda, A.; Fukui, K.; Akashi, Y.; Ako, J.; Ikari, Y.; Ebina, T.; Tamura, K.; Namiki, A.; et al. A Japanese Dose of Prasugrel versus a Standard Dose of Clopidogrel in Patients with Acute Myocardial Infarction from the K-ACTIVE Registry. *J. Clin. Med.* **2022**, *11*, 2016. https://doi.org/10.3390/jcm11072016

Academic Editors: Atsushi Tanaka, Koichi Node and Ignatios Ikonomidis

Received: 19 February 2022
Accepted: 31 March 2022
Published: 4 April 2022

Keywords: aspirin; clopidogrel; prasugrel; P2Y12 inhibitor; bleeding

1. Introduction

Dual antiplatelet therapy (DAPT) with aspirin and a P2Y12 inhibitor is essential for contemporary percutaneous coronary intervention (PCI) with drug-eluting stents (DESs) in patients with acute myocardial infarction (AMI). Clopidogrel had been widely used as the P2Y12 inhibitor of choice in DAPT since 2006 in Japan. However, a considerable proportion of Japanese patients are reported to be CYP2C19 poor metabolizers (PMs), who can only attain a low concentration of the active metabolite of clopidogrel [1,2].

Prasugrel is a newer P2Y12 inhibitor with a more consistent, rapid, and pronounced inhibition of platelet activity than clopidogrel [3–5]. In an initial study from the Trial to Assess Improvement in Therapeutic Outcomes by Optimizing Platelet Inhibition with Prasugrel-Thrombolysis in Myocardial Infarction (TRITON-TIMI38) in patients with acute coronary syndrome (ACS) undergoing PCI, which included a very low proportion of East Asian patients (<1%), prasugrel at a standard dose (loading dose (LD)/maintenance dose (MD): 60/10 mg) showed significantly fewer ischemic events but a higher incidence of bleeding than clopidogrel (LD/MD: 300/75 mg) [6]. Because East Asians are known to have a higher bleeding risk than Western populations, a reduced dose of prasugrel (LD/MD: 20/3.75 mg), compared with the standard dose of clopidogrel (LD/MD: 300/75 mg) in the prasugrel group compared with clopidogrel group for Japanese patients with ACS undergoing PCI (PRASFIT-ACS) showed efficacy and safety [7,8]. Accordingly, a reduced dose of prasugrel was approved in 2014 in Japan, and the Japanese Circulation Society (JCS) guideline recommends a reduced dose of prasugrel (LD/MD: 20/3.75 mg) and standard dose of clopidogrel (LD/MD: 300/75 mg) as class I for both ACS and chronic coronary syndrome (CCS) [9]. However, despite this unique dose setting of prasugrel, little real-world clinical data regarding ischemic and bleeding events in Japanese AMI patients have been collected.

Therefore, we tried to assess the efficacy and safety between prasugrel and clopidogrel using the K-ACTIVE (Kanagawa-Acute Cardiovascular Registry) registry.

2. Materials and Methods

2.1. Study Subjects

The K-ACTIVE is an observational multicenter registry of AMI that enrolled patients from 52 PCI-capable hospitals in Kanagawa Prefecture, Japan, beginning in October 2015, including large and small, urban and rural, and educational and non-educational hospitals. This registry was approved by the local institutional review board and was registered in the University Hospital Medical Information Network (UMIN) in October 2015 (UMIN000019156). AMI was diagnosed as a ST-elevation myocardial infarction (STEMI) or non-STEMI (NSTEMI) based on the Third Universal Definition of Myocardial Infarction Consensus Document [10]. All consecutive AMI patients who presented to hospitals within 24 h of the onset of symptoms were registered. Each attending hospital was required to submit data to an online database on consecutive patients. A follow-up study of patients was performed based on the medical information available at each study site.

2.2. Study Endpoint

Patients treated between October 2015 and December 2019 were included in this study. Based on the initial DAPT regimen, patients were divided into a prasugrel group (prasugrel and aspirin) and a clopidogrel group (clopidogrel and aspirin). The selection and duration of medication, including the DAPT, was left to the attending cardiologist based on the JCS guideline [11]. As patients were included before the focused update of the JCS guideline, the duration of the DAPT was likely to be 1 year for most patients [9]. Oral anticoagulation therapy included both warfarin and direct oral anticoagulation therapy. Atrial fibrillation included paroxysmal, persistent, and continuous types. The efficacy endpoint was a composite of cardiovascular death, non-fatal MI, and non-fatal stroke including both ischemic and hemorrhagic. The safety endpoint was type 3 or 5 bleeding based on the Bleeding Academic Research Consortium (BARC) criteria. Secondary endpoints included a composite of ischemic events (cardiovascular death, non-fatal MI, and non-fatal stroke) and bleeding events (BARC type 3 or 5 bleeding).

2.3. Statistical Analysis

Continuous variables were expressed as the mean ± standard deviation or median value (25th–75th percentile), as appropriate. The normality of data was tested with the Anderson–Darling test. Categorical variables were expressed as percentages. Continuous variables were compared using a *t*-test or Wilcoxon test. Categorical variables were analyzed by a Fisher's exact test or the chi-squared test, as appropriate. The age, sex, Killip classification, creatine, use of oral anticoagulation therapy (OAC), body weight, trans-radial approach, type of AMI, previous MI, use of intra-aortic balloon pumping (IABP), and presence of multivessel disease were included in the adjusted model as confounders. Propensity scores for all patients were estimated using multivariable logistic regression models with the above-mentioned confounders. A propensity analysis was conducted using the inverse probability of treatment weights (IPTW) [12]. The cumulative incidence of efficacy endpoint, safety endpoint, and composited ischemic and bleeding events were expressed by a Kaplan–Meier curve without and with adjustment using IPTW. A subgroup analysis was also performed. The JMP 15 (SAS Institute, Cary, NC, USA) or R (version 3.6.1, R Foundation for Statistical Computing, Vienna, Austria) software programs were used to perform the statistical analyses. p-values of <0.05 were considered statistically significant.

3. Results

3.1. Study Population

Between October 2015 and December 2019, a total of 7583 patients were registered in the K-ACTIVE registry. After excluding 3179 patients with missing data regarding antiplatelet therapy and 728 patients without dual antiplatelet therapy, a total of 3676 patients who had received prasugrel (n = 2786) and clopidogrel (n = 890) were included in the study population.

3.2. Patient Characteristics

Table 1 shows the patient characteristics in each group. The clopidogrel group was older and had more comorbidities, including hypertension; diabetes; dyslipidemia; hemodialysis; and a history of MI, atrial fibrillation, and OAC therapy, than the prasugrel group. The prevalence of male gender and smoking was lower in the clopidogrel group than in the prasugrel group. Among the laboratory data, significant differences were observed in the low-density lipoprotein (LDL) cholesterol, serum creatinine, and albumin levels; the high-density lipoprotein (HDL) cholesterol and HbA1c values did not differ markedly between the groups. The height and body weight values were lower in the clopidogrel group than in the prasugrel group.

3.3. AMI Characteristics

Table 2 shows the characteristics of AMI. The prevalence of STEMI and peak creatine kinase levels were lower in the clopidogrel group than in the prasugrel group. There was no significant difference in the culprit vessel, presence of multi-vessel disease, approach site, use of thrombolysis, extracorporeal membrane oxygenation, or out-of-hospital cardiac arrest between the groups. Coronary artery bypass graft and intra-aorta balloon pumping were selected more frequently in the clopidogrel group, while PCI was selected more frequently in the prasugrel group.

Table 1. Patient characteristics.

	Prasugrel Group (n = 2786)	Clopidogrel Group (n = 890)	p-Value
Age, years	67 ± 16	71 ± 13	<0.01
Male, n (%)	2220 (79.7%)	654 (73.5%)	<0.01
Hypertension, n (%)	1779 (63.9%)	618 (69.4%)	<0.01
Diabetes, n (%)	912 (32.7%)	334 (37.5%)	<0.01
Dyslipidemia, n (%)	1052 (37.8%)	363 (40.8%)	0.11
Smoking, n (%)	1878 (67.4%)	531 (59.7%)	<0.01
Hemodialysis, n (%)	52 (1.9%)	29 (3.3%)	0.02
Previous MI, n (%)	225 (8.1%)	126 (14.2%)	<0.01
Atrial fibrillation, n (%)	165 (5.9%)	88 (9.9%)	<0.01
Previous hospital visit, n (%)	1940 (69.6%)	656 (73.7%)	0.02
Oral anticoagulation therapy, n (%)	112 (4.0%)	80 (9.0%)	<0.01
Creatine, mg/dL	0.86 (0.72–1.03)	0.91 (0.76–1.10)	<0.01
LDL, mg/dL	124 (100–151)	114 (90–43)	<0.01
HDL, mg/dL	47 (40–57)	48 (50–58)	0.14
A1c, %	5.9 (5.6–6.6)	6.0 (5.6–6.7)	0.38
Alb, g/dL	4.1 (3.7–4.4)	3.9 (3.6–4.3)	<0.01
Height, cm	165 (158–170)	163 (155–169)	<0.01
Body weight, Kg	65 (56–74)	62 (53–71)	<0.01

Data are expressed as the mean ± standard mediation or median (interquartile) or number (%). MI = myocardial infarction, LDL = low-density lipoprotein cholesterol, HDL = high-density lipoprotein cholesterol, Alb = albumin.

Table 2. AMI characteristics.

	Prasugrel Group (n = 2786)	Clopidogrel Group (n = 890)	p-Value
Systolic blood pressure	143 (123–164)	138 (119–162)	<0.01
Heart rate	78 (65–91)	79 (66–92)	0.2
Type of AMI			<0.01
STEMI	2201 (79.0%)	612 (68.8%)	
NSTEMI	585 (21.0%)	278 (31.2%)	
Peak creatine kinase	1503 (601–3224)	1141 (411–2687)	<0.01
Culprit			0.29
LMT	277 (9.9%)	107 (12.0%)	
LAD	1428 (51.3%)	437 (49.1%)	
LCX	151 (5.4%)	51 (5.7%)	
RCA	928 (33.3%)	293 (32.9%)	
Multi-vessel disease	1318 (48.9%)	409 (48.1%)	0.69
Approach			0.41
Radial	1955 (72.4%)	631 (74.3%)	
Femoral	720 (26.7%)	208 (24.5%)	
Brachial	26 (1.0%)	10 (1.2%)	
Percutaneous coronary intervention	2772 (99.5%)	861 (96.7%)	<0.01
Thrombolysis	35 (1.3%)	7 (0.8%)	0.36
CABG	22 (0.8%)	17 (1.9%)	<0.01
IABP	292 (10.5%)	116 (13.1%)	0.04
ECMO	45 (1.7%)	16 (1.8%)	0.76
OHCA	87 (3.1%)	35 (3.9%)	0.24

Table 2. *Cont.*

	Prasugrel Group (n = 2786)	Clopidogrel Group (n = 890)	p-Value
Killip classification			<0.01
1	2344 (84.1%)	697 (78.3%)	
2	136 (4.9%)	74 (8.3%)	
3	131 (4.7%)	55 (6.2%)	
4	175 (6.3%)	64 (7.2%)	

Data are expressed as median (interquartile) or number (%). AMI = acute myocardial infarction, LM = left main, LAD = left anterior descending artery, RCA = right coronary artery, LCX = left circumflex artery, TIMI = thrombolysis in myocardial infarction, PCI = percutaneous coronary intervention, CK = creatine kinase, IABP = intra-aortic balloon pumping, ECMO = extracorporeal membrane oxygenation, CABG = coronary artery bypass grafting.

3.4. Clinical Outcome

Table 3 shows the in-hospital mortality and unadjusted ischemic and bleeding events. Most of the events had a greater prevalence in the clopidogrel group than in the prasugrel group. The cumulative incidence rate of ischemic events, BARC type 3 or 5 bleeding, and composite events, which were unadjusted and adjusted by IPWT, is shown in Figure 1A–C. Ischemic events and composite events were significantly more frequent in the clopidogrel group than in the prasugrel group before adjustment (p = 0.007, p = 0.002, respectively), while bleeding events were comparable between the groups (p = 0.131). All differences became non-significant after adjustment by IPWT. The results of the subgroup analyses are shown in Figure 2A–C. Significant interactions were observed in the radial approach and hemodialysis for composite events.

Table 3. Clinical outcomes.

	Prasugrel Group (n = 2786)	Clopidogrel Group (n = 890)	p-Value
In-hospital mortality	33 (1.2%)	15 (1.7%)	0.24
Ischemic events at 1 year	69 (2.5%)	40 (4.5%)	<0.01
Cardiac death	42 (1.5%)	26 (3.0%)	<0.01
Myocardial infarction	15 (0.5%)	2 (0.2%)	0.39
Stroke	12 (0.4%)	12 (1.4%)	<0.01
Bleeding events at 1 year	24 (0.9%)	14 (1.6%)	0.08

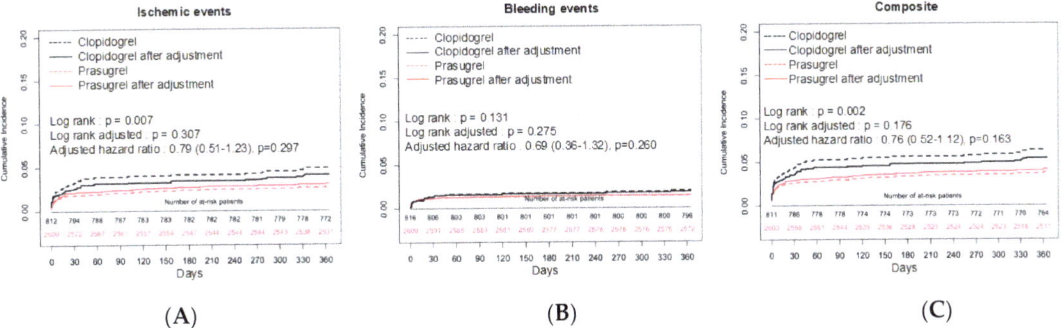

Figure 1. Kaplan–Meier survival curves showing the efficacy endpoint (ischemic events, (**A**)), safety endpoint (bleeding events, (**B**)), and composite endpoint (composite of ischemic and bleeding events, (**C**)) before and after adjustment using the inverse propensity of treatment weights.

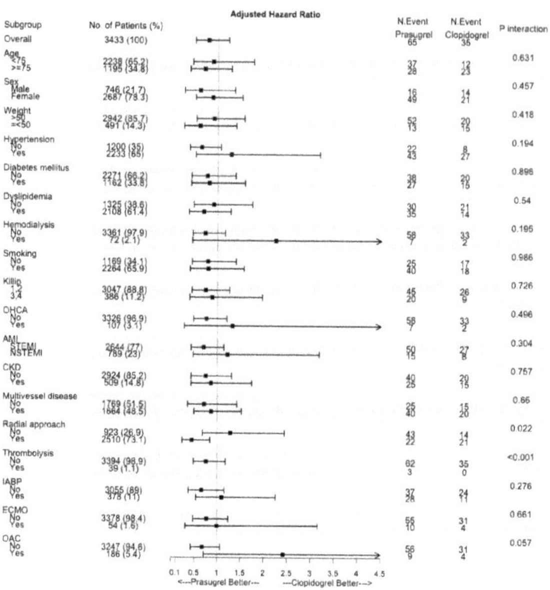

(A)

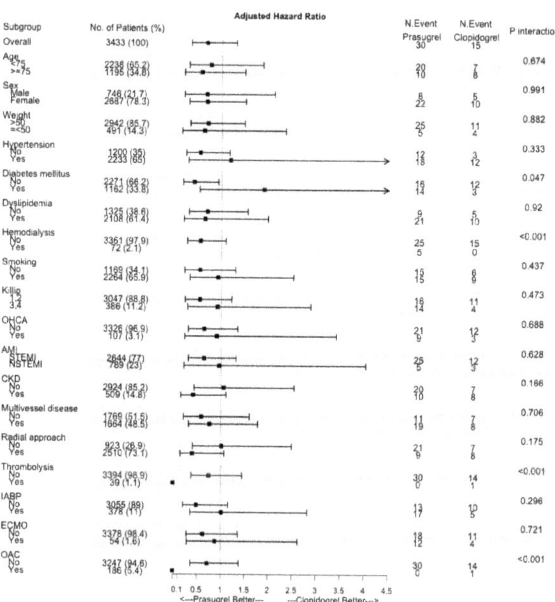

(B)

Figure 2. *Cont.*

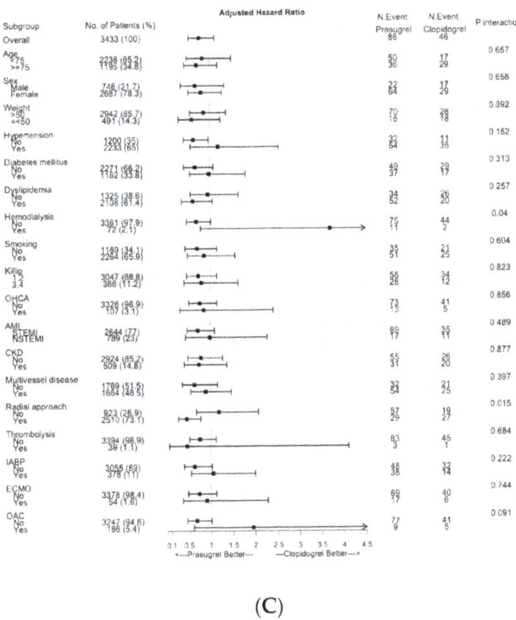

(C)

Figure 2. Results of a subgroup analysis of the efficacy endpoint (ischemic events, (**A**)), safety endpoint (bleeding events, (**B**)), and composite endpoint (composite of ischemic and bleeding events, (**C**)).

4. Discussion

Regarding the main findings of this study, a substantial number of patients with AMI were treated with prasugrel in a Japanese real-world registry. Prasugrel was used largely in younger, male STEMI patients with fewer comorbidities than clopidogrel-treated patients. Ischemic and bleeding events were observed to have a similar incidence in both groups, with a numerically greater tendency seen in the clopidogrel group.

Globally, clopidogrel is the most frequently used P2Y12 inhibitor in both ACS and CCS, accounting for about 50% to 80% of cases of P2Y12 inhibitor use worldwide [13–17]. However, our data showed that clopidogrel was used only in 24% of patients, while prasugrel was used in 76% of patients in the Japanese ACS registry. This trend was similarly observed in other Japanese registries [18–22]. According to a study by Akita et al. that investigated 62,737 Japanese ACS patients, 68.1% of patients received prasugrel, while 31.9% received clopidogrel [18]. The dose of prasugrel was basically reduced (LD/MD: 20/3.75 mg) in contrast to the standard dose of clopidogrel (LD/MD: 300/75 mg) in these Japanese real-world practice settings [18–23]. The findings of such clinical studies comparing a Japanese dose of prasugrel and a standard dose of clopidogrel in CAD patients are inconsistent among Japanese registry studies [18–23]. Some studies have reported that bleeding events are more frequent among patients that have received a Japanese dose of prasugrel, while others have reported that bleeding events are less frequent among patients that have received a Japanese dose of prasugrel [19–23]. The relatively low 1-year cardiac mortality rates of our study as compared to the JAMIR data (1.8%, 3.8%, respectively) may be due to a difference in the AMI condition, as the proportions of patients with Killip grade 2 or greater were different (17.2%, 23.9%, respectively). In terms of the efficacy, these two P2Y12 inhibitors seem to be equivalent [18–23]. Our study does not seem to show greatly different results from those of these previous studies. Globally, however, the standard dose of prasugrel is likely to be more efficient than a standard dose of clopidogrel at the cost of safety, as reported in the TRITON-TIMI38 [6]. One of the largest network meta-analyses involving 52,816 patients from 12 randomized trials showed that prasugrel reduced the risk of MI (hazard ratio (HR) 0.81, 95% confidence interval (CI) (0.67–0.98)) and stent thrombosis (HR 0.50, 95% CI (0.38–0.64)), but increased the major bleeding risk (HR 1.26, 95% CI (1.01–1.56)) [24].

The East Asian paradox is a well-known phenomenon wherein East Asian patients have a similar or even lower rate of ischemic events than white patients, despite having a higher level of platelet reactivity during DAPT [7]. Thus, a Japanese dose of prasugrel may be reasonable, as shown in the present and previous studies [8,19]. Ohya et al. reported a further reduced maintenance dose of prasugrel (2.5 mg) for patients with a low body weight ($\leq$50 kg), elderly age ($\geq$75 years old), or renal insufficiency (eGFR $\leq$ 30 mL/min/1.73 m^2) [25]. The rate of out-of-hospital definite or probable stent thrombosis was 0% in patients receiving prasugrel at 2.5 mg/day (n = 284) and 3.75 mg/day (n = 487), while the cumulative 1-year incidence of out-of-hospital major bleeding was not significantly different for either of the groups [25]. This strategy seems reasonable [25]. However, the question of whether a single dose or single strategy fits all Japanese patients remains, as about 65% of East Asian individuals carry a CYP2C19 loss-of-function allele, whereas only 30% of white individuals are carriers.

Tailor-made prescriptions have been attempted in prasugrel treatment. Stent thrombosis is reportedly due in part to a CYP polymorphism underuse of prasugrel [26,27]. For patients with the CYP2C19 loss-of-function (LoF) genotype or intermediate/poor metabolizers, a Japanese dose of prasugrel (LD/MD: 20/3.75 mg) or further reduced dose of prasugrel (LD/MD: 20/2.5 mg) might not be sufficient. A recent international meta-analysis assessed the risk of major adverse cardiovascular events (MACEs) following CYP2C19 LoF genotype-guided prasugrel/ticagrelor versus clopidogrel therapy for ACS patients undergoing PCI (n = 16132) [28]. Patients treated with prasugrel or ticagrelor showed a significantly reduced risk of MACEs (risk ratio 0.58; 95% CI 0.45–0.76; $p < 0.0001$) compared with those treated with clopidogrel, despite both groups carrying CYP2C19 LoF alleles [28]. Notably, no significant differences in the risk of MACE were found for the patients carrying CYP2C19 non-LoF alleles (risk ratio 0.91; 95% CI 0.81–1.02; $p = 0.11$). Bleeding events were not significantly different between the groups carrying CYP2C19 LoF alleles (Risk ratio 1.06; 95% CI 0.88–1.28; $p = 0.55$) [28]. The VerifyNow-P2Y12® rapid analyzer, which is a rapid assay that tests platelet activity over 3 min and uses of a combination of ADP and prostaglandin E1 (PGE1) to directly measure the effect of P2Y12 inhibitor on the P2Y12 receptor, is now widely available [29]. Monitoring platelet inhibition helped researchers to decide whether or not to use a reduced dose of prasugrel in the initial Japanese Phase II trial [8,30]. A VerifyNow-P2Y12 value of >208 reaction units (PRU) is generally defined as a high on-treatment platelet reactivity (HPR) and has been shown to be related to stent thrombosis and MI, while a VerifyNow-P2Y12 value of <85 PRU is considered to indicate low on-treatment platelet reactivity [31]. These kinds of precision medicines may be ideal, although they are associated with financial issues [32].

Several limitations associated with the present study warrant mention. First, nearly half of the patients in the K-ACTIVE registry were not included in the current analysis due to a lack of information regarding antiplatelet therapy. Second, our registry lacked information regarding the dose and duration of antiplatelet drugs and P2Y12 inhibitor switching after discharge, which influences both ischemic and bleeding events. Because our study population was gathered from 2015 to 2019, which is before the announcement of the focused update of the JCS guideline, it is highly possible that the duration for DAPT was 1 year in most subjects [9]. Similarly, the prasugrel dose was likely to be 3.75 mg in most of the patients, as the further reduced dose of prasugrel (2.5 mg) was only published in 2018 [25]. Third, this was an observational study, and residual or unmeasured confounding factors are likely to persist. For instance, the baseline characteristics differed considerably between the prasugrel and clopidogrel groups. Ischemic and bleeding events may potentially be related to selective prescribing. Although we performed an IPTW analysis to adjust for potential confounders, this method may not be sufficient to abolish this limitation. Fourth, bleeding and ischemic events might be underreported in registries, but this would have been similar for both groups, and severe and ischemic bleeding events are less likely to be missed. Fifth, information regarding the type of stents (drug-eluting stents or bare-metal stents) which can influence the duration of DAPT was not recorded. Finally, the present study was conducted in 52 institutions in Kanagawa, Japan, so the generalization of our finding to other parts of Japan is unreasonable.

5. Conclusions

A Japanese dose of prasugrel was frequently used in AMI patients from the real-world database of the K-ACTIVE registry in Kanagawa, Japan. Both the prasugrel and clopidogrel groups showed comparable rates of 1-year ischemic and bleeding events. Further studies are needed to establish optimized antiplatelet therapy for Japanese AMI patients.

Author Contributions: Data curation, T.M., A.M., K.F., Y.A., J.A., Y.I., T.E., K.T., A.N., I.M. and K.K.; Investigation, H.M.; Supervision, H.S.; Statistics, T.M. All authors have read and agreed to the published version of the manuscript.

Funding: This work was supported in part by a Grant-in-Aid for Scientific Research (15K09101) from the Ministry of Education, Science, and Culture, Japan, and financially supported by Daiichi Sankyo Co., LTD., Terumo, Abott Vascular Japan, and Boston Scientific Japan.

Institutional Review Board Statement: The study was conducted in accordance with the Declaration of Helsinki, and approved by the Institutional Review Board (or Ethics Committee) of Showa University Fujigaoka Hospital (protocol code 2014139 and date of approval 1 April 2015).

Informed Consent Statement: Informed consent was obtained from all subjects involved in the study.

Acknowledgments: We thank all of the investigators, clinical research coordinators, and data managers involved in the K-ACTIVE study for their contributions.

Conflicts of Interest: The authors declare no conflict of interest.

References

1. Yamamoto, K.; Hokimoto, S.; Chitose, T.; Morita, K.; Ono, T.; Kaikita, K.; Tsujita, K.; Abe, T.; Deguchi, M.; Miyagawa, H.; et al. Impact of CYP2C19 polymorphism on residual platelet reactivity in patients with coronary heart disease during antiplatelet therapy. *J. Cardiol.* **2011**, *57*, 194–201. [CrossRef] [PubMed]
2. Jinnai, T.; Horiuchi, H.; Makiyama, T.; Tazaki, J.; Tada, T.; Akao, M.; Ono, K.; Hoshino, K.; Naruse, Y.; Takahashi, K.; et al. Impact of CYP2C19 polymorphisms on the antiplatelet effect of clopidogrel in an actual clinical setting in Japan. *Circ. J.* **2009**, *73*, 1498–1503. [CrossRef] [PubMed]
3. Sugidachi, A.; Ogawa, T.; Kurihara, A.; Hagihara, K.; Jakubowski, J.A.; Hashimoto, M.; Niitsu, Y.; Asai, F. The greater in vivo antiplatelet effects of prasugrel as compared to clopidogrel reflect more efficient generation of its active metabolite with similar antiplatelet activity to that of clopidogrel's active metabolite. *J. Thromb. Haemost.* **2007**, *5*, 1545–1551. [CrossRef] [PubMed]
4. Jernberg, T.; Payne, C.D.; Winters, K.J.; Darstein, C.; Brandt, J.T.; Jakubowski, J.A.; Naganuma, H.; Siegbahn, A.; Wallentin, L. Prasugrel achieves greater inhibition of platelet aggregation and a lower rate of non-responders compared with clopidogrel in aspirin-treated patients with stable coronary artery disease. *Eur. Heart J.* **2006**, *27*, 1166–1173. [CrossRef]
5. Wallentin, L.; Varenhorst, C.; James, S.; Erlinge, D.; Braun, O.Ö.; Jakubowski, J.A.; Sugidachi, A.; Winters, K.J.; Siegbahn, A. Prasugrel achieves greater and faster P2Y12receptor-mediated platelet inhibition than clopidogrel due to more efficient generation of its active metabolite in aspirin-treated patients with coronary artery disease. *Eur. Heart J.* **2008**, *29*, 21–30. [CrossRef] [PubMed]
6. Wiviott, S.D.; Braunwald, E.; McCabe, C.H.; Montalescot, G.; Ruzyllo, W.; Gottlieb, S.; Neumann, F.-J.; Ardissino, D.; De Servi, S.; Murphy, S.A.; et al. Prasugrel versus Clopidogrel in Patients with Acute Coronary Syndromes. *N. Engl. J. Med.* **2007**, *357*, 2001–2015. [CrossRef]
7. Levine, G.N.; Jeong, Y.H.; Goto, S.; Anderson, J.L.; Huo, Y.; Mega, J.L.; Taubert, K.; Smith, S.C., Jr. Expert consensus document: World Heart Federation expert consensus statement on antiplatelet therapy in East Asian patients with ACS or undergoing PCI. *Nat. Rev. Cardiol.* **2014**, *11*, 597–606. [CrossRef]
8. Saito, S.; Isshiki, T.; Kimura, T.; Ogawa, H.; Yokoi, H.; Nanto, S.; Takayama, M.; Kitagawa, K.; Nishikawa, M.; Miyazaki, S.; et al. Efficacy and safety of adjusted-dose prasugrel compared with clopidogrel in Japanese patients with acute coronary syndrome-The PRASFIT-ACS study. *Circ. J.* **2014**, *78*, 1684–1692. [CrossRef]
9. Nakamura, M.; Kimura, K.; Kimura, T.; Ishihara, M.; Otsuka, F.; Kozuma, K.; Kosuge, M.; Shinke, T.; Nakagawa, Y.; Natsuaki, M.; et al. JCS 2020 guideline focused update on antithrombotic therapy in patients with coronary artery disease. *Circ. J.* **2020**, *84*, 831–865. [CrossRef]

10. Thygesen, K.; Alpert, J.S.; Jaffe, A.S.; Simoons, M.L.; Chaitman, B.R.; White, H.D.; Thygesen, K.; Alpert, J.S.; White, H.D.; Jaffe, A.S.; et al. Third universal definition of myocardial infarction. *Eur. Heart J.* **2012**, *33*, 2551–2567. [CrossRef]
11. Kimura, K.; Kimura, T.; Ishihara, M.; Nakagawa, Y.; Nakao, K.; Miyauchi, K.; Sakamoto, T.; Tsujita, K.; Hagiwara, N.; Miyazaki, S.; et al. JCS 2018 Guideline on Diagnosis and Treatment of Acute Coronary Syndrome. *Circ. J.* **2019**, *83*, 1085–1196. [CrossRef]
12. Heinze, G.; Jüni, P. An overview of the objectives of and the approaches to propensity score analyses. *Eur. Heart J.* **2011**, *32*, 1704–1708. [CrossRef]
13. Dayoub, E.J.; Nathan, A.S.; Khatana, S.A.M.; Seigerman, M.; Tuteja, S.; Kobayashi, T.; Kolansky, D.M.; Groeneveld, P.W.; Giri, J. Use of prasugrel and ticagrelor in stable ischemic heart disease after percutaneous coronary intervention, 2009–2016. *Circ. Cardiovasc. Interv.* **2019**, *12*, e007434. [CrossRef]
14. Dayoub, E.J.; Seigerman, M.; Tuteja, S.; Kobayashi, T.; Kolansky, D.M.; Giri, J.; Groeneveld, P.W. Trends in platelet adenosine diphosphate P2Y12 receptor inhibitor use and adherence among antiplatelet-naive patients after percutaneous coronary intervention, 2008–2016. *JAMA Intern. Med.* **2018**, *178*, 943–950. [CrossRef]
15. Cimminiello, C.; Dondi, L.; Pedrini, A.; Ronconi, G.; Calabria, S.; Piccinni, C.; Friz, H.P.; Martini, N.; Maggioni, A.P. Patterns of treatment with antiplatelet therapy after an acute coronary syndrome: Data from a large database in a community setting. *Eur. J. Prev. Cardiol.* **2019**, *26*, 836–846. [CrossRef]
16. Sim, D.S.; Jeong, M.H.; Kim, H.S.; Gwon, H.C.; Seung, K.B.; Rha, S.W.; Chae, S.C.; Kim, C.J.; Cha, K.S.; Park, J.S.; et al. Association of potent P2Y12 blockers with ischemic and bleeding outcomes in non-ST-segment elevation myocardial infarction. *J. Cardiol.* **2019**, *73*, 142–150. [CrossRef]
17. Ahn, K.T.; Seong, S.W.; Choi, U.L.; Jin, S.A.; Kim, J.H.; Lee, J.H.; Choi, S.W.; Jeong, M.H.; Chae, S.C.; Kim, Y.J.; et al. Comparison of 1-year clinical outcomes between prasugrel and ticagrelor versus clopidogrel in type 2 diabetes patients with acute myocardial infarction underwent successful percutaneous coronary intervention. *Medicine* **2019**, *98*, e14833. [CrossRef]
18. Akita, K.; Inohara, T.; Yamaji, K.; Kohsaka, S.; Numasawa, Y.; Ishii, H.; Amano, T.; Kadota, K.; Nakamura, M.; Maekawa, Y. Impact of reduced-dose prasugrel vs. standard-dose clopidogrel on in-hospital outcomes of percutaneous coronary intervention in 62 737 patients with acute coronary syndromes: A nationwide registry study in Japan. *Eur. Heart J. Cardiovasc. Pharmacother.* **2020**, *6*, 231–238. [CrossRef]
19. Yasuda, S.; Honda, S.; Takegami, M.; Nishihira, K.; Kojima, S.; Asaumi, Y.; Suzuki, M.; Kosuge, M.; Takahashi, J.; Sakata, Y.; et al. Contemporary Antiplatelet Therapy and Clinical Outcomes of Japanese Patients with Acute Myocardial Infarction–Results from the Prospective Japan Acute Myocardial Infarction Registry (JAMIR). *Circ. J.* **2019**, *83*, 1633–1643. [CrossRef]
20. Hagiwara, H.; Fukuta, H.; Hashimoto, H.; Niimura, T.; Zamami, Y.; Ishizawa, K.; Kamiya, T.; Ohte, N. A comparison of the safety and effectiveness of prasugrel and clopidogrel in younger population undergoing percutaneous coronary intervention: A retrospective study using a Japanese claims database. *J. Cardiol.* **2021**, *77*, 285–291. [CrossRef]
21. Sakamoto, K.; Sato, R.; Tabata, N.; Ishii, M.; Yamashita, T.; Nagamatsu, S.; Motozato, K.; Yamanaga, K.; Hokimoto, S.; Sueta, D.; et al. Temporal trends in coronary intervention strategies and the impact on one-year clinical events: Data from a Japanese multi-center real-world cohort study. *Cardiovasc. Interv. Ther.* **2021**, *37*, 66–77. [CrossRef] [PubMed]
22. Shoji, S.; Sawano, M.; Sandhu, A.T.; Heidenreich, P.A.; Shiraishi, Y.; Ikemura, N.; Ueno, K.; Suzuki, M.; Numasawa, Y.; Fukuda, K.; et al. Ischemic and Bleeding Events among Patients with Acute Coronary Syndrome Associated with Low-Dose Prasugrel vs. Standard-Dose Clopidogrel Treatment. *JAMA Netw. Open* **2020**, *3*, e202004. [CrossRef] [PubMed]
23. Tokimasa, S.; Kitahara, H.; Nakayama, T.; Fujimoto, Y.; Shiba, T.; Shikama, N.; Nameki, M.; Himi, T.; Fukushima, K.-I.; Kobayashi, Y. Multicenter research of bleeding risk between prasugrel and clopidogrel in Japanese patients with coronary artery disease undergoing percutaneous coronary intervention. *Heart Vessels* **2019**, *34*, 1581–1588. [CrossRef] [PubMed]
24. Navarese, E.P.; Khan, S.U.; Kołodziejczak, M.; Kubica, J.; Buccheri, S.; Cannon, C.P.; Gurbel, P.A.; De Servi, S.; Budaj, A.; Bartorelli, A.; et al. Comparative Efficacy and Safety of Oral P2Y12Inhibitors in Acute Coronary Syndrome: Network Meta-Analysis of 52 816 Patients from 12 Randomized Trials. *Circulation* **2020**, *142*, 150–160. [CrossRef]
25. Ohya, M.; Shimada, T.; Osakada, K.; Kuwayama, A.; Miura, K.; Murai, R.; Amano, H.; Kubo, S.; Otsuru, S.; Habara, S.; et al. In-hospital bleeding and utility of a maintenance dose of prasugrel 2.5 mg in high bleeding risk patients with acute coronary syndrome. *Circ. J.* **2018**, *82*, 1874–1883. [CrossRef]
26. Ohno, Y.; Okada, S.; Kitahara, H.; Nishi, T.; Nakayama, T.; Fujimoto, Y.; Kobayashi, Y. Repetitive stent thrombosis in a patient who had resistance to both clopidogrel and prasugrel. *J. Cardiol. Cases* **2016**, *13*, 139–142. [CrossRef]
27. Yamagata, Y.; Koga, S.; Ikeda, S.; Maemura, K. Acute thrombosis of everolimus-eluting platinum chromium stent caused by impaired prasugrel metabolism due to cytochrome P450 enzyme 2B6*2 (C64T) polymorphism: A case report. *Eur. Heart J. Case Rep.* **2020**, *4*, 1–7. [CrossRef]
28. Biswas, M.; Kali, M.S.K.; Biswas, T.K.; Ibrahim, B. Risk of major adverse cardiovascular events of CYP2C19 loss-of-function genotype guided prasugrel/ticagrelor vs clopidogrel therapy for acute coronary syndrome patients undergoing percutaneous coronary intervention: A meta-analysis. *Platelets* **2020**, *32*, 1–10. [CrossRef]
29. Malinin, A.; Pokov, A.; Spergling, M.; Defranco, A.; Schwartz, K.; Schwartz, D.; Mahmud, E.; Atar, D.; Serebruany, V. Monitoring platelet inhibition after clopidogrel with the VerifyNow-P2Y12®rapid analyzer: The VERIfy Thrombosis Risk ASsessment (VERITAS) study. *Thromb. Res.* **2007**, *119*, 277–284. [CrossRef]

30. Yokoi, H.; Kimura, T.; Isshiki, T.; Ogawa, H.; Ikeda, Y. Pharmacodynamic assessment of a novel P2Y 12 receptor antagonist in Japanese patients with coronary artery disease undergoing elective percutaneous coronary intervention. *Thromb. Res.* **2012**, *129*, 623–628. [CrossRef]
31. Stone, G.W.; Witzenbichler, B.; Weisz, G.; Rinaldi, M.J.; Neumann, F.J.; Metzger, D.C.; Henry, T.D.; Cox, D.A.; Duffy, P.L.; Mazzaferri, E.; et al. Platelet reactivity and clinical outcomes after coronary artery implantation of drug-eluting stents (ADAPT-DES): A prospective multicentre registry study. *Lancet* **2013**, *382*, 614–623. [CrossRef]
32. AlMukdad, S.; Elewa, H.; Al-Badriyeh, D. Economic Evaluations of CYP2C19 Genotype-Guided Antiplatelet Therapy Compared to the Universal Use of Antiplatelets in Patients with Acute Coronary Syndrome: A Systematic Review. *J. Cardiovasc. Pharmacol. Ther.* **2020**, *25*, 201–211. [CrossRef] [PubMed]

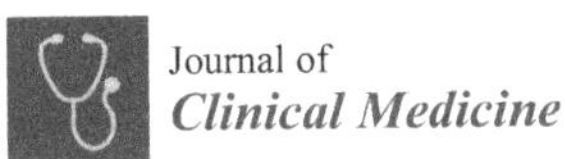
Journal of
Clinical Medicine

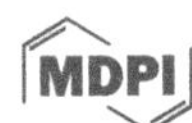

Article

Nitrates vs. Other Types of Vasodilators and Clinical Outcomes in Patients with Vasospastic Angina: A Propensity Score-Matched Analysis

Hyun-Jin Kim [1], Sang-Ho Jo [2,*], Min-Ho Lee [3], Won-Woo Seo [4], Hack-Lyoung Kim [5], Kwan Yong Lee [6], Tae-Hyun Yang [7], Sung-Ho Her [8], Byoung-Kwon Lee [9], Keun-Ho Park [10], Youngkeun Ahn [11], Seung-Woon Rha [12], Hyeon-Cheol Gwon [13], Dong-Ju Choi [14] and Sang Hong Baek [6]

1 Division of Cardiology, Department of Internal Medicine, Hanyang University College of Medicine, Seoul 04763, Korea; titi8th@hanyang.ac.kr
2 Division of Cardiology, Department of Internal Medicine, Hallym University Sacred Heart Hospital, Anyang-si 14068, Korea
3 Division of Cardiology, Department of Internal Medicine, Soonchunhyang University Seoul Hospital, Seoul 04401, Korea; neoich@gmail.com
4 Division of Cardiology, Department of Internal Medicine, Kangdong Sacred Heart Hospital, Hallym University College of Medicine, Seoul 05355, Korea; wonwooda@gmail.com
5 Cardiovascular Center, Seoul National University Boramae Medical Center, Seoul 07061, Korea; khl2876@gmail.com
6 Division of Cardiology, Seoul St. Mary's Hospital, The Catholic University of Korea, Seoul 06591, Korea; cycle210@catholic.ac.kr (K.Y.L.); whitesh@catholic.ac.kr (S.H.B.)
7 Department of Cardiovascular Medicine, Busan Paik Hospital, Inje University, Busan 04551, Korea; yangthmd@naver.com
8 Department of Cardiovascular Medicine, St. Vincent's Hospital, The Catholic University of Korea, Suwon 16249, Korea; hhhsungho@naver.com
9 Department of Cardiovascular Medicine, Gangnam Severance Hospital, Yonsei University, Seoul 06273, Korea; cardiobk@gmail.com
10 Division of Cardiology, Department of Internal Medicine, Chosun Medical Center, Gwangju 61453, Korea; keuno21@naver.com
11 Department of Cardiology, Chonnam National University Hospital, Chonnam National University Medical School, Gwangju 61469, Korea; cecilyk@hanmail.net
12 Department of Cardiovascular Medicine, Guro Hospital, Korea University, Seoul 08308, Korea; swrha617@yahoo.co.kr
13 Department of Cardiovascular Medicine, Samsung Medical Center, Sungkyunkwan University, Seoul 06351, Korea; hcgwon@naver.com
14 Division of Cardiology, Department of Internal Medicine, Seoul National University Bundang Hospital, Seongnam 13620, Korea; djchoi@snubh.org
* Correspondence: sophi5neo@gmail.com; Tel.: +82-031-380-3722

Abstract: Although vasodilators are widely used in patients with vasospastic angina (VA), few studies have compared the long-term prognostic effects of different types of vasodilators. We investigated the long-term effects of vasodilators on clinical outcomes in VA patients according to the type of vasodilator used. Study data were obtained from a prospective multicenter registry that included patients who had symptoms suggestive of VA. Patients were classified into two groups according to use of nitrates (n = 239) or other vasodilators (n = 809) at discharge. The composite clinical events rate, including acute coronary syndrome (ACS), cardiac death, new-onset arrhythmia (including ventricular tachycardia and ventricular fibrillation), and atrioventricular block, was significantly higher in the nitrates group (5.3% vs. 2.2%, p = 0.026) during one year of follow-up. Specifically, the prevalence of ACS was significantly more frequent in the nitrates group (4.3% vs. 1.5%, p = 0.024). After propensity score matching, the adverse effects of nitrates remained. In addition, the use of nitrates at discharge was independently associated with a 2.69-fold increased risk of ACS in VA patients. In conclusion, using nitrates as a vasodilator at discharge can increase the adverse clinical outcomes in VA patients at one year of follow-up. Clinicians need to be aware of the prognostic value and consider prescribing other vasodilators.

Citation: Kim, H.-J.; Jo, S.-H.; Lee, M.-H.; Seo, W.-W.; Kim, H.-L.; Lee, K.Y.; Yang, T.-H.; Her, S.-H.; Lee, B.-K.; Park, K.-H.; et al. Nitrates vs. Other Types of Vasodilators and Clinical Outcomes in Patients with Vasospastic Angina: A Propensity Score-Matched Analysis. *J. Clin. Med.* **2022**, *11*, 3250. https://doi.org/10.3390/jcm11123250

Academic Editors: Koichi Node and Atsushi Tanaka

Received: 4 April 2022
Accepted: 5 June 2022
Published: 7 June 2022

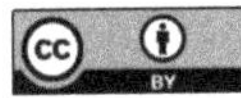

Keywords: vasospastic angina; nitrate; vasodilator; acute coronary syndrome

1. Introduction

Vasospastic angina (VA) is a functional disorder caused by the focal or diffuse spasm of the smooth muscle layer of the coronary arterial wall, resulting in a high grade of obstruction and transient myocardial ischemia [1,2]. Overall, the long-term prognosis of VA is known to be good [3]. However, once a serious heart condition occurs with VA, it may lead to sudden cardiac death following myocardial infarction or fatal ventricular arrhythmia [4,5]. Treatment with calcium channel blockers (CCBs) is recommended as first-line therapy for patients with VA according to current guidelines, since CCBs are highly effective for preventing coronary spasm [1]. Along with CCBs, nitrates or nicorandil are often used as concomitant therapy for the prevention of coronary artery spasm (Class IIa recommendation). Nitrates are metabolized to nitric oxide (NO), which activates NO-cyclic guanosine-3′, -5′-monophasphate (cGMP) signaling pathways within vascular smooth muscle cells, resulting in vasodilation [1,6]. Nicorandil has the properties of nitrates and also acts as a K_{ATP} channel agonist, which could result in vasodilation without intracellular cGMP accumulation [7,8]. Additionally, the vasodilatory effects of other nitrate agents, including molsidomine, involve the main mechanism of NO production and secretion [9]. While these vasodilators can improve vasospastic symptoms acutely, their effects on long-term prognosis in VA patients have been controversial. Some studies suggested that long-term nitrate therapy was neutral to clinical outcomes in patients with VA [10]. Meanwhile, a Japanese multicenter registry [11] demonstrated that long-term nitrate therapy did not improve the clinical prognosis (median follow-up duration 32 months) compared with non-nitrate therapy in patients with VA. Korean data from single-center registry [12] also demonstrated that long-term nitrate therapy worsened prognosis (median follow-up duration 54.7 months). However, these prior research studies have limitations as they included retrospective populations, which may make it unclear whether nitrate promotes poor prognosis or serves as a surrogate marker for more serious heart disease. Indeed, despite the widespread use of nitrates and other vasodilators in patients with VA, there has been no study comparing the effects on long-term prognosis according to vasodilator type. This study investigated the actual prescribing status of vasodilators in VA patients at discharge and effects on prognosis according to the type of vasodilator used in a large-scale nationwide prospective registry.

2. Materials and Methods

2.1. Study Population

Study data were obtained from a prospective nationwide Vasospastic Angina in Korea registry (VA-Korea). The study design of VA-Korea has been published previously [3,13,14]. Between May 2010 and June 2015, 11 tertiary hospitals in Korea participated in this registry. Patient's inclusion criteria were: patients were 18 years of age or older, with suspected symptoms of vasospastic angina, and those who underwent invasive coronary angiography (CAG) with ergonovine (EG) provocation test, all of which were satisfied. The exclusion criteria were: end-stage renal disease on continuous dialysis, known malignancy, inflammatory disease, or catheter-induced spasm at baseline. Of 2960 initially enrolled patients with suspected VA (Figure 1), 1987 patients had intermediate or significant spasm after intracoronary EG injection during CAG. Among them, only 1302 patients were prescribed vasodilators when they were discharged: 254 patients were prescribed two or more types of vasodilators as discharge medications and 1048 patients were prescribed one vasodilator. We included the 1048 patients using a single vasodilator in the final analysis and classified the patients into two groups depending on the type of vasodilator used at discharge: nitrates group and other vasodilators group. The other vasodilator group was defined as patients who used nicorandil, molsidomine, or trimetazidine at discharge. This study protocol complied with the Declaration of Helsinki and was reviewed and approved by the Institutional Review Board of Hallym University Sacred Heart Hospital (Approved No. 2010-I007). All patients provided written informed consent prior to study entry.

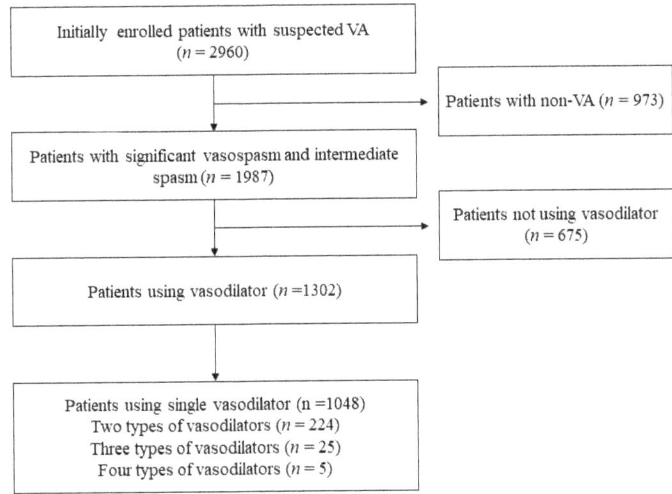

Figure 1. Study population selection process.

2.2. Data Collection

The patient data were collected through the VA-Korea database via a web-based electronic data capture system containing an electronic case report form. The following patient clinical and demographical characteristics were collected from this database: age, sex, body mass index (BMI; kg/m^2), blood pressure, cardiovascular risk factors, and previous cardiovascular medications. Laboratory data related with cardiovascular disease were also obtained. We also collected left ventricular ejection fraction from echocardiography data at admission. In addition, we extracted information on the types of vasodilator prescribed at discharge (nitrates, nicorandil, molsidomine, and trimetazidine).

2.3. Invasive CAG and EG Provocation Test

The baseline CAG and EG provocation tests were performed according to the Guidelines for Diagnosis and Treatment of Patients with VA of the Japanese Circulation Society [1]. The baseline CAG was performed by a well-trained interventional cardiologist; vasoactive medications were discontinued at least 48 h before the procedure. Intracoronary EG was injected in incremental doses of 20 (E1), 40 (E2), and 60 (E3) µg into the left coronary artery (LCA) for the test of provocation [1,15]. Incremental doses of 10 (E1), 20 (E2), and 40 (E3) µg were injected into the right coronary artery (RCA) when LCA did not induce coronary spasm. When spasm was induced, 200 µg of nitroglycerine was injected. Chest pain, location of spasm and electrocardiography (ECG) change were recorded during the provocation test. ECG change was defined as ST segment depression (≥1 mm) or elevation or T-wave inversion in at least 2 consecutive leads [12]. We defined significant vasospasm as total or luminal diameter narrowing by more than 90% of the coronary arteries accompanied by ECG changes and/or chest pain after EG injection [1]. Intermediate spasm was defined as 50% to 90% luminal diameter stenosis of the coronary arteries. All patients who had spasms on the EG provocation test or spontaneous spasm were treated with medication during follow-up according to the clinician's discretion.

2.4. Study Outcomes

The primary outcome was rate of composite clinical events for one year of follow-up (median duration, 365 days; mean 345.0 ± 60.5 days). The composite clinical events included acute coronary syndrome (ACS), cardiac death, new-onset arrhythmia including ventricular fibrillation (VF) and ventricular tachycardia (VT), and atrioventricular (AV) block. VT was defined as sustained VT resulting in hemodynamic instability, and AV block was defined as a high-degree AV block resulting in hemodynamic instability. All-cause death was also noted during the one-year follow-up. Occurrence of death and the timing of death were confirmed through medical records review or telephone interviews. In addition, readmission or emergency room visits due to angina was investigated for one year after diagnosis with vasospastic angina. To investigate whether patients were taking medication continuously, drug compliance was also assessed for one year after diagnosis. Good compliance was defined as maintaining a vasodilator for one year without any change and interruption, and poor compliance was as discontinuation of a vasodilator within one year.

2.5. Statistical Analyses

All categorical data are presented as frequencies and percentages, and continuous variables are expressed as means and standard deviations. For continuous variables, the Shapiro–Wilk test was used for confirming the normal distribution of each dataset. Pearson's chi-squared test was used to compare categorical variables, the Student's t-test was used to compare normal distributed continuous variables, and the Mann–Whitney U-test was used to compared non-normal distributed continuous variables. In addition, we also used propensity scores and 1:1 matching analysis to adjust the uneven distribution of baseline characteristics between the nitrate group and other vasodilator groups. A multiple logistic regression model was constructed to represent the propensity score, which was the probability of the nitrates group. The adjusted variables were as follows: age, sex, history of coronary artery disease, hypertension, and diabetes, current smoking status, alcohol drinking, and cardiovascular medications. The 174 patients in the nitrates group were matched to 174 patients in the other vasodilators group. McNemar's test was used to compare categorical variables between matched patient groups, and a paired t-test was used for continuous variables. Kaplan–Meier survival analysis and log-rank test were used to compare the ACS-free survival rates and cumulative composite clinical events-free survival rates between the nitrates group and the other vasodilators group. In addition, univariate analysis and multivariate logistic regression analysis were performed to evaluate the risk of ACS after adjustment for individual risk factors. Variables with predictive significance ($p < 0.05$) of ACS in univariate analysis were included in the regression analysis. A p-value less than 0.05 was considered statistically significant. All analyses were performed using SPSS 21.0 software (IBM Corp., Armonk, NY, USA).

3. Results

3.1. Baseline Characteristics

Among 1048 patients with VA using a single vasodilator at discharge who underwent CAG and EG provocation test, there were 239 patients who were prescribed a nitrate at discharge (nitrates group) and 809 patients who were prescribed another vasodilator (other vasodilators group: 521 patients used nicorandil, 177 patients used molsidomine, and 111 patients used trimetazidine). Patients' baseline characteristics according to vasodilator type are shown in Table 1. Patients in the nitrates group were significantly older than patients in the other vasodilators group, and significantly more patients in the nitrates group reported alcohol drinking and current smoking than patients in the other vasodilators group. Previous use of antiplatelet agents and statins was more frequent in the other vasodilators group than in the nitrates group. Table 1 also shows the laboratory findings of the two groups: there were no significant differences between the two groups. Likewise, there were no significant differences in other histories or medications related to traditional cardiovascular risk factors or diseases between the two groups. Supplementary Table S1 (Supplementary Materials online) shows the comparison of coronary angiographic characteristics after EG provocation test between the two groups. There were no significant differences in location of spasm between the two groups, but provocation-associated chest pain was more frequent in the nitrates group than in the other vasodilators group. In addition, there was no significant difference in multi-vessel involvement in which spam occurred in two or more coronary arteries after EG provocation test: 23.1% in the nitrates group and 26.7% in the other type of vasodilator group (p = 0.308).

Table 1. Baseline Characteristics.

	All (n = 1048)	Nitrates (n = 239)	Other Types of Vasodilator (n = 809)	p Value
Age, years	54.8 ± 11.2	52.6 ± 11.4	55.5 ± 11.1	0.001
Male, n (%)	666 (63.5)	160 (66.9)	5056 (62.5)	0.214
BMI, kg/m^2	24.7 ± 3.3	24.9 ± 4.1	24.7 ± 3.1	0.450
SBP, mmHg	126.0 ± 18.0	126.8 ± 18.7	125.7 ± 17.8	0.404
DBP, mmHg	77.2 ± 12.2	78.3 ± 13.3	76.9 ± 11.8	0.118
Previous CAD, n (%)	108 (10.3)	19 (7.9)	89 (11.0)	0.171
Diabetes mellitus, n (%)	101 (9.6)	20 (8.4)	81 (10.0)	0.446
Hypertension, n (%)	386 (36.9)	98 (41.0)	288 (35.6)	0.131
Dyslipidemia, n (%)	183 (17.5)	46 (19.4)	137 (17.0)	0.382
Alcohol drinking, n (%)	455 (43.4)	137 (57.3)	318 (39.3)	<0.001
Current smoking, n (%)	304 (29.5)	91 (38.1)	213 (26.9)	0.001
Laboratory finding				
Hemoglobin, g/dL	13.9 ± 1.9	13.9 ± 1.8	13.9 ± 1.9	0.945
Creatinine, mg/dL	0.8 ± 0.2	0.8 ± 0.2	0.8 ± 0.2	0.294
Glucose, mg/dL	111.3 ± 35.8	112.8 ± 46.4	110.9 ± 32.1	0.565
hs-CRP, mg/dL	0.9 ± 5.8	1.1 ± 7.0	0.8 ± 5.3	0.453
Total cholesterol, mg/dL	173.6 ± 35.6	175.3 ± 35.2	173.0 ± 35.7	0.406
LDL cholesterol, mg/dL	103.1 ± 31.8	103.6 ± 31.4	103.0 ± 31.9	0.811
Triglyceride, mg/dL	145.7 ± 105.4	151.5 ± 94.7	143.9 ± 108.6	0.349
HDL cholesterol, mg/dL	46.3 ±12.7	42.2 ± 11.9	46.7 ± 13.0	0.126
LV EF, %	64.6 ± 6.6	65.1 ± 6.1	64.4 ± 6.8	0.167
Previous cardiovascular medication				
Antiplatelet, n (%)	222 (21.3)	37 (15.5)	186 (23.0)	0.042
Statin, n (%)	163 (15.6)	26 (10.9)	137 (16.9)	0.025
CCB, n (%)	191 (18.2)	40 (16.7)	151 (18.7)	0.166
Discharge medication				
CCB, n (%)	959 (91.5)	220 (92.1)	739 (91.3)	0.732
Clinical diagnosis before ergonovine				
Angina, n (%)	962 (92.1)	226 (94.6)	736 (91.4)	0.114
Myocardial infarction, n (%)	18 (1.7)	3 (1.3)	15 (1.9)	0.777
Cardiac arrest, n (%)	11 (1.1)	6 (2.5)	5 (0.6)	0.022
Syncope, n (%)	11 (1.1)	4 (1.7)	7 (0.9)	0.286
VT or VF, n (%)	5 (0.5)	1 (0.4)	4 (0.5)	1.000
AV block, n (%)	1 (0.1)	0 (0.0)	1 (0.1)	1.000

AV, atrioventricular; BMI, body mass index; CAD, coronary artery disease; CCB, calcium channel blocker; DBP, diastolic blood pressure; HDL, high-density lipoprotein; hs-CRP, high sensitive-C reactive protein; LDL, low-density lipoprotein; LV EF, left ventricular ejection fraction; SBP, systolic blood pressure; VF, ventricular fibrillation; VT, ventricular tachycardia.

3.2. Clinical Outcomes according to Vasodilator Type

Among 1048 patients, 780 patients had one year of follow-up data, and the composite clinical events of ACS, cardiac death, VT or VF, or AV block occurred in 23 patients. The one-year composite clinical events rate was significantly higher in the nitrates group than in the other vasodilators group (5.3% vs. 2.2%, p = 0.026) (Table 2). Specifically, the prevalence of one-year ACS was significantly more frequent in the nitrates group than in the other vasodilators group (4.3% vs. 1.5%, $p = 0.024$). However, one-year all-cause death rates did not differ significantly according to the vasodilator type. There was also no significant difference between the two groups in terms of readmission or emergency room visits for one year. Based on whether the VA patients received a nitrate or other vasodilators at discharge, the cumulative composite clinical events rate and the cumulative ACS-free survival rate were analyzed, and results are shown in Figure 2A,B. Patients in the nitrates group had a significantly lower cumulative event-free survival rate than patients in the other vasodilators group at the one-year follow-up (89.2% vs. 96.1%, log-rank $p = 0.026$) (Figure 2A). Patients in the nitrates group also had a significantly lower cumulative ACS-free survival rate (90.4% vs. 97.1%, log-rank $p = 0.023$) (Figure 2B) (Supplementary Table S2 showed the time to event of each individuals). Additionally, there was no significant difference in the rate of the one-year composite clinical events among nicorandil group, molsidomine group, and trimetazidine group (Supplementary Table S3). The prevalence of one-year ACS showed also no significant difference among three groups.

Table 2. One-year clinical event rate of patients with VA according to types of vasodilators.

	All (n = 780)	Nitrates (n = 187)	Other Types of Vasodilator (n = 593)	p Value
Composite events	23 (2.9)	10 (5.3)	13 (2.2)	0.026
ACS	17 (2.2)	8 (4.3)	9 (1.5)	0.024
Cardiac death	1 (0.1)	0 (0.0)	1 (0.1)	0.567
VT or VF	2 (0.3)	1 (0.5)	1 (0.2)	0.422
AV block	3 (0.4)	1 (0.5)	2 (0.3)	0.561
All-cause death	3 (0.4)	1 (0.5)	2 (0.3)	0.561
Readmission or emergency room visits due to angina	88 (11.3)	23 (12.3)	65 (11.0)	0.614

ACS, acute coronary syndrome; AV, atrioventricular; VA, vasospastic angina; VF, ventricular fibrillation; VT, ventricular tachycardia.

3.3. Clinical Outcomes in Propensity Score-Matched Population

After propensity score matching, 174 patients in the nitrates group were successfully matched to an equal number of patients in the other vasodilators group. Baseline characteristics were not significantly different between groups after propensity score matching (Supplementary Table S4). The rate of one-year composite clinical events of the matched population was significantly higher in the nitrates group (5.7% vs. 1.1%, $p = 0.035$) (Table 3). In addition, the one-year ACS events rate of the matched population was significantly higher in the nitrates group (4.6% vs. 0.6%, $p = 0.037$). Figure 3 shows the cumulative composite clinical events rate and cumulative ACS-free survival rate between the matched groups. Patients in the nitrates group had a significantly lower cumulative event-free survival rate than patients in the other vasodilators group (94.2% vs. 98.9%, log-rank $p = 0.021$) (Figure 3A), as well as a lower cumulative ACS-free survival rate (95.4% vs. 99.4%, log-rank $p = 0.019$) (Figure 3B).

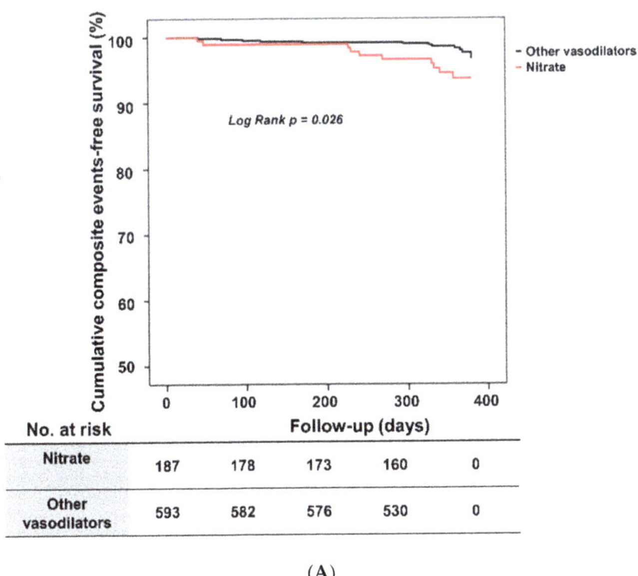

(A)

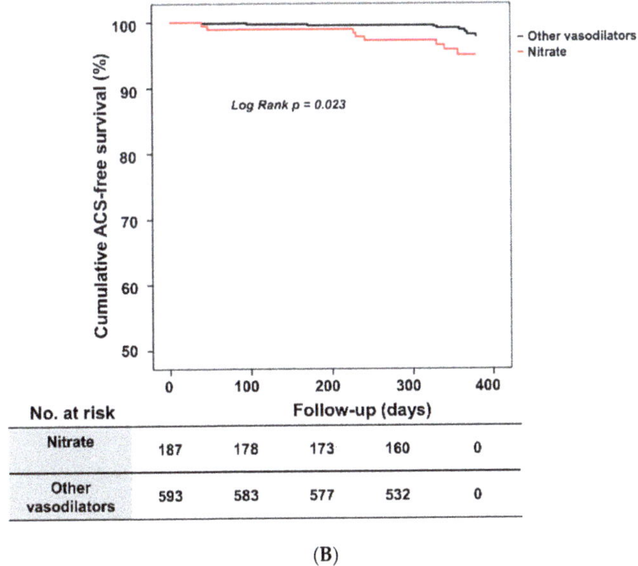

(B)

Figure 2. Kaplan–Meier survival curves of the entire population. (**A**) Cumulative composite events-free survival according to vasodilator. (**B**) Cumulative ACS-free survival according to vasodilator. ACS, acute coronary syndrome.

Table 3. One-year clinical event rate of patients with VA according to types of vasodilators after 1:1 propensity-matching.

	All (n = 348)	Nitrates (n = 174)	Other Types of Vasodilator (n = 174)	p Value
Composite events	12 (3.4)	10 (5.7)	2 (1.1)	0.035
ACS	9 (2.6)	8 (4.6)	1 (0.6)	0.037
Cardiac death	0 (0.0)	0 (0.0)	0 (0.0)	-
VT or VF	1 (0.3)	1 (0.6)	0 (0.0)	1.000
AV block	2 (0.6)	1 (0.6)	1 (0.6)	1.000
All-cause death	2 (0.6)	1 (0.6)	1 (0.6)	1.000
Readmission or emergency room visits due to angina	43 (12.4)	22 (12.6)	21 (12.1)	0.871

ACS, acute coronary syndrome; AV, atrioventricular; VA, vasospastic angina; VF, ventricular fibrillation; VT, ventricular tachycardia.

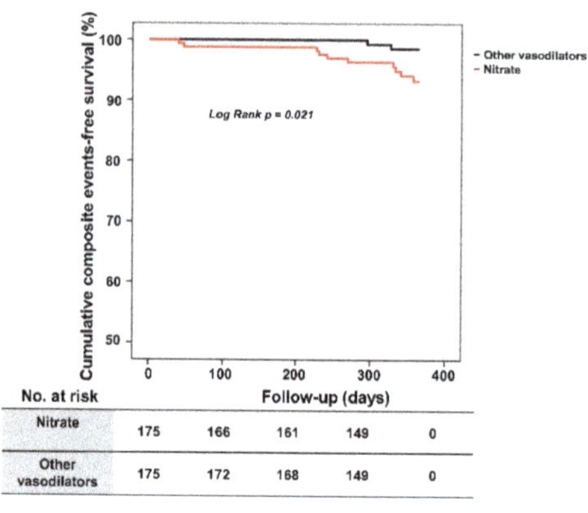

(**A**)

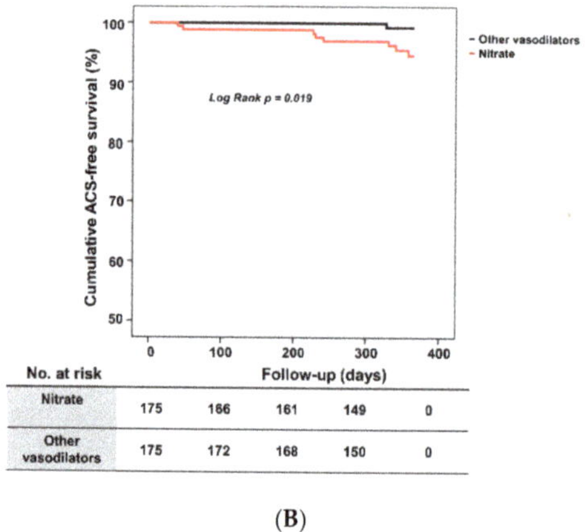

(**B**)

Figure 3. Kaplan–Meier survival curves in propensity score-matched population. (**A**) Cumulative composite events-free survival according to vasodilator. (**B**) Cumulative ACS-free survival according to vasodilator. ACS, acute coronary syndrome.

3.4. Effect of Nitrate Type on One-Year ACS Rate in VA Patients

According to univariate analysis (Table 4), the following factors were associated with ACS events at one-year follow-up in VA patients: use of nitrates at discharge (odds ratio (OR), 2.86; 95% confidence interval (CI), 1.104–7.420; $p = 0.031$) and age. After adjusting for age, the Cox regression analysis showed that the use of nitrates at discharge was independently associated with a 2.69-fold increased hazard for ACS in VA patients (OR, 2.69; 95% CI, 1.035–6.979; $p = 0.042$). However, the use of other vasodilators, including nicorandil, molsidomine, and trimetazidine, at discharge was not an independent predictor of ACS in VA patients.

Table 4. Predictors of ACS in patients with VA.

	Univariate			Multivariate		
	OR	95% CI	*p*	OR	95% CI	*p*
Nitrate	2.86	1.104–7.420	0.031	2.69	1.035–6.979	0.042
Nicorandil	1.10	0.424–2.847	0.847	-	-	-
Molsidomine	0.04	0.000–11.521	0.263	-	-	-
Trimetazidine	0.04	0.000–41.670	0.368	-	-	-
Age	0.96	0.914–1.000	0.049	0.96	0.915–1.003	0.067
Previous CAD	1.06	0.242–4.641	0.938	-	-	-
Hypertension	0.85	0.315–2.307	0.754	-	-	-
Diabetes	1.43	0.328–6.276	0.632	-	-	-
Current smoking	1.51	0.665–3.406	0.327	-	-	-
Alcohol drinking	1.01	0.452–2.242	0.987	-	-	-
LDL-cholesterol	1.01	0.995–1.026	0.193	-	-	-
CCB at index admission	1.49	0.198–11.268	0.697	-	-	-

ACS = acute coronary syndrome; CAD = coronary artery disease; CCB = calcium-channel blocker; CI = confidence interval; LDL = low-density lipoprotein; OR = odds ratio; VA = vasospastic angina.

3.5. Subgroup Analysis

A subgroup analysis of the one-year clinical events rate of patients with VA according to drug compliance was performed. There were 776 patients with confirmed one-year drug compliance: 55.9% of patients in the nitrates group maintained the nitrate for one year, and 65.6% of patients in the other vasodilators group maintained the vasodilator for one year. Among patients with good drug compliance during one year, there were no significant differences in composite clinical events rate or all-cause death rate between the two groups (Supplementary Table S5). However, among patients with poor compliance, the one-year ACS rate was significantly higher in the nitrates group than in the other vasodilators group (7.3% vs. 2.0%, $p = 0.036$) (Supplementary Table S6).

4. Discussion

According to results from this nationwide prospective large-scale registry, the incidence of one-year composite clinical events including ACS was significantly higher in VA patients who used nitrates at discharge than in those who used other vasodilators at discharge; the adverse effects of nitrates were consistent after propensity score matching. Specifically, the use of nitrates at discharge was independently associated with a 2.69-fold increased risk of ACS in patients with VA. The nitrates group had lower drug compliance during one year of follow-up compared to the other vasodilators group, which affected one-year clinical events rates. Indeed, in patients with poor compliance, the one-year ACS rate in the group who used nitrates at discharge was significantly higher than in the group who used other vasodilators at discharge.

Nitrates, nicorandil, and other types of vasodilators are widely used for relieving acute angina symptoms in ischemic heart disease, including VA [16]. Long-acting nitrates are metabolized to NO within vascular smooth muscle cells, resulting in dilation of the coronary vasculature [1,6]. Nitrates including isosorbide dinitrate or isosorbide mononitrate ER have been proven to suppress acute angina symptoms and prevent recurrent attacks [17]. However, the frequent and continued use of nitrates can cause reduced vasodilatory effects due to the development of nitrate tolerance, which is caused by multiple factors [18,19]. In addition, during periods of nitrate withdrawal or nitrate-free periods, "rebound angina" may occur, in which the frequency of angina increases suddenly [16,20]. Increased sensitivity to vasoconstriction has been known to be a possible mechanism to explain rebound angina, while the vasodilating effect of NO decreases during the nitrate-free periods [20,21]. This is consistent with our results that the nitrates group had an increased risk of ACS during one year of follow-up, especially VA patients with poor drug compliance. On the contrary, nicorandil, which has properties similar to those of nitrates and acts as a K_{ATP} channel agonist, does not cause tolerance or rebound angina [16]. This is because nicorandil opens up potassium channels in the plasma membrane with the hyperpolarization of plasma smooth muscle cells, which can cause vascular relaxation without cGMP accumulation in the cells [22]. The role of K_{ATP} channels is to inhibit the formation of cGMP, which is associated with nitrate tolerance [22]. Another vasodilator, molsidomine, is a NO donor and delivers NO directly to vascular smooth muscle cells, activating the soluble guanylate cyclase, which synthesizes vasodilating cGMP from guanosine triphosphate [23,24]. This may also be the reason for the lower levels of tolerance to molsidomine compared to other nitrates. Since the mechanisms involved in vasodilation differ according to the type of drug, rebound angina or drug tolerance can occur differently in patients with VA. In this study, the composite clinical events rate including ACS was significantly higher in the nitrates group than in the other vasodilators group during one year of follow-up, which was maintained even after propensity score matching. Moreover, other vasodilators, including nicorandil, molsido-mine, and trimetazidine, did not raise ACS risk. Although the exact mechanism for different clinical outcomes according to type of vasodilator in VA patients is unclear, it may be related to the different endothelium-dependent responsiveness of vascular smooth muscle cell, which is an important pathogenesis of VA. To the best of our knowledge, there have been no clinical or experimental studies of direct comparison of this issue; a large-scale study will be needed in the future.

There was a small study that evaluated the long-term effects of nitrate treatment on cardiac events including cardiac death and readmission for ACS in VA patients who were treated with CCBs in a single Japanese center [25]. There were 48 patients who were treated with nitrates, 38 who were treated with nicorandil, and 145 patients who did not use vasodilators. The results showed that nitrates independently increased the risk of cardiac events by 5.18 times during 70 months of follow-up, but nicorandil did not increase the risk. In a recent multicenter study in Japan, Takahashi et al. [11] showed a long-term effect of nitrate therapy on major adverse cardiac events (MACE), including non-fatal myocardial infarction, cardiac death, heart failure, hospitalization due to unstable angina, and appropriate implantable cardioverter defibrillator shocks in 1492 VA patients. When they were followed for a median 32 months, the nitrates group did not have a significantly decreased or increased risk of MACE compared with the group not using nitrates. Even when nitrates and nicorandil were analyzed separately, neither of them affected MACE. In another recent study in Korea, Kim et al. [26] revealed that nitrates increased the risk of MACE, including cardiac death, myocardial infarction, any revascularization, or readmission due to recurrent angina, by 1.32-fold compared with not using nitrates in patients with VA during a median 55 months of follow-up. Specifically, patients treated with nitrates had a significantly higher risk of MACE by 1.70-fold, but nicorandil did not show any association with an increased risk of MACE. Although the clinical outcomes of each previous study were different from the outcomes of our study, which was composite clinical events including ACS, cardiac death, new-onset arrhythmia including VT and VF, and AV block, they showed that nicorandil had a neutral effect on adverse clinical outcomes and nitrates had a neutral effect or a tendency to increase the risk of adverse clinical outcomes. The most recent study using this VA-Korea registry [27] also showed that the risk of ACS at 2 years was significantly increased in the nitrate group compared with the non-vasodilator group (HR 2.49, 95% CI 1.01–6.14, $p = 0.047$) and that was not increased in the non-nitrate other type vasodilator group compared with the non-vasodilator group (HR 0.92, 95% CI 0.39–2.13, $p = 0.841$). However, composite clinical outcome including ACS, cardiac death, and new-onset arrhythmia at 2 years showed no significant differences between the nitrate, non-nitrate other type vasodilator, or non-vasodilator groups. This is not a direct comparison study of nitrate and non-nitrate other types of vasodilators. In this regard, it is notable that our study directly compared nitrates to other vasodilators and also presented and analyzed drug compliance.

The results of this study can be helpful in real-world practice. When VA patients are prescribed nitrates at discharge, their drug compliance may be poor owing to the side effects such as headache or dizziness. In the nitrates group, 55.9% maintained the drug for one year, and in the other vasodilators group, 65.6% maintained the drug. Poor drug compliance with nitrates will increase the occurrence of rebound angina and may also be associated with an increased risk of adverse clinical events compared to other vasodilators. Clinicians should be able to select a differentiated drug for each individual considering the effect of drug compliance to vasodilators on the prognosis in VA patients. In addition, vasospasm was confirmed by using EG in this study, but acetylcholine also can induce spasm, and that effect is promptly dissolved by intracoronary nitroglycerin. Since this study is about the vasodilator effect on clinical outcome in vasospastic patients, further studies are needed, but it is carefully suggested that the results can be applied to vasospastic angina patients who have been diagnosed with acetylcholine.

Several limitations of this study should be considered. First, this is a prospective multicenter cohort study, and it may have inevitable bias that can affect the results unlike a randomized controlled trial. However, to avoid bias as much as possible, propensity score matching and multivariate logistic regression analysis were attempted. Second, regardless of the type of vasodilator prescribed, just over half of the VA patients maintained the use of a vasodilator for one year; this may have affected our results because patients may not have had sufficient effectiveness of the nitrates or other vasodilators. Third, the patients in this study included both intermediate spasm or significant spasm after EG provocation test, and it was not a study targeting only definite vasospastic angina, but all patients with vasospasm of 50% or more who needed vasodilator therapy under the judgment of the clinician. However, even if the EG provocation test shows intermediate vasospasm results, it does not mean that vasodilator is not used in real clinical practice. This study showed the prescription patterns of vasodilator and its effects on prognosis according to the type of vasodilator in all vasospastic angina patients who need vasodilator in real clinical settings. Finally, subgroup analysis results were obtained from a much smaller sample size that was analyzed according to drug compliance, and this may limit the interpretation of this results.

5. Conclusions

In conclusion, prescribing nitrates as a vasodilator at discharge in VA patients can increase the adverse clinical outcomes including ACS during one year; poor compliance with nitrates is also associated with adverse clinical outcomes. This is an emphatic real clinical practice and prognosis for patients with symptoms suspected of VA who underwent CAG and EG tests. Thus, in the management of VA patients, clinicians should choose a vasodilator in consideration of a patient's compliance, as well as the drug mechanism, and they should consider prescribing vasodilators other than nitrates in order to achieve better clinical outcomes. In addition to this study, landmark trials that can provide a guide for prescribing vasodilators in VA patients will be needed in the future, and if these evidences are accumulated, it will form the basis for the management of VA patients.

Supplementary Materials: The following supporting information can be downloaded at https://www.mdpi.com/article/10.3390/jcm11123250/s1, Table S1: Coronary artery spasm and associated characteristics after provocation test according to vasodilator; Table S2: Time to composite clinical outcome in nitrate group and other types of vasodilator group; Table S3: One-year clinical event rate of patients with VA according to types of vasodilator in other types of vasodilator; Table S4: Baseline characteristics after propensity matching; Table S5: One-year clinical event rate of patients with good drug compliance; Table S6: One-year clinical event rate of patients with poor-compliance during 1 year.

Author Contributions: Conceptualization, H.-J.K. and S.-H.J.; Data curation, M.-H.L., W.-W.S., H.-L.K., H.-C.G. and D.-J.C.; Investigation, S.-H.J., W.-W.S., T.-H.Y., S.-H.H., B.-K.L., K.-H.P. and S.H.B.; Methodology, H.-J.K.; Software, H.-J.K., S.-H.J. and M.-H.L.; Validation, K.Y.L., Y.A., S.-W.R. and S.H.B.; Visualization, S.-H.J. and H.-J.K.; Writing—original draft, H.-J.K.; Writing—review and editing, S.-H.J. and M.-H.L. All authors have read and agreed to the published version of the manuscript.

Funding: This work was supported by grants from the Hallym University (HURF-2020-12) and the Ministry of SMEs and Startups of Korea (no. S2722143).

Institutional Review Board Statement: The study was conducted in accordance with the Declaration of Helsinki and approved by the Institutional Review Board of Hallym University Sacred Heart Hospital (Approved No. 2010-I007).

Informed Consent Statement: Written informed consent has been obtained from the patient(s) to publish this paper.

Data Availability Statement: Not applicable.

Conflicts of Interest: The authors declare no conflict of interest. The funders had no role in the design of the study; in the collection, analyses, or interpretation of data; in the writing of the manuscript, or in the decision to publish the results.

References

1. JCS Joint Working Group. Guidelines for diagnosis and treatment of patients with vasospastic angina (Coronary Spastic Angina) (JCS 2013). *Circ. J.* **2014**, *78*, 2779–2801. [CrossRef]
2. Yamagishi, M.; Tamaki, N.; Akasaka, T.; Ikeda, T.; Ueshima, K.; Uemura, S.; Otsuji, Y.; Kihara, Y.; Kimura, K.; Kimura, T.; et al. JCS 2018 Guideline on Diagnosis of Chronic Coronary Heart Diseases. *Circ. J.* **2021**, *85*, 402–572. [CrossRef] [PubMed]
3. Shin, D.I.; Baek, S.H.; Her, S.H.; Han, S.H.; Ahn, Y.; Park, K.H.; Kim, D.S.; Yang, T.H.; Choi, D.J.; Suh, J.W.; et al. The 24-Month Prognosis of Patients With Positive or Intermediate Results in the Intracoronary Ergonovine Provocation Test. *JACC Cardiovasc. Interv.* **2015**, *8*, 914–923. [CrossRef] [PubMed]
4. Matsue, Y.; Suzuki, M.; Nishizaki, M.; Hojo, R.; Hashimoto, Y.; Sakurada, H. Clinical implications of an implantable cardioverter-defibrillator in patients with vasospastic angina and lethal ventricular arrhythmia. *J. Am. Coll. Cardiol.* **2012**, *60*, 908–913. [CrossRef]
5. Ong, P.; Athanasiadis, A.; Borgulya, G.; Voehringer, M.; Sechtem, U. 3-year follow-up of patients with coronary artery spasm as cause of acute coronary syndrome: The CASPAR (coronary artery spasm in patients with acute coronary syndrome) study follow-up. *J. Am. Coll. Cardiol.* **2011**, *57*, 147–152. [CrossRef]
6. Parker, J.D.; Parker, J.O. Nitrate therapy for stable angina pectoris. *N. Engl. J. Med.* **1998**, *338*, 520–531. [CrossRef] [PubMed]
7. Aizawa, T.; Ogasawara, K.; Nakamura, F.; Hirosaka, A.; Sakuma, T.; Nagashima, K.; Kato, K. Effect of nicorandil on coronary spasm. *Am. J. Cardiol.* **1989**, *63*, 75J–79J. [CrossRef]
8. Krumenacker, M.; Roland, E. Clinical profile of nicorandil: An overview of its hemodynamic properties and therapeutic efficacy. *J. Cardiovasc. Pharmacol.* **1992**, *20* (Suppl. S3), S93–S102.
9. Majid, P.A.; DeFeyter, P.J.; Van der Wall, E.E.; Wardeh, R.; Roos, J.P. Molsidomine in the treatment of patients with angina pectoris. *N. Engl. J. Med.* **1980**, *302*, 1–6. [CrossRef]
10. Gori, T.; Parker, J.D. Nitrate-induced toxicity and preconditioning: A rationale for reconsidering the use of these drugs. *J. Am. Coll. Cardiol.* **2008**, *52*, 251–254. [CrossRef]
11. Takahashi, J.; Nihei, T.; Takagi, Y.; Miyata, S.; Odaka, Y.; Tsunoda, R.; Seki, A.; Sumiyoshi, T.; Matsui, M.; Goto, T.; et al. Prognostic impact of chronic nitrate therapy in patients with vasospastic angina: Multicentre registry study of the Japanese coronary spasm association. *Eur. Heart J.* **2015**, *36*, 228–237. [CrossRef]
12. Kim, D.W.; Her, S.H.; Ahn, Y.; Shin, D.I.; Han, S.H.; Kim, D.S.; Choi, D.J.; Kwon, H.M.; Gwon, H.C.; Jo, S.H.; et al. Clinical outcome according to spasm type of single coronary artery provoked by intracoronary ergonovine tests in patients without significant organic stenosis. *Int. J. Cardiol.* **2018**, *252*, 6–12. [CrossRef] [PubMed]
13. Lee, M.H.; Jo, S.H.; Kwon, S.; Park, B.W.; Bang, D.W.; Hyon, M.S.; Baek, S.H.; Han, S.H.; Her, S.H.; Shin, D.I.; et al. Impact of Overweight/Obesity on Clinical Outcomes of Patient with Vasospastic Angina: From the Vasospastic Angina in Korea Registry. *Sci. Rep.* **2020**, *10*, 4954. [CrossRef]
14. Cho, S.S.; Jo, S.H.; Han, S.H.; Lee, K.Y.; Her, S.H.; Lee, M.H.; Seo, W.W.; Kim, S.E.; Yang, T.H.; Park, K.H.; et al. Clopidogrel plus Aspirin Use is Associated with Worse Long-Term Outcomes, but Aspirin Use Alone is Safe in Patients with Vasospastic Angina: Results from the VA-Korea Registry, A Prospective Multi-Center Cohort. *Sci. Rep.* **2019**, *9*, 17783. [CrossRef] [PubMed]

15. Takagi, Y.; Yasuda, S.; Takahashi, J.; Tsunoda, R.; Ogata, Y.; Seki, A.; Sumiyoshi, T.; Matsui, M.; Goto, T.; Tanabe, Y.; et al. Clinical implications of provocation tests for coronary artery spasm: Safety, arrhythmic complications, and prognostic impact: Multicentre registry study of the Japanese Coronary Spasm Association. *Eur. Heart J.* **2013**, *34*, 258–267. [CrossRef] [PubMed]
16. Tarkin, J.M.; Kaski, J.C. Vasodilator Therapy: Nitrates and Nicorandil. *Cardiovasc. Drugs Ther.* **2016**, *30*, 367–378. [CrossRef]
17. Conti, C.R.; Hill, J.A.; Feldman, R.L.; Conti, J.B.; Pepine, C.J. Isosorbide dinitrate and nifedipine in variant angina pectoris. *Am. Heart J.* **1985**, *110*, 251–256. [CrossRef]
18. Munzel, T.; Gori, T. Nitrate therapy and nitrate tolerance in patients with coronary artery disease. *Curr. Opin. Pharmacol.* **2013**, *13*, 251–259. [CrossRef]
19. Thadani, U. Challenges with nitrate therapy and nitrate tolerance: Prevalence, prevention, and clinical relevance. *Am. J. Cardiovasc. Drugs* **2014**, *14*, 287–301. [CrossRef]
20. Munzel, T.; Mollnau, H.; Hartmann, M.; Geiger, C.; Oelze, M.; Warnholtz, A.; Yehia, A.H.; Forstermann, U.; Meinertz, T. Effects of a nitrate-free interval on tolerance, vasoconstrictor sensitivity and vascular superoxide production. *J. Am. Coll. Cardiol.* **2000**, *36*, 628–634. [CrossRef]
21. Munzel, T.; Kurz, S.; Heitzer, T.; Harrison, D.G. New insights into mechanisms underlying nitrate tolerance. *Am. J. Cardiol.* **1996**, *77*, 24C–30C. [CrossRef]
22. O'Rourke, S.T. KATP channel activation mediates nicorandil-induced relaxation of nitrate-tolerant coronary arteries. *J. Cardiovasc. Pharmacol.* **1996**, *27*, 831–837. [CrossRef]
23. Rosenkranz, B.; Winkelmann, B.R.; Parnham, M.J. Clinical pharmacokinetics of molsidomine. *Clin. Pharm.* **1996**, *30*, 372–384. [CrossRef] [PubMed]
24. Messin, R.; Opolski, G.; Fenyvesi, T.; Carreer-Bruhwyler, F.; Dubois, C.; Famaey, J.P.; Geczy, J. Efficacy and safety of molsidomine once-a-day in patients with stable angina pectoris. *Int. J. Cardiol.* **2005**, *98*, 79–89. [CrossRef]
25. Kosugi, M.; Nakagomi, A.; Shibui, T.; Kato, K.; Kusama, Y.; Atarashi, H.; Mizuno, K. Effect of long-term nitrate treatment on cardiac events in patients with vasospastic angina. *Circ. J.* **2011**, *75*, 2196–2205. [CrossRef] [PubMed]
26. Kim, C.H.; Park, T.K.; Cho, S.W.; Oh, M.S.; Lee, D.H.; Seong, C.S.; Gwag, H.B.; Lim, A.Y.; Yang, J.H.; Song, Y.B.; et al. Impact of different nitrate therapies on long-term clinical outcomes of patients with vasospastic angina: A propensity score-matched analysis. *Int. J. Cardiol.* **2018**, *252*, 1–5. [CrossRef] [PubMed]
27. Lim, Y.; Kim, M.C.; Ahn, Y.; Cho, K.H.; Sim, D.S.; Hong, Y.J.; Kim, J.H.; Jeong, M.H.; Baek, S.H.; Her, S.H.; et al. Prognostic Impact of Chronic Vasodilator Therapy in Patients With Vasospastic Angina. *J. Am. Heart Assoc.* **2022**, *11*, e023776. [CrossRef] [PubMed]

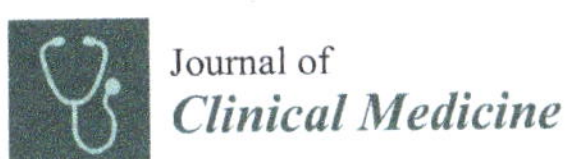

Journal of
Clinical Medicine

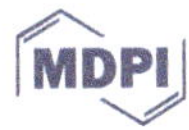

Article

Development of a Laboratory Risk-Score Model to Predict One-Year Mortality in Acute Myocardial Infarction Survivors

Yuhei Goriki [1,2], Atsushi Tanaka [2,*], Goro Yoshioka [2], Kensaku Nishihira [3], Nehiro Kuriyama [3], Yoshisato Shibata [3] and Koichi Node [2]

1 Department of Cardiovascular Medicine, National Hospital Organization Ureshino Medical Center, Ureshino 843-0393, Japan; i03.eou2@gmail.com
2 Department of Cardiovascular Medicine, Saga University, Saga 849-8501, Japan; s04211090s@gmail.com (G.Y.); node@cc.saga-u.ac.jp (K.N.)
3 Miyazaki Medical Association Hospital Cardiovascular Center, Miyazaki 880-0834, Japan; nishihira@med.miyazaki-u.ac.jp (K.N.); n-kuriyama@cure.or.jp (N.K.); yshibata@cure.or.jp (Y.S.)
* Correspondence: tanakaa2@cc.saga-u.ac.jp; Tel.: +81-952-34-2364; Fax: +81-952-34-2089

Abstract: The high post-discharge mortality rate of acute myocardial infarction (AMI) survivors is concerning, indicating a need for reliable, easy-to-use risk prediction tools. We aimed to examine if a combined pre-procedural blood testing risk model predicts one-year mortality in AMI survivors. Overall, 1355 consecutive AMI patients who received primary coronary revascularization were divided into derivation (n = 949) and validation (n = 406) cohorts. A risk-score model of parameters from pre-procedural routine blood testing on admission was generated. In the derivation cohort, multivariable analysis demonstrated that hemoglobin < 11 g/dL (odds ratio (OR) 4.01), estimated glomerular filtration rate < 30 mL/min/1.73 m^2 (OR 3.75), albumin < 3.8 mg/dL (OR 3.37), and high-sensitivity troponin I > 2560 ng/L (OR 3.78) were significantly associated with one-year mortality after discharge. An increased risk score, assigned from 0 to 4 points according to the counts of selected variables, was significantly associated with higher one-year mortality in both cohorts (p < 0.001). Receiver-operating characteristics curve analyses of risk models demonstrated adequate discrimination between patients with and without one-year death (area under the curve (95% confidence interval) 0.850 (0.756–0.912) in the derivation cohort; 0.820 (0.664–0.913) in the validation cohort). Our laboratory risk-score model can be useful for predicting one-year mortality in AMI survivors.

Keywords: biomarker; mortality; myocardial infarction; risk-score model

Citation: Goriki, Y.; Tanaka, A.; Yoshioka, G.; Nishihira, K.; Kuriyama, N.; Shibata, Y.; Node, K. Development of a Laboratory Risk-Score Model to Predict One-Year Mortality in Acute Myocardial Infarction Survivors. *J. Clin. Med.* **2022**, *11*, 3497. https://doi.org/10.3390/jcm11123497

Academic Editor: Jasper Boeddinghaus

Received: 15 May 2022
Accepted: 16 June 2022
Published: 17 June 2022

1. Introduction

Acute myocardial infarction (AMI) is a major cause of poor outcomes and clinical concerns worldwide [1]. Over the past two decades, in-hospital death rates from AMI have decreased dramatically, partly due to advances in the clinical management of the acute phase of AMI and guideline-directed medical therapy [2]. However, long-term prognosis of AMI survivors is still unfavorable. In this regard, post-discharge mortality remains a clinical concern [2,3]. Therefore, there is a need for reliable and easy-to-use risk prediction tools for early identification of at-risk patients, which may help with timely prevention and well-tailored treatment.

Several risk-score models to predict prognosis after acute coronary syndrome (ACS), including AMI, are currently available [4,5]. The Global Registry of Acute Coronary Events (GRACE) 2.0 score is one of the most established risk-score models for determining mortality risk in AMI patients [4]. This model was created prior to the contemporary era of optimal medical therapy and increased usage of percutaneous coronary intervention (PCI) for AMI patients [2,6]. In addition, this model requires several clinical variables: age, systolic blood pressure (BP), heart rate, creatinine, cardiac arrest at admission, ST-segment deviation, abnormal cardiac enzyme, and Killip classification. However, in the emergency setting of AMI, several variables, such as heart rate and systolic BP, often fluctuate significantly, which could compromise the prediction value of the GRACE 2.0 model, resulting in a requirement for reassessment. Unlike these clinical measurements, blood parameters can be rapidly obtained in a non-subjective fashion, even in the emergent setting of AMI, suggesting that a blood-parameter-based model may be easy to use for AMI mortality risk prediction.

Several models of combined blood variables have been used as predictive indicators of AMI mortality risk [7,8]. We have also previously reported a risk-score model combining pre-procedural laboratory variables to predict the risk of in-hospital death in ST-segment elevation myocardial infarction (STEMI), comparable to the GRACE 2.0 model [9]. However, whether combined-blood-parameter-based models could predict post-discharge mortality in AMI survivors remains largely unknown. Herein, we aimed to create a risk-score model based on a combination of pre-procedural laboratory parameters for one-year mortality after discharge in AMI survivors and compare its predictive ability with a conventional model (GRACE 2.0 model).

2. Materials and Methods

2.1. Design and Participants

This was a retrospective observational study conducted in Miyazaki Medical Association Hospital. The study population comprised 1852 consecutive patients hospitalized for ACS between Apr 2012 and Jan 2018, were included in the present study. Patients who did not undergo primary PCI, recurrent ACS or unstable angina pectoris, who died during hospitalization, lost to follow-up one year after discharge, and lack of laboratory information on admission were excluded from the analyses. Thus, 1355 patients were included in the present study. Patients were randomly classified into either derivation (n = 949) or validation cohorts (n = 406) [10,11] (Figure 1). This study was approved by the Institutional Review Board of Miyazaki Medical Association Hospital and complied with the latest Helsinki Declaration. Nevertheless, written informed consent was waived due to the retrospective of the study.

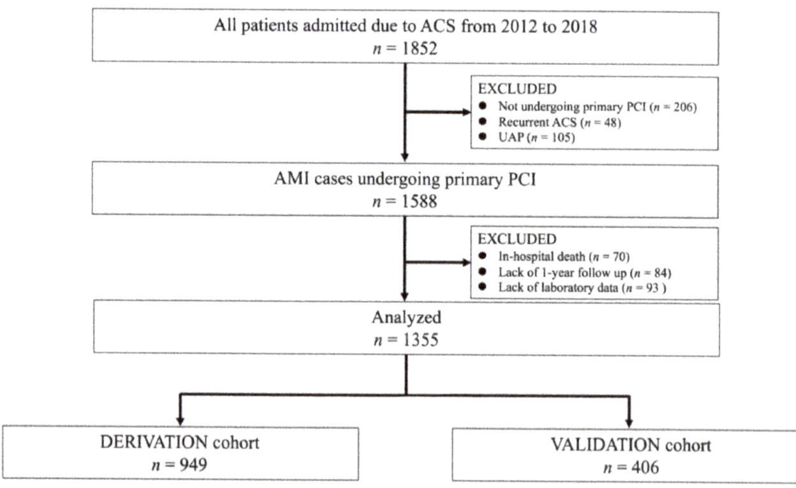

Figure 1. Flow chart of study participant selection. ACS, acute coronary syndrome; PCI, percutaneous coronary intervention; UAP, unstable angina pectoris.

2.2. Definition of STEMI and NSTEMI

STEMI and non-ST-segment elevation myocardial infarction (NSTEMI) were diagnosed by cardiologists based on the universal definitions [12]. Treatment and management depend on the latest domestic guidelines released by the Japanese Circulation Society (Diagnosis and Treatment of Acute Coronary Syndrome).

2.3. Data Acquisition

Participants' baseline characteristics and clinical manifestations, vital signs, medical history, usual laboratory data, high-sensitivity troponin I (hsTnI), type of AMI, Killip classification and left ventricular ejection fraction were collected on admission. Hs-TnI levels were measured on a chemiluminescence immunoassay (ARCHITECT® high sensitive troponin I (Abbott Japan, Tokyo, Japan)) with a coefficient of variation < 10% at 32 ng/L and 99th percentile reference limit < 34.2 or 15.6 ng/L (male or female). For the procedure-related parameters, clinical information on peak creatine kinase (CK), culprit lesion and mechanical support were collected during coronary procedure. Medications at discharge were also collected. Information on post-discharge death was collected by medical records or telephone calls. The estimated glomerular filtration rate (eGFR) was calculated with the revised equation for the Japanese population [13].

2.4. Statistics

Continuous variables are expressed as mean ± standard deviation for normal distribution or median [interquartile range] for non-normal distribution values. Categorical variables are shown as numbers (%). Comparisons of continuous variables between both cohorts were done with Student's *t*-test or Wilcoxon test, where appropriate. Categorical variables were compared using the chi-squared test.

The laboratory variables significantly associated with post-discharge death selected by the univariate analysis were categorized based on the cutoff values reported previously [14–21] and then applied for the multivariable analysis to develop the risk-score model. Those variables were further selected using a multivariable logistic regression model using the backward factor elimination method. Finally, the remaining variables were given an equivalent point to calculate the risk score for one-year mortality. The subjects were classified into three groups based on the total scores, as follows: low risk (0–1 point), moderate risk (2 points) and high risk (3–4 points). Cochran-Armitage trend analysis was used to assess statistical trends among three risk groups. The predictive abilities of the risk models for predicting post-discharged death were assessed for their discrimination and calibration, and which were analyzed by the receiver operating characteristic curve and Hosmer–Lemeshow goodness-of-fit test, respectively. The risk score for predicting one-year mortality was also calculated using the GRACE 2.0 ACS Risk Calculator app. We estimated the area under the curve (AUC) of the GRACE 2.0 model and compared it with that of the present model derived from the validation cohort. Differences in those AUCs were appraised by the DeLong method [22]. Statistical analyses were conducted using the JMP version 15 (SAS Institute Inc., Cary, NC, USA), and statistical significance was set at p-value < 0.05 (2-tailed), except for the Hosmer–Lemeshow goodness-of-fit test.

3. Results

3.1. Baseline Demographics and Characteristics

The study population consisted of 1355 subjects (derivation 949; validation 406). Baseline demographics and characteristics of the two cohorts are listed in Table 1. There were no significant differences in the clinical information on admission and during hospitalization between the derivation and validation cohorts. Medications at discharge were comparable between the two cohorts. Post-discharge deaths were observed in 30 patients (3.2%) in the derivation cohort and 14 (3.5%) in the validation cohort.

Table 1. Demographics and characteristics in both cohorts.

	Derivation (n = 949)	Validation (n = 405)	p-Value
Age, years	69.2 ± 12.1	68.6 ± 12.6	0.435
Female, n (%)	250 (26.3)	111 (27.4)	0.635
Body mass index, kg/m^2	24.0 ± 3.7	24.0 ± 4.1	0.789
Systolic blood pressure, mmHg	142.1 ± 28.5	141.0 ± 28.0	0.464
Pulse rate, bpm	77.1 ± 19.7	77.3 ± 17.8	0.863
Medical history			
Hypertension, n (%)	687 (72.4)	277 (68.4)	0.149
Dyslipidemia, n (%)	508 (53.5)	211 (52.1)	0.628
Diabetes mellitus, n (%)	264 (27.8)	102 (25.2)	0.317
Smoking, n (%)	467 (49.2)	189 (46.7)	0.391
Previous myocardial infarction, n (%)	70 (7.4)	23 (5.7)	0.274
Peripheral artery disease, n (%)	29 (3.1)	13 (3.2)	0.855
Malignancy, n (%)	45 (4.7)	14 (3.5)	0.288
Laboratory parameters			
White blood cell, ×10^2/μL	96.4 ± 37.1	96.8 ± 33.3	0.857
Hemoglobin, g/dL	13.8 ± 2.1	13.8 ± 2.1	0.845
Platelet, ×10^4/μL	21.7 ± 6.2	22.1 ± 6.3	0.246
Glycated hemoglobin A1c, %	6.0 (5.7, 6.6)	5.9 (5.6, 6.5)	0.168
Glucose, mg/dL	148 (107, 189)	141 (102, 181)	0.196
eGFR, mL/min/1.73 m^2	66.2 ± 22.7	67.9 ± 24.1	0.899
LDL-cholesterol, mg/dL	122.8 ± 35.1	123.6 ± 37.7	0.698
HDL-cholesterol, mg/dL	46.8 ± 12.0	48.8 ± 13.2	0.097
Albumin, g/dL	4.0 ± 0.5	4.0 ± 0.5	0.648
Creatine kinase, U/L	156 (96, 356)	169 (100, 395)	0.286
hs-TnI, ng/L	300 (50, 3180)	380 (60, 3010)	0.653
STEMI, n (%)	640 (67.4)	278 (68.5)	0.709
Killip classification ≥ 3, n (%)	64 (6.7)	19 (4.7)	0.146
LVEF (on admission), %	52.4 ± 11.7	52.5 ± 10.6	0.550
Peak creatine kinase, IU/L	1231 (358, 2950)	1185 (299, 2687)	0.337
IABP, n (%)	93 (9.8)	28 (6.9)	0.086
ECMO, n (%)	9 (1.0)	2 (0.5)	0.166
Medication at discharge			
Antiplatelet therapy, n (%)	940 (99.0)	404 (99.5)	0.214
Aspirin (100 mg daily), n (%)	899 (94.7)	391 (96.5)	0.131
Prasugrel (3.75 mg daily), n (%)	208 (21.9)	73 (18.0)	0.221
Clopidogrel (75 mg daily), n (%)	670 (70.6)	308 (76.0)	0.089
Dual antiplatelet therapy, n (%)	857 (90.3)	377 (93.0)	0.165
Statin, n (%)	860 (90.6)	370 (91.1)	0.844
β-Blocker, n (%)	424 (44.9)	195 (48.0)	0.326
ACE inhibitor, n (%)	390 (41.1)	147 (36.2)	0.091
ARB, n (%)	296 (31.2)	147 (36.2)	0.074
Diuretic, n (%)	177 (18.7)	68 (16.8)	0.401
Post-discharge death during one-year follow-up, n (%)	30 (3.2)	14 (3.5)	0.785

Categorical variables are shown as numbers (%); data for continuous variables are shown as mean ± standard deviation for normal distribution or median (interquartile range) for non-normal distribution. ACE, angiotensin-converting enzyme; ARB, angiotensin receptor blocker; ECMO, extracorporeal membrane oxygenation; eGFR, estimated glomerular filtration rate; HDL, high-density lipoprotein; hs-TnI, high-sensitivity troponin I; IABP, intra-aortic balloon pumping; LDL, low-density lipoprotein; LVEF, left ventricular ejection fraction; STEMI, ST-segment elevation myocardial infarction.

3.2. Laboratory Parameters Associated with Post-Discharge Death

Table 2 shows the univariate analysis of blood variables between survivors and non-survivors at one-year post-discharge in the derivation cohort. Significant variables detected in the univariate analysis were subjected to a multivariable stepwise backward logistic regression analysis. In that analysis, hemoglobin level < 11 g/dL, eGFR < 30 mL/min/1.73 m^2, albumin level < 3.8 mg/dL, and hs-TnI > 2560 ng/L (normal upper limit × 80) were significantly associated with post-discharge death in the derivation cohort (Table 3). The odds ratio for one-year mortality ranged from 3.37 to 4.01. Zero to four points were assigned to each patient according to the number of risk factors they had.

Table 2. Univariate analysis of laboratory variables associated with post-discharge death.

	Survivors	Non-Survivors (Post-Discharge Death)	p-Value
White blood cell, $\times 10^3/\mu L$	9.6 ± 3.5	9.4 ± 4.2	0.656
Hemoglobin, g/dL	13.9 ± 2.0	11.7 ± 2.1	<0.001
Platelet, $\times 10^4/\mu L$	21.8 ± 6.1	18.1 ± 7.3	0.001
Glycated hemoglobin A1c, %	6.0 (5.4, 6.6)	6.3 (5.4, 6.7)	0.688
Glucose, mg/dL	148 (123, 187)	154 (119, 212)	0.531
eGFR, mL/min/1.73 m^2	66.9 ± 22.1	43.7 ± 28.1	<0.001
LDL-cholesterol, mg/dL	123.7 ± 34.8	93.9 ± 32.9	<0.001
HDL-cholesterol, mg/dL	47.0 ± 12.1	41.8 ± 10.7	0.020
Albumin, mg/dL	4.1 ± 0.5	3.4 ± 0.5	<0.001
Creatine kinase, U/L	152 (96, 355)	232 (77, 855)	0.128
hs-TnI, ng/L	280 (50, 2030)	5900 (560, 21300)	<0.001

Data for continuous variables are expressed as mean ± standard deviation for normal distribution or median (interquartile range) for non-normal distribution. See Table 1 for abbreviation definitions.

Table 3. Independent predictors for post-discharge death and given risk-score.

	Odds Ratio	95% Confidence Interval	p-Value	Risk-Score
Hemoglobin < 11 g/dL	4.01	1.65–9.72	0.002	1
eGFR < 30 mL/min/1.73 m^2	3.75	1.53–9.19	0.004	1
Albumin < 3.8 mg/dL	3.37	1.31–8.67	0.012	1
hs-TnI > 2560 ng/L (normal upper limit × 80)	3.78	1.64–8.72	0.002	1

See Table 1 for abbreviation definitions.

3.3. Predictive Model of Post-Discharge Death

The incidence of post-discharge death during one-year follow-up increased significantly as the total risk score elevated in both cohorts (Figure 2A,B). The risk-score model demonstrated adequate discrimination between subjects who died or not after discharge in the validation (AUC, 95% confidence interval (CI): 0.850, 0.756–0.913) and derivation (0.820, 0.664–0.913) cohorts (Figure 3). The Hosmer–Lemeshow test indicated a favorable fit in both cohorts ($\chi^2 = 0.328$, $p = 0.849$ for the derivation; $\chi^2 = 0.556$, $p = 0.757$ for the validation). When patients were further classified into three subgroups based on their risk score: 0–1 point (defined as low-risk), 2 points (moderate-risk), and 3–4 points (high-risk), a similar trend for post-discharge mortality during one-year follow-up was also observed in those subgroups (Figure 4A,B).

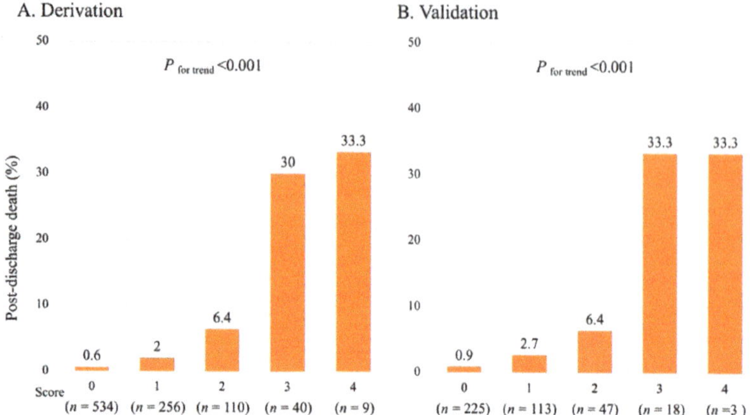

Figure 2. Post-discharge death rates according to the risk-score estimated by the laboratory model.

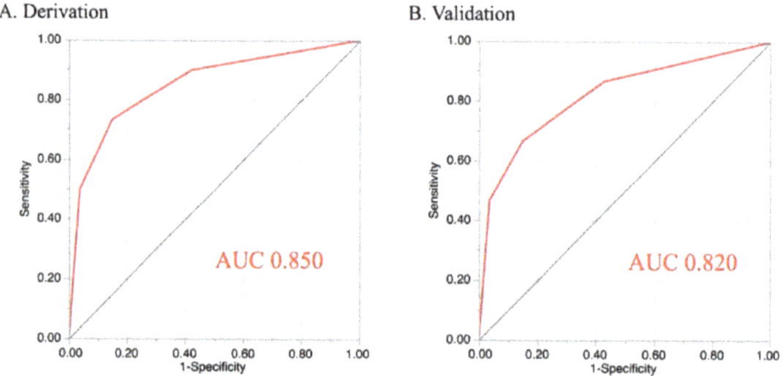

Figure 3. Receiver operating characteristic curves of the present model. AUC, area under the curve.

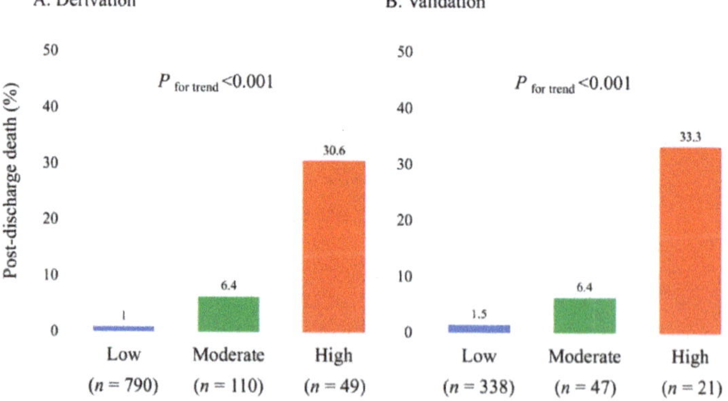

Figure 4. Incidence of post-discharge death in the risk-based subgroups. A total risk score of 0–1 point was defined as low-risk, 2 points as moderate-risk, and 3–4 points as high-risk.

3.4. Comparison with GRACE 2.0 Model

The AUCs of the present and GRACE 2.0 models in the validation cohort were 0.820 (95% CI, 0.664–0.913) and 0.806 (95% CI, 0.681–0.890). The predictive power was similar between the two models (Figure 5). Additionally, we compared the predictive ability between these risk models based on the type of AMI and gender. In all cases, the predictive power was not significantly different between these models (Table 4). Furthermore, the laboratory model was able to stratify the possible risk of post-discharge death, especially in the high-risk subgroup from the GRACE 2.0 model (risk-score > 8.0%) [23], but not in the low–intermediate-risk groups from the GRACE 2.0 model (risk-score ≤ 8.0%) (Figure 6).

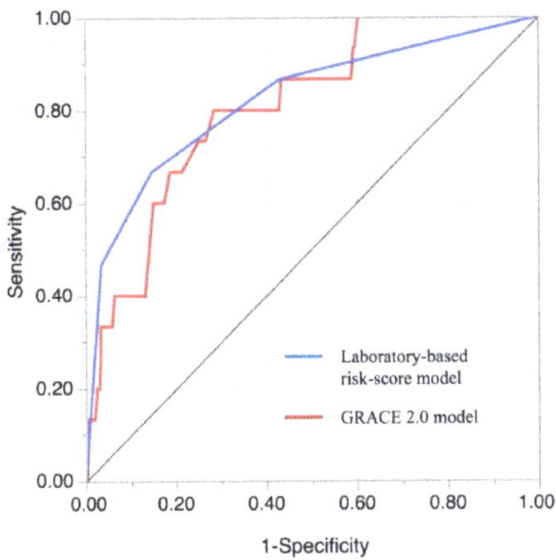

Risk score	AUC	ΔAUC	P value
Laboratory-based risk-score model	0.820	Reference	
GRACE 2.0 model	0.806	0.014	0.742

Figure 5. Comparison of the predictive abilities for one-year mortality between the laboratory and GRACE 2.0 models. AUCs of the laboratory (blue) and GRACE 2.0 (red) models in the validation cohort were 0.820 (95% CI, 0.664–0.913) and 0.810 (95% CI, 0.681–0.890). AUC, area under the curve; GRACE, Global Registry of Acute Coronary Events.

Table 4. Comparisons of AUCs between the two models according to AMI and sex statuses.

		AUC of the Laboratory-Based Risk-Score Model	AUC of the GRACE 2.0 Model	ΔAUC	p-Value
Type of AMI	STEMI	0.820	0.866	−0.046	0.124
	NSTEMI	0.871	0.855	0.016	0.738
Sex	Male	0.831	0.861	−0.036	0.397
	Female	0.836	0.840	−0.005	0.905

AMI, acute myocardial infarction; AUC, area under the curve; NSTEMI, non-ST-segment elevation myocardial infarction; STEMI, ST-segment elevation myocardial infarction. For other abbreviations, see Table 1.

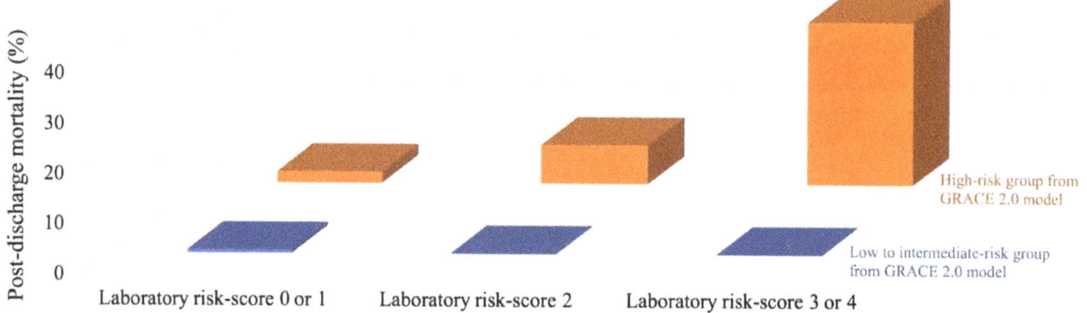

	Laboratory risk-score 0 or 1	Laboratory risk-score 2	Laboratory risk-score 3 or 4	*P* value
Mortality in the high-risk group from GRACE 2.0 model	2.2 % (9/408)	7.7 % (9/117)	32.4 % (22/68)	< 0.001
Mortality in the low to intermediate-risk group from GRACE 2.0 model	0.2 % (4/702)	0 % (0/34)	0 % (0/2)	0.653

Figure 6. Dual-stratification by the laboratory model × the GRACE 2.0 model. All subjects from both study cohorts were stratified by the GRACE 2.0 model (high-risk > 8.0%, low to intermediate-risk ≤ 8.0%) and further subdivided into three subgroups by the laboratory model (low risk: 0–1 points, moderate risk: 2 points, and high risk: 3–4 points). The table below the graph shows the post-discharge one-year mortality for each subgroup. GRACE, The Global Registry of Acute Coronary Events.

4. Discussion

The main findings of this investigation were as follows: (i) individual blood variables measured on admission (hemoglobin < 11 g/dL, eGFR < 30 mL/min/1.73 m^2, albumin < 3.8 mg/dL, and hs-TnI > 2560 ng/L) were independently related with an augmented risk of post-discharge mortality rates at one-year; (ii) a simple model, using a combination of pre-procedural laboratory measures, can be useful for assessing the risk of post-discharge death at one-year follow-up; (iii) the predictive ability of our model was similar to that of the GRACE 2.0 model; and (iv) our model provided predictive power to further subdivide the high-risk population estimated by the GRACE 2.0 model. Therefore, these results may indicate that our novel model with pre-procedural laboratory parameters can help predict one-year mortality in AMI survivors.

Some risk stratification models for estimating the risk of post-discharge death rates have been developed for patients with AMI. Among these risk prediction models, the GRACE 2.0 system has been recommended for stratifying AMI mortality risk according to guidelines [24]. However, cohorts enrolled from the GRACE model were patients in the 2000s, while medical management of AMI has developed beyond the clinical surroundings of the 2000s [2]. Moreover, some of the hemodynamic statuses required to calculate the GRACE score often fluctuate widely, especially in the emergency clinical phase of AMI. Therefore, the risk estimated by the GRACE model may also vary. While the measurements of blood parameters can be performed readily and objectively, this study sought to create a laboratory-based model to estimate the risk of one-year death in AMI survivors.

Individual blood parameters considered for the risk assessment in the present study are useful markers for predicting the prognosis in patients with AMI [14–21]. In particular, the presence of anemia or renal dysfunction is a powerful predictor of poor outcomes in post-AMI patients [7–10]. Actually, several risk calculators for predicting long-term mortality need renal functional parameters and hemoglobin levels [4,5]. Besides anemia-

and chronic kidney disease (CKD)-related parameters, our model found two new individual blood parameters as possible candidates to predict post-discharge death: albumin and hsTnI levels.

Albumin is a marker of nutrition, frailty, and inflammation [25], all of which have been individually reported to contribute to the cardiovascular disease prognosis [26,27]. Recently, the relationship between albumin level and post-discharge prognosis of AMI has been reported [28,29]. Thus, serum albumin levels are affected by various aspects of clinical situations and may represent a predictive marker for clinical outcomes in post-AMI patients.

Our study also demonstrated a relationship between hsTnI and one-year death rates in AMI survivors. The biological kinetics of troponin on admission due to AMI was associated with ischemic time, infarct size and death during hospitalization [21,30]. Additionally, left ventricular dysfunction and onset-to-balloon time were predictors of cardiovascular events after AMI [31]. Therefore, the severity of myocardial damage, as measured by hsTnI on admission, has the potential to predict the incidence of post-discharge death in AMI survivors. In our study, the multivariable logistic regression analysis eventually selected those four parameters and co-included them in our model, which provided the predictive power of post-discharge death in AMI survivors, similarly to the GRACE 2.0 model.

In 2015, Pocock et al. created a predictive model for one-year mortality in AMI [5]. That model comprised 12 clinical parameters and discriminated the risk of post-discharge death within one year after AMI. However, calculating risk may be complicated, because as many as 12 factors are required, hampering the dissemination to clinical practice, especially in the emergency setting. Furthermore, the predictive ability of that model in comparison with other models was also unknown. In contrast, our model is easy to calculate only with four variables immediately obtained at admission for AMI. Additionally, our model was able to predict the risk of post-AMI death one year after discharge, being comparable to that of the GRACE 2.0 model. Notably, the present model was useful for stratifying risk in the high-risk subpopulation classified by the GRACE 2.0 model. These findings suggest that our model is clinically helpful in improving the predictive value for the risk of post-discharge death after AMI, specifically in the high-risk population derived from the GRACE 2.0 model, simply and objectively.

Compared to those existing models, our study's strengths and novelty were that we developed the risk-score model showing the predictive ability comparable to the GRACE 2.0 model by combining only four blood parameters, each of which has prognostic evidence in patients with AMI. Considering that each blood parameter can reflect different aspects of a patient's medical conditions, combining those parameters could provide a comprehensive and integrated approach to risk stratification and predicting prognosis. Several models based on the combined blood parameters have predicted short-term clinical outcomes in patients with AMI [7,8,32]. To the best of our knowledge, we first show that a risk-score model based on the combination of blood parameters on admission for AMI can predict the mid-term prognosis in AMI survivors.

Our study has some potential limitations. Firstly, this study was not a multi-center, prospective design. Secondly, since the cohorts included only Japanese and in relatively small numbers, the generalizability of our findings to other ethnicities remains uncertain. Thirdly, the current analyses assessed the predictive power of a risk-score model composed of only pre-procedural blood parameters upon admission for AMI. In addition, our predictive model did not account for the laboratory parameters obtained at post-procedure and/or discharge. Therefore, we cannot determine whether the selected parameters dominantly reflect acutely evoked pathophysiological reactions due to AMI or the chronic clinical conditions of the patients. Fourthly, the platelet count was lower in non-survivors than in the survivors in the univariate analysis. Actually, the risk of bleeding complications may be augmented in patients with a lower level of platelet count by receiving antiplatelet therapy, adversely affecting prognosis. Conversely, the patients who underwent PCI for coronary artery disease should receive antiplatelet therapy according to the relevant guidelines to reduce the risk of stent thrombosis [33]. Accordingly, most subjects received that therapy upon discharge, and their prognoses with and without it were not compared in this study. Therefore, the possibility that the antiplatelet therapy upon discharge had affected prognosis to some extent in this study cohort cannot be excluded. Finally, the study focused only on the laboratory variables to develop the current risk-score model. Therefore, non-laboratory variables, such as age, vital signs and cardiac function, related to the prognosis after AMI were not considered to predict the risk of post-discharge death. Nevertheless, our laboratory-based model showed comparable performance to the GRACE 2.0 model in predicting post-discharge death and partly improved the risk stratification, specifically in the high-risk population derived from the conventional model. As the present study sought to create a laboratory-based model to predict one-year mortality after AMI, further research is required to assess whether our model can predict longer-term prognosis and/or other clinical outcomes after AMI.

5. Conclusions

Our findings suggest that the present risk-score model is useful for predicting one-year mortality in AMI survivors who underwent primary PCI simply and objectively.

Author Contributions: Conceptualization, Y.G., A.T. and K.N. (Koichi Node); methodology, Y.G., A.T. and G.Y.; software, Y.G.; validation, Y.G., A.T. and G.Y.; formal analysis, Y.G.; investigation, Y.G. and G.Y.; resources, Y.G., G.Y., K.N. (Kensaku Nishihira), N.K. and Y.S.; data curation, Y.G.; writing: original draft preparation, Y.G. and A.T.; writing: review and editing, all authors; visualization, Y.G. and A.T.; supervision, A.T., Y.S. and K.N. (Koichi Node); project administration, A.T. and K.N. (Koichi Node); funding acquisition, A.T. All authors have read and agreed to the published version of the manuscript.

Funding: This work was supported by the Japan Society for the Promotion of Science KAKENHI Grant Number JP21K08130 and the Takeda Science Foundation.

Institutional Review Board Statement: The study was approved by the Institutional Review Board of Miyazaki Medical Association Hospital (2019-30).

Informed Consent Statement: Written informed consent was waived because of the retrospective nature.

Data Availability Statement: The raw data for the study will not be shared.

Acknowledgments: We would like to thank Aya Yamada (Saga University) for her dedicated study support.

Conflicts of Interest: The authors declare no conflict of interest related to the study.

References

1. Ibanez, B.; James, S.; Agewall, S.; Antunes, M.J.; Bucciarelli-Ducci, C.; Bueno, H.; Caforio, A.L.P.; Crea, F.; Goudevenos, J.A.; Halvorsen, S.; et al. 2017 ESC Guidelines for the management of acute myocardial infarction in patients presenting with ST-segment elevation: The Task Force for the management of acute myocardial infarction in patients presenting with ST-segment elevation of the European Society of Cardiology (ESC). *Eur. Heart J.* **2018**, *39*, 119–177. [PubMed]
2. Puymirat, E.; Simon, T.; Cayla, G.; Cottin, Y.; Elbaz, M.; Coste, P.; Lemesle, G.; Motreff, P.; Popovic, B.; Khalife, K.; et al. Acute Myocardial Infarction: Changes in Patient Characteristics, Management, and 6-Month Outcomes over a Period of 20 Years in the FAST-MI Program (French Registry of Acute ST-Elevation or Non-ST-Elevation Myocardial Infarction) 1995 to 2015. *Circulation* **2017**, *136*, 1908–1919. [CrossRef] [PubMed]
3. Fox, K.A.; Carruthers, K.F.; Dunbar, D.R.; Graham, C.; Manning, J.R.; De Raedt, H.; Buysschaert, I.; Lambrechts, D.; Van de Werf, F. Underestimated and under-recognized: The late consequences of acute coronary syndrome (GRACE UK-Belgian Study). *Eur. Heart J.* **2010**, *31*, 2755–2764. [CrossRef] [PubMed]
4. Fox, K.A.; Fitzgerald, G.; Puymirat, E.; Huang, W.; Carruthers, K.; Simon, T.; Coste, P.; Monsegu, J.; Gabriel Steg, P.; Danchin, N.; et al. Should patients with acute coronary disease be stratified for management according to their risk? Derivation, external validation and outcomes using the updated GRACE risk score. *BMJ Open* **2014**, *4*, e004425. [CrossRef] [PubMed]
5. Pocock, S.; Bueno, H.; Licour, M.; Medina, J.; Zhang, L.; Annemans, L.; Danchin, N.; Huo, Y.; Van de Werf, F. Predictors of one-year mortality at hospital discharge after acute coronary syndromes: A new risk score from the EPICOR (long-term follow up of antithrombotic management patterns in acute Coronary syndrome patients) study. *Eur. Heart J. Acute Cardiovasc. Care* **2015**, *4*, 509–517. [CrossRef]

6. Simonsson, M.; Wallentin, L.; Alfredsson, J.; Erlinge, D.; Hellström Ängerud, K.; Hofmann, R.; Kellerth, T.; Lindhagen, L.; Ravn-Fischer, A.; Szummer, K.; et al. Temporal trends in bleeding events in acute myocardial infarction: Insights from the SWEDEHEART registry. *Eur. Heart J.* **2020**, *41*, 833–843. [CrossRef]
7. O'Donoghue, M.L.; Morrow, D.A.; Cannon, C.P.; Jarolim, P.; Desai, N.R.; Sherwood, M.W.; Murphy, S.A.; Gerszten, R.E.; Sabatine, M.S. Multimarker Risk Stratification in Patients with Acute Myocardial Infarction. *J. Am. Heart Assoc.* **2016**, *5*, e002586. [CrossRef]
8. Damman, P.; Beijk, M.A.; Kuijt, W.J.; Verouden, N.J.; van Geloven, N.; Henriques, J.P.; Baan, J.; Vis, M.M.; Meuwissen, M.; van Straalen, J.P.; et al. Multiple biomarkers at admission significantly improve the prediction of mortality in patients undergoing primary percutaneous coronary intervention for acute ST-segment elevation myocardial infarction. *J. Am. Coll. Cardiol.* **2011**, *57*, 29–36. [CrossRef]
9. Goriki, Y.; Tanaka, A.; Nishihira, K.; Kawaguchi, A.; Natsuaki, M.; Watanabe, N.; Ashikaga, K.; Kuriyama, N.; Shibata, Y.; Node, K. A Novel Predictive Model for In-Hospital Mortality Based on a Combination of Multiple Blood Variables in Patients with ST-Segment-Elevation Myocardial Infarction. *J. Clin. Med.* **2020**, *9*, 852. [CrossRef]
10. Tsai, T.T.; Patel, U.D.; Chang, T.I.; Kennedy, K.F.; Masoudi, F.A.; Matheny, M.E.; Kosiborod, M.; Amin, A.P.; Weintraub, W.S.; Curtis, J.P.; et al. Validated contemporary risk model of acute kidney injury in patients undergoing percutaneous coronary interventions: Insights from the National Cardiovascular Data Registry Cath-PCI Registry. *J. Am. Heart Assoc.* **2014**, *3*, e001380. [CrossRef]
11. Goriki, Y.; Yoshioka, G.; Natsuaki, M.; Shinzato, K.; Nishihira, K.; Kuriyama, N.; Shimomura, M.; Inoue, Y.; Nishikido, T.; Kaneko, T.; et al. Simple risk-score model for in-hospital major bleeding based on multiple blood variables in patients with acute myocardial infarction. *Int. J. Cardiol.* **2022**, *346*, 1–7. [CrossRef]
12. Thygesen, K.; Alpert, J.S.; White, H.D. Universal definition of myocardial infarction. *J. Am. Coll. Cardiol.* **2007**, *50*, 2173–2195. [CrossRef] [PubMed]
13. Matsuo, S.; Imai, E.; Horio, M.; Yasuda, Y.; Tomita, K.; Nitta, K.; Yamagata, K.; Tomino, Y.; Yokoyama, H.; Hishida, A. Revised equations for estimated GFR from serum creatinine in Japan. *Am. J. Kidney Dis.* **2009**, *53*, 982–992. [CrossRef] [PubMed]
14. Ducrocq, G.; Puymirat, E.; Steg, P.G.; Henry, P.; Martelet, M.; Karam, C.; Schiele, F.; Simon, T.; Danchin, N. Blood transfusion, bleeding, anemia, and survival in patients with acute myocardial infarction: FAST-MI registry. *Am. Heart J.* **2015**, *170*, 726–734.e2. [CrossRef] [PubMed]
15. Kunadian, V.; Mehran, R.; Lincoff, A.M.; Feit, F.; Manoukian, S.V.; Hamon, M.; Cox, D.A.; Dangas, G.D.; Stone, G.W. Effect of anemia on frequency of short- and long-term clinical events in acute coronary syndromes (from the Acute Catheterization and Urgent Intervention Triage Strategy Trial). *Am. J. Cardiol.* **2014**, *114*, 1823–1829. [CrossRef] [PubMed]
16. Saltzman, A.J.; Stone, G.W.; Claessen, B.E.; Narula, A.; Leon-Reyes, S.; Weisz, G.; Brodie, B.; Witzenbichler, B.; Guagliumi, G.; Kornowski, R.; et al. Long-term impact of chronic kidney disease in patients with ST-segment elevation myocardial infarction treated with primary percutaneous coronary intervention: The HORIZONS-AMI (Harmonizing Outcomes with Revascularization and Stents in Acute Myocardial Infarction) trial. *JACC Cardiovasc. Interv.* **2011**, *4*, 1011–1019. [PubMed]
17. Kotwal, S.; Ranasinghe, I.; Brieger, D.; Clayton, P.A.; Cass, A.; Gallagher, M. The influence of chronic kidney disease and age on revascularization rates and outcomes in acute myocardial infarction—A cohort study. *Eur. Heart J. Acute Cardiovasc. Care* **2017**, *6*, 291–298. [CrossRef]
18. Yadav, M.; Généreux, P.; Giustino, G.; Madhavan, M.V.; Brener, S.J.; Mintz, G.; Caixeta, A.; Xu, K.; Mehran, R.; Stone, G.W. Effect of Baseline Thrombocytopenia on Ischemic Outcomes in Patients with Acute Coronary Syndromes Who Undergo Percutaneous Coronary Intervention. *Can. J. Cardiol.* **2016**, *32*, 226–233. [CrossRef]
19. Liu, R.; Hu, Y.; Yang, J.; Wang, Q.; Yang, H.; Wang, Z.; Su, S.; Yuan, J.; Yang, Y. Effect of Baseline Thrombocytopenia on Long-Term Outcomes in Patients with Acute ST-Segment Elevated Myocardial Infarction—A Large Propensity Score-Matching Analysis from the China Acute Myocardial Infarction (CAMI) Registry. *Circ. J.* **2021**, *85*, 150–158. [CrossRef]
20. Yoshioka, G.; Tanaka, A.; Nishihira, K.; Natsuaki, M.; Kawaguchi, A.; Watanabe, N.; Shibata, Y.; Node, K. Prognostic impact of follow-up serum albumin after acute myocardial infarction. *ESC Heart Fail.* **2021**, *8*, 5456–5465. [CrossRef]
21. Wanamaker, B.L.; Seth, M.M.; Sukul, D.; Dixon, S.R.; Bhatt, D.L.; Madder, R.D.; Rumsfeld, J.S.; Gurm, H.S. Relationship between Troponin on Presentation and in-Hospital Mortality in Patients with ST-Segment-Elevation Myocardial Infarction Undergoing Primary Percutaneous Coronary Intervention. *J. Am. Heart Assoc.* **2019**, *8*, e013551. [CrossRef] [PubMed]
22. DeLong, E.R.; DeLong, D.M.; Clarke-Pearson, D.L. Comparing the areas under two or more correlated receiver operating characteristic curves: A nonparametric approach. *Biometrics* **1988**, *44*, 837–845. [CrossRef] [PubMed]
23. Hung, J.; Roos, A.; Kadesjö, E.; McAllister, D.A.; Kimenai, D.M.; Shah, A.S.V.; Anand, A.; Strachan, F.E.; Fox, K.A.A.; Mills, N.L.; et al. Performance of the GRACE 2.0 score in patients with type 1 and type 2 myocardial infarction. *Eur. Heart J.* **2021**, *42*, 2552–2561. [CrossRef] [PubMed]
24. Collet, J.P.; Thiele, H.; Barbato, E.; Barthélémy, O.; Bauersachs, J.; Bhatt, D.L.; Dendale, P.; Dorobantu, M.; Edvardsen, T.; Folliguet, T.; et al. 2020 ESC Guidelines for the management of acute coronary syndromes in patients presenting without persistent ST-segment elevation. *Eur. Heart J.* **2021**, *42*, 1289–1367. [CrossRef] [PubMed]
25. Fanali, G.; di Masi, A.; Trezza, V.; Marino, M.; Fasano, M.; Ascenzi, P. Human serum albumin: From bench to bedside. *Mol. Asp. Med.* **2012**, *33*, 209–290. [CrossRef] [PubMed]

26. Patel, A.; Goodman, S.G.; Yan, A.T.; Alexander, K.P.; Wong, C.L.; Cheema, A.N.; Udell, J.A.; Kaul, P.; D'Souza, M.; Hyun, K.; et al. Frailty and Outcomes after Myocardial Infarction: Insights from the CONCORDANCE Registry. *J. Am. Heart Assoc.* **2018**, *7*, e009859. [CrossRef] [PubMed]
27. Cheng, Y.L.; Sung, S.H.; Cheng, H.M.; Hsu, P.F.; Guo, C.Y.; Yu, W.C.; Chen, C.H. Prognostic Nutritional Index and the Risk of Mortality in Patients with Acute Heart Failure. *J. Am. Heart Assoc.* **2017**, *6*, e004876. [CrossRef]
28. Xia, M.; Zhang, C.; Gu, J.; Chen, J.; Wang, L.C.; Lu, Y.; Huang, C.Y.; He, Y.M.; Yang, X.J. Impact of serum albumin levels on long-term all-cause, cardiovascular, and cardiac mortality in patients with first-onset acute myocardial infarction. *Clin. Chim. Acta* **2018**, *477*, 89–93. [CrossRef]
29. Yoshioka, G.; Tanaka, A.; Nishihira, K.; Shibata, Y.; Node, K. Prognostic impact of serum albumin for developing heart failure remotely after acute myocardial infarction. *Nutrients* **2020**, *12*, 2637. [CrossRef]
30. Mahmoud, K.D.; Hillege, H.L.; Jaffe, A.S.; Lennon, R.J.; Holmes, D.R., Jr. Biochemical Validation of Patient-Reported Symptom Onset Time in Patients With ST-Segment Elevation Myocardial Infarction Undergoing Primary Percutaneous Coronary Intervention. *JACC Cardiovasc. Interv.* **2015**, *8*, 778–787. [CrossRef]
31. Shimizu, A. What are the most useful predictors of cardiac mortality in patients post myocardial infarction? *Circ. J.* **2013**, *77*, 319–320. [CrossRef] [PubMed]
32. Goriki, Y.; Tanaka, A.; Nishihira, K.; Kuriyama, N.; Shibata, Y.; Node, K. A novel prediction model of acute kidney injury based on combined blood variables in STEMI. *JACC Asia* **2021**, *1*, 372–381. [CrossRef]
33. Kimura, K.; Kimura, T.; Ishihara, M.; Nakagawa, Y.; Nakao, K.; Miyauchi, K.; Sakamoto, T.; Tsujita, K.; Hagiwara, N.; Miyazaki, S.; et al. JCS 2018 Guideline on Diagnosis and Treatment of Acute Coronary Syndrome. *Circ. J.* **2019**, *83*, 1085–1196. [CrossRef] [PubMed]

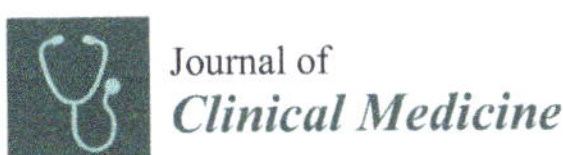

Journal of
Clinical Medicine

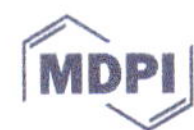

Article

Predictive and Prognostic Value of Serum Neutrophil Gelatinase-Associated Lipocalin for Contrast-Induced Acute Kidney Injury and Long-Term Clinical Outcomes after Percutaneous Coronary Intervention

Jaeho Byeon †, Ik Jun Choi †, Dongjae Lee, Youngchul Ahn, Mi-Jeong Kim and Doo Soo Jeon *

Division of Cardiology, Department of Internal Medicine, Incheon St. Mary's Hospital, College of Medicine, The Catholic University of Korea, Seoul 06591, Korea
* Correspondence: jeondoosoo@hanmail.net; Tel.: +82-32-280-2139; Fax: +82-32-280-5164
† These authors contributed equally to this work.

Abstract: Neutrophil gelatinase-associated lipocalin (NGAL) has been proposed as an early marker for estimating the risk of contrast-induced acute kidney injury (CI-AKI). However, the predictive value of baseline serum NGAL levels for CI-AKI remains unclear. Serum NGAL was measured before percutaneous coronary intervention in 633 patients with coronary artery disease. The primary clinical endpoints were a composite of major adverse cardiac and cerebrovascular events (MACCEs; cardiac death, myocardial infarction, stroke, and any revascularization). The mean follow-up duration was 29.4 months. Ninety-eight (15.5%) patients developed CI-AKI. Compared with patients without CI-AKI, baseline serum NGAL was higher in patients with CI-AKI (149.6 ± 88.8 ng/mL vs. 138.0 ± 98.6 ng/mL, $p = 0.0279$), although serum creatinine and estimated glomerular filtration rate were not different between groups. Patients in the highest tertile of baseline serum NGAL showed a significantly higher rate of MACCEs (10.5% vs. 3.8%, $p = 0.02$). Using the first tertile as a reference, the adjusted hazard ratios for MACCEs in patients in the second and third tertiles of NGAL were 2.151 (confidence interval (CI) 0.82 to 5.59, $p = 0.116$) and 2.725 (CI 1.05 to 7.05, $p = 0.039$), respectively. Baseline serum NGAL is a reliable marker for predicting CI-AKI, and high serum NGAL levels are associated with a higher incidence rate of long term MACCEs.

Keywords: NGAL; contrast-induced acute kidney injury; coronary artery disease; percutaneous coronary intervention

Citation: Byeon, J.; Choi, I.J.; Lee, D.; Ahn, Y.; Kim, M.-J.; Jeon, D.S. Predictive and Prognostic Value of Serum Neutrophil Gelatinase-Associated Lipocalin for Contrast-Induced Acute Kidney Injury and Long-Term Clinical Outcomes after Percutaneous Coronary Intervention. *J. Clin. Med.* **2022**, *11*, 5971. https://doi.org/10.3390/jcm11195971

Academic Editors: Koichi Node and Atsushi Tanaka

Received: 17 September 2022
Accepted: 7 October 2022
Published: 10 October 2022

1. Introduction

Contrast-induced acute kidney injury (CI-AKI) is a major complication of coronary artery disease (CAD) treated by percutaneous coronary intervention (PCI) [1] and is associated with increased mortality and cardiovascular outcomes [2–4]. CI-AKI is characterized by a decline in kidney function that occurs within days after the intravascular administration of contrast medium [5]. The mechanisms involved in CI-AKI include ischemic injury to the renal medulla, oxidative damage, and direct toxicity involving the renal tubules. The prediction and prevention of CI-AKI are important in the management of the periprocedural period. Many studies have identified some biomarkers that may be used to anticipate the development of acute kidney injury in various clinical situations. Neutrophil gelatinase-associated lipocalin (NGAL) is a well-known marker of kidney tubular injury [6]. The predictive power of changes in NGAL for AKI after contrast use has been widely reported [7–10]. However, the predictive value of baseline serum NGAL for CI-AKI after PCI remains controversial. We sought to evaluate the ability of baseline serum NGAL to predict the incidence of CI-AKI and the prognostic performance in patients with CAD undergoing PCI.

2. Materials and Methods

2.1. Study Populations

We screened 796 consecutive patients with CAD scheduled for PCI at Incheon St. Mary's Hospital between September 2015 and November 2017. Patients with cardiogenic shock, end-stage renal disease requiring dialysis, or insufficient blood samples and those who did not undergo PCI were excluded. Of the 796 patients, 633 had samples available for the measurement of the serum level of NGAL. All participants provided written informed consent to participate before PCI and blood sampling. The study protocol was reviewed and approved by the appropriate institutional review board.

2.2. PCI Procedure and Medical Treatments

Coronary angiography and PCI were performed according to standard techniques at the operator's discretion. The contrast medium used was iodixanol (Visipaque, GE Healthcare, Chicago, IL, USA). Antiplatelet therapy and periprocedural anticoagulation were administered according to standard regimens. All patients were recommended for guideline-directed medical therapy, including antiplatelets, statins, beta-blockers, or renin-angiotensin-aldosterone blockades, following standard European and American guidelines [11,12]. Clinical follow-up was performed every 3 months after the index procedure.

2.3. Laboratory Measurements

Blood samples were drawn upon arrival at the catheterization laboratory and were collected immediately after sheath insertion and before PCI. After the blood was centrifuged, plasma was subsequently stored at −80 °C. Serum NGAL levels were measured by a Human Lipocalin-2/NGAL Quantikine ELISA kit (Catalog #DLCN20) from R&D Systems (Minneapolis, MN, USA). The measurement of NGAL levels was performed in the Clinical Research Laboratory, Incheon St. Mary's Hospital, The Catholic University of Korea.

2.4. Study Endpoints and Definitions

The primary endpoint was major adverse cardiac and cerebrovascular events (MACCEs), including cardiovascular death, nonfatal myocardial infarction, nonfatal stroke, and any revascularization. Patient follow-up information, including survival and clinical events, was collected through hospital chart review and telephone interviews with patients by trained reviewers who were blinded to the study results. In addition, the mortality data were verified by the database of the National Health Insurance Corporation, Korea, using a unique personal identification number.

CI-AKI occurring within 72 h of contrast use is defined by the International Kidney Disease Improving Global Outcomes classification as follows: an increase in serum creatinine of $\geq$0.3 mg/dL, an increase in serum creatinine of $\geq$1.5 times baseline, a urine volume $\leq$0.5 mL/kg/h for 6 h. [13]

2.5. Statistical Analysis

Continuous variables are expressed as the mean ± standard deviation and were analyzed by independent sample t test or the Mann-Whitney U test. Categorical variables are presented as percentages or rates and were analyzed by the chi-square test or Fisher's exact test. Serum NGAL levels are expressed as a continuous variable or by groups, categorized into three groups by tertiles. Differences in baseline characteristics between the different tertiles of serum NGAL levels were evaluated using one-way analysis of variance for continuous variables and the chi-square test for categorical variables. Traditional cardiovascular risk factors and CI-AKI risk factors were used for univariate analysis, and only variables with $p < 0.1$ in univariate analysis were analyzed with multivariate analysis for association with the risk of contrast-induced acute kidney injury. Multivariable analysis was performed to assess the prognostic value of serum NGAL and MACCEs after adjusting for age, sex, estimated glomerular filtration rate, body mass index, hypertension, diabetes mellitus, smoking, family history of coronary artery disease, chronic kidney disease, dyslipidemia, prior stroke, prior myocardial infarction, acute myocardial infarction, hypotension, multivessel disease, and left ventricular ejection fraction. Hazard ratios (HR) were estimated with multivariable adjusted Cox proportional hazards models, using the first tertile of NGAL as a reference. Kaplan-Meier curves were used to analyze the clinical outcomes and overall survival rate of patients. All analyses were 2-tailed, and $p < 0.05$ was considered indicative of statistical significance. All statistical analyses were performed using SPSS 27 statistical software (SPSS Inc., Chicago, IL, USA) and R version 4.2.1 (R Foundation for Statistical Computing, Vienna, Austria).

3. Results

3.1. Patient Characteristics

Overall, 633 patients with CAD treated by PCI were analyzed. The baseline characteristics of the total patient population per tertile are shown in Table 1. The mean age of all 633 patients was 65.5 ± 11.7 years old, and 66.0% of the patients were men. Among them, 225 patients (35.5%) had a history of chronic kidney disease, defined by an estimated glomerular filtration rate (eGFR) of less than 60 mL/min/1.73 m^2. When categorized into three groups according to the tertile of baseline serum NGAL (NGAL tertiles, 1st: 25.4 to 83.7 ng/mL, 2nd: 83.8 to 143.8 ng/mL, 3rd: 143.9 to 567.9 ng/mL), there was a significant trend toward higher serum NGAL levels with older age, hypertension, diabetes, chronic kidney disease, low ejection fraction, high C-reactive protein, higher contrast volume, multivessel coronary disease, larger number of stents, and longer stent length. There were no significant differences with regard to sex, body mass index, dyslipidemia, or culprit coronary lesions among the three tertiles.

3.2. Serum NGAL Levels and Contrast-Induced Acute Kidney Injury

Among all patients, 98 (15.5%) patients developed CI-AKI (Table S1). Those subjects who suffered from CI-AKI had higher baseline NGAL levels than those without CI-AKI (149.6 ± 88.8 ng/mL vs. 138.0 ± 98.6 ng/mL, $p = 0.0279$). However, the serum creatinine level (1.14 ± 1.53 mg/dL vs. 1.09 ± 0.63 mg/dL, $p = 0.737$) and eGFR (73.0 ± 34.2.4 mL/min/1.73 m^2 vs. 71.5 ± 26.9 mL/min/1.73 m^2, $p = 0.685$) were not different between the two groups. Additionally, there was no difference in the infused contrast volume (217.9 ± 121.0 mL vs. 220.8 ± 115.6 mL, $p = 0.831$). Patients who required renal replacement therapy were not reported during in-hospital periods or overall follow-up.

There was an increase in the incidence of CI-AKI with increasing tertiles of NGAL (Figure 1). Compared with the reference group (1st tertile), the adjusted odds ratios for CI-AKI were 2.7 (CI 1.391–5.239, $p = 0.003$) for the 2nd tertile of NGAL and 3.57 (CI 1.788–7.141, $p < 0.001$) for the 3rd tertile of NGAL (Table 2).

3.3. Serum NGAL Levels and Cardiac and Cerebrovascular Outcomes

The median follow-up duration was 29.4 months (IQR 23.8 to 37.2). During the overall follow-up, MACCEs occurred in 43 patients (6.8%). Cardiovascular death, nonfatal myocardial infarction, nonfatal stroke, and any revascularization occurred in 24 (3.79%), 2 (0.31%), 6 (0.94%), and 16 (2.52%) patients, respectively. The individual components of MACCEs and all-cause death are presented in Table 3, and Kaplan-Meier curves for serum NGAL levels according to tertiles and primary outcomes are shown in Figure 2. Patients in the highest tertile showed significantly higher rates of MACCEs (10.5% vs. 3.8%, $p = 0.02$) and all-cause death (11.0% vs. 1.4%, $p < 0.001$) than patients in the first tertile. Using the first tertile as a reference, the adjusted HRs for those in the second and third tertiles of NGAL were 2.151 (CI 0.827–5.592, $p = 0.116$) and 2.725 (CI 1.052–7.058, $p = 0.039$) for MACCEs and 3.692 (CI 0.938–14.522, $p = 0.062$) and 6.172 (CI 1.650–23.077, $p = 0.007$) for all-cause death (Table 4).

Table 1. Baseline clinical and angiographic characteristics.

Variables	NGAL Tertile 1 (n = 212)	NGAL Tertile 2 (n = 212)	NGAL Tertile 3 (n = 209)	p Value
Age (years)	63.8 ± 10.8	65.1 ± 11.4	67.8 ± 12.7	0.002
Male	131 (61.8%)	136 (64.2%)	151 (72.2%)	0.060
Body mass index (kg/m^2)	24.9 ± 3.1	24.7 ± 3.9	24.7 ± 3.5	0.834
Hypertension	139 (65.6%)	156 (73.6%)	161 (77.0%)	0.027
Diabetes mellitus	80 (37.7%)	70 (33.0%)	98 (46.9%)	0.012
Dyslipidemia	70 (33.0%)	76 (35.8%)	75 (35.9%)	0.777
Current smoking	53 (25.0%)	64 (30.2%)	64(30.6%)	0.363
Family history of coronary artery disease	20 (9.4%)	19 (9.0%)	15 (7.2%)	0.683
Prior stroke	17 (8.0%)	19 (9.0%)	31 (14.8%)	0.049
Prior myocardial infarction	19 (9.0%)	19 (9.0%)	16 (7.7%)	0.858
Prior percutaneous coronary intervention	29 (13.7%)	29 (13.7%)	27 (12.9%)	0.966
Prior statin use	59 (27.8%)	67 (31.6%)	66 (31.6%)	0.624
Clinical presentation				<0.001
Stable angina pectoris	73 (34.4%)	59 (27.8%)	41 (19.6%)	
Unstable angina pectoris	61 (28.8%)	51 (24.1%)	33(15.8%)	
NSTEMI	48 (22.6%)	60 (28.3%)	89 (42.6%)	
STEMI	27 (12.7%)	38 (17.9%)	40 (19.1%)	
Silent myocardial ischemia	3 (1.4%)	4 (1.9%)	6 (2.9%)	
Ejection fraction (%)	57.1 ± 10.5	54.5 ± 12.8	52.6 ± 13.0	0.001
Total cholesterol (mg/dL)	135.2 ± 34.9	137.2 ± 31.6	131.4 ± 30.8	0.414
Triglyceride (mg/dL)	135.2 ± 80.3	144.1 ± 75.9	194.5 ± 306.3	0.032
HDL cholesterol (mg/dL)	47.0 ± 11.2	45.1 ± 10.5	41.0 ± 10.0	<0.001
LDL cholesterol (mg/dL)	72.2 ± 24.4	74.6 ± 22.7	71.4 ± 21.3	0.558
High-sensitivity C-reactive protein (mg/L)	5.2 ± 17.3	7.3 ± 20.5	17.8 ± 39.5	<0.001
Creatinine (mg/dL)	0.89 ± 0.22	1.02 ± 0.32	1.46 ± 2.40	<0.001
eGFR (mL/min/1.73 m^2)	83.1 ± 31.5	72.3 ± 27.0	58.5 ± 26.6	<0.001
eGFR <60 mL/min/1.73 m^2	41 (19.3%)	78 (36.8%)	106 (50.7%)	<0.001
Hemoglobin (mg/dL)	13.7 ± 2.9	13.5 ± 2.0	13.2 ± 2.4	0.167
Medications at discharge				
Aspirin	210 (99.1%)	207 (97.6%)	198 (94.7%)	0.025
Clopidogrel	150 (70.8%)	131 (61.8%)	115 (55.0%)	0.004
Potent P2Y12 inhibitor	62 (29.2%)	80 (37.7%)	94 (45.0%)	0.004
Statins	210 (99.1%)	210 (99.1%)	206 (98.6%)	0.856
Beta-blocker	134 (63.2%)	151 (71.2%)	160 (76.6%)	0.011
Renin angiotensin system inhibitor	124 (58.5%)	113 (53.3%)	107 (51.2%)	0.302
Hypotension	13 (6.1%)	26 (12.3%)	26 (12.4%)	0.052
IABP or ECMO	0 (0%)	2 (0.9%)	2 (1.0%)	0.363
Culprit coronary lesion				0.215
Left anterior descending	114 (54.5%)	101 (48.1%)	91 (45.0%)	
Left circumflex	30 (14.4%)	41 (19.5%)	49 (24.3%)	
Right	53 (25.4%)	59 (28.1%)	54 (26.7%)	
Left main	12 (5.7%)	9 (4.3%)	7 (3.5%)	
Multivessel	55 (25.9%)	67 (31.6%)	82 (39.2%)	0.014
Contrast volume (mL)	198.9 ± 103.6	221.1 ± 127.9	233.1 ± 124.1	0.020
Number of total stents	1.56 ± 0.92	1.71 ± 1.00	1.89 ± 1.16	0.006
Mean diameter of stents (mm)	3.13 ± 0.43	3.12 ± 0.44	3.07 ± 0.39	0.255
Total length of stents (mm)	39.1 ± 26.9	42.9 ± 29.7	51.1 ± 36.1	<0.001

Note: Values are number (%) or mean ± standard deviation. Abbreviation: NSTEMI, non-ST-segment elevation myocardial infarction; STEMI, ST-segment elevation myocardial infarction; HDL, high-density lipoprotein; LDL, low-density lipoprotein; eGFR, estimated glomerular filtration rate; IABP, intra-aortic balloon pump; ECMO, extracorporeal membrane oxygenation.

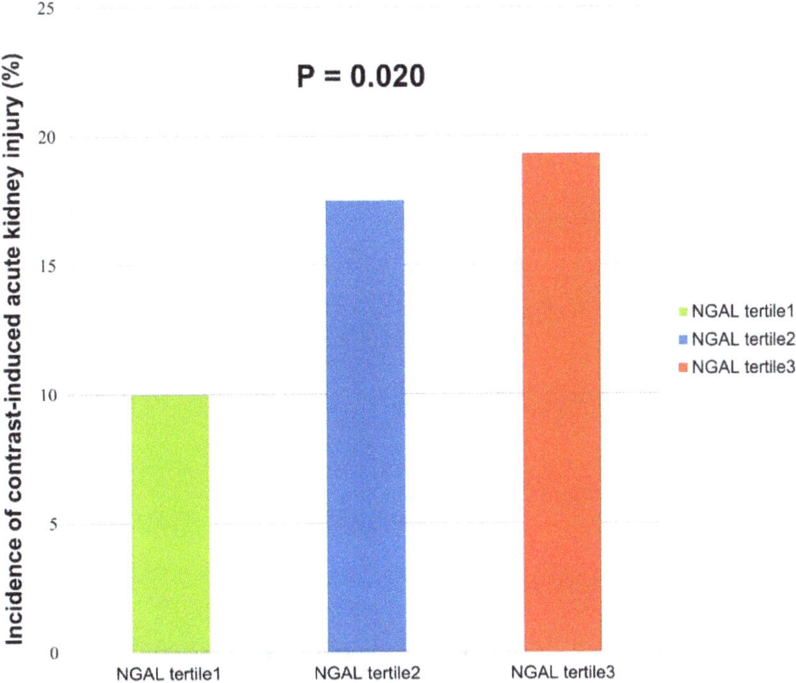

Figure 1. The incidence of contrast-induced acute kidney injury according to tertiles of baseline serum NGAL.

Table 2. Associations between clinical characteristics and the risk of contrast-induced acute kidney injury according to univariate and multivariate logistic regression models.

	Univariate		Multivariate	
	OR (95% CI)	***p* Value**	**OR (95% CI)**	***p* Value**
Age	1.025 (1.005–1.044)	0.012	1.041 (1.014–1.068)	0.003
Female	1.556 (1.003–2.415)	0.048	0.337 (0.151–0.751)	0.008
Body mass index	0.953 (0.879–0.994)	0.030	0.987 (0.919–1.060)	0.716
Hypertension	1.245 (0.757–2.046)	0.388		
Diabetes mellitus	1.714 (1.111–2.644)	0.015	1.787 (1.082–2.952)	0.023
Dyslipidemia	0.560 (0.342–0.918)	0.021	0.361 (0.076–1.701)	0.198
Smoking	1.134 (0.709–1.813)	0.599		
Family history of CAD	0.813 (0.356–1.857)	0.623		
Chronic kidney disease	1.730 (0.759–3.942)	0.192		
Prior stroke	1.261 (0.647–2.458)	0.496		
Prior statin use	0.622 (0.374–1.034)	0.067	1.952 (0.395–9.648)	0.412
Acute myocardial infarction	1.752 (1.131–2.714)	0.012	1.618 (0.962–2.721)	0.069
Left ventricular ejection fraction	0.963 (0.948–0.979)	<0.001	0.961 (0.943–0.980)	<0.001
eGFR	1.012 (1.005–1.018)	0.001	1.035 (1.023–1.047)	<0.001
Hemoglobin	0.900 (0.810–0.999)	0.048	0.932 (0.814–1.068)	0.310
Multivessel disease	1.258 (0.803–1.972)	0.317		
LAD lesion	1.451 (0.930–2.262)	0.101		
Hypotension	0.877 (0.418–1.839)	0.728		
Contrast volume	1.000 (0.998–1.002)	0.816		
NGAL tertile 2	1.913 (1.078–3.394)	0.027	2.700 (1.391–5.239)	0.003
NGAL tertile 3	2.167 (1.228–3.823)	0.008	3.573 (1.788–7.141)	<0.001

OR indicates odds ratio; CI, confidence interval; CAD, coronary artery disease; eGFR, estimated glomerular filtration rate; LAD, left anterior descending.

Table 3. Clinical outcomes according to NGAL tertiles.

	NGAL			*p* Value
	Tertile 1	Tertile 2	Tertile 3	
MACCEs	8 (3.8%)	13 (6.1%)	22 (10.5%)	0.020
All-cause death	3 (1.4%)	9 (4.2%)	23 (11.0%)	<0.001
Cardiovascular death	2 (0.9%)	7 (3.3%)	15 (7.2%)	0.003
Nonfatal myocardial infarction	1 (0.5%)	1 (0.5%)	0 (0%)	0.610
Nonfatal stroke	2 (0.9%)	2 (0.9%)	2 (1.0%)	0.999
Any revascularization	5 (2.4%)	5 (2.4%)	6 (2.9%)	0.928

MACCEs, major adverse cardiac and cerebrovascular events; NGAL, neutrophil gelatinase-associated lipocalin.

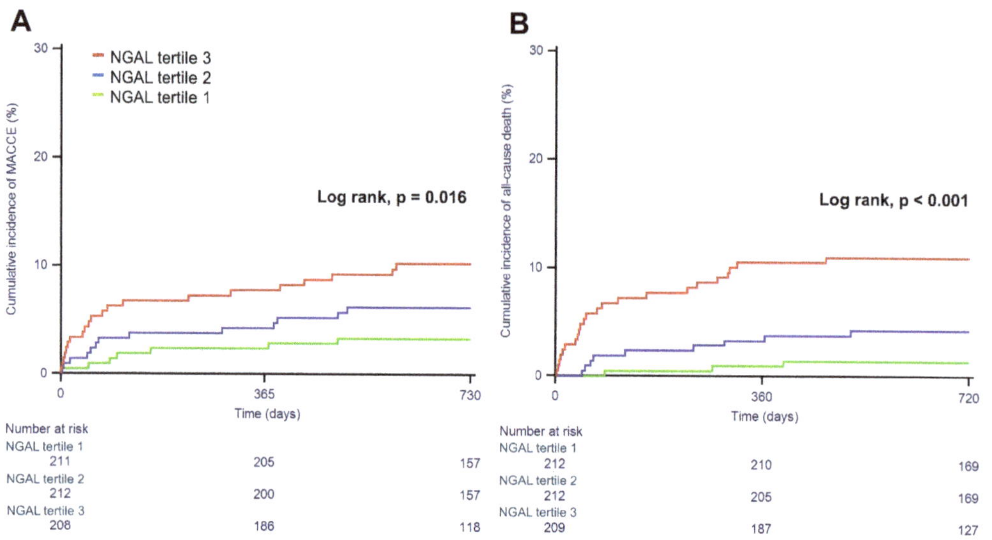

Figure 2. Kaplan-Meier curves for major adverse cardiac and cerebrovascular events (**A**) and all-cause death (**B**) according to tertiles of baseline serum NGAL.

Table 4. Hazard ratios of baseline serum NGAL tertiles for MACCEs and all-cause death.

	Model 1		Model 2		Model 3		Model 4	
	HR (95% CI)	*p* Value	HR (95% CI)	*p* Value	HR (95% CI)	*p* Value	HR (95% CI)	*p* Value
MACCEs								
Tertile 1	1		1		1		1	
Tertile 2	1.652 (0.685–3.986)	0.264	1.600 (0.662–3.868)	0.297	1.545 (0.633–3.775)	0.340	2.151 (0.827–5.592)	0.116
Tertile 3	2.984 (1.328–6.704)	0.008	2.781 (1.211–6.386)	0.016	2.596 (1.093–6.167)	0.031	2.725 (1.052–7.058)	0.039
All-cause death								
Tertile 1	1		1		1		1	
Tertile 2	3.039 (0.823–11.227)	0.095	2.631 (0.710–9.752)	0.148	2.437 (0.650–9.142)	0.187	3.692 (0.938–14.522)	0.062
Tertile 3	8.260 (2.480–27.512)	0.001	5.879 (1.721–20.078)	0.005	5.077 (1.416–18.201)	0.013	6.172 (1.650–23.077)	0.007

Model 1 is the univariate analysis. Model 2 is adjusted for age and sex. Model 3 is adjusted for age, sex, and estimated glomerular filtration rate. Model 4 is adjusted for age, sex, estimated glomerular filtration rate, body mass index, hypertension, diabetes mellitus, smoking, family history of coronary artery disease, chronic kidney disease, dyslipidemia, prior stroke, prior myocardial infarction, acute myocardial infarction, hypotension, multivessel disease, and left ventricular ejection fraction. MACCEs, major adverse cardiac and cerebrovascular events, HR, hazard ratio, CI, confidence interval.

4. Discussion

The present study demonstrates that baseline serum NGAL levels can be used to predict the occurrence of CI-AKI independent of potential confounding factors such as serum creatinine, eGFR, and infused contrast volume. In addition, baseline serum NGAL levels are associated with MACCEs and all-cause mortality in patients with CAD treated with PCI. According to these findings, baseline serum NGAL might serve as a predictor of the development of CI-AKI and cardiac and cerebrovascular outcomes in patients with CAD undergoing PCI before the administration of contrast medium.

NGAL is a protein in the lipocalin family and is expressed by neutrophils and various epithelial cells [14]. NGAL is well known to exert a bacteriostatic effect by depleting siderophores, and on the other hand, increased serum NGAL levels have been reported in the setting of systemic disease in the absence of overt bacterial infection. Expression of NGAL increases 25- to 100-fold in humans in response to renal tubular injury and appears very rapidly in urine and serum [15]. Although the clinical usefulness of NGAL is well known in kidney injury, elevated NGAL has also been recently reported in heart failure, coronary artery disease, and cerebrovascular disease. NGAL is upregulated under conditions of failing myocardium, atherosclerotic plaques, and systemic inflammation [16]. Some investigators have suggested that serum NGAL may be of prognostic value in patients with myocardial infarction [17,18]. Here, our study has shown that baseline serum NGAL also has prognostic value in patients with CAD. Moreover, a serum NGAL level in the highest tertile was a risk factor for the occurrence of CI-AKI.

Contrast-induced AKI is an important complication of any procedure using intravascular contrast. In a retrospective analysis of the Mayo Clinic PCI registry, Rihal et al. reported the incidence among patients undergoing PCI to be 3.3%, and the 5-year estimated mortality rate in survivors with AKI was 44.6% [19]. In another large-scale PCI registry, Tsai et al. showed that 7.1% of patients experienced AKI and 0.3% required the initiation of dialysis. The risks of in-hospital myocardial infarction, bleeding, and death were greater for patients who had AKI after undergoing PCI than for those who did not have AKI [1]. To date, there have been no clinical trials demonstrating the prevention of CI-AKI. N-acetylcysteine (NAC) is a pharmacological drug that has been most widely studied in randomized controlled trials. Recent work by Weisbord et al. showed no benefit of oral NAC over placebo for the prevention of CI-AKI in the PRESERVE trial [20]. In previous studies, older age, left ventricular systolic dysfunction, chronic kidney disease (CKD), diabetes, acute coronary syndrome, and cardiogenic shock were associated with AKI after PCI [1,21]. In patients with high-risk factors, as mentioned above, adequate intravascular volume expansion with isotonic saline before and after contrast media exposure along with the avoidance of nephrotoxic drugs is the only recommended prophylactic strategy to date [22,23]. Our study shows that old age, female sex, diabetes, LV systolic dysfunction, CKD, and baseline NGAL levels are independent risk factors for CI-AKI. Even after adjustment for well-established risk factors, baseline serum NGAL was found to be a strong risk factor for CI-AKI. In addition to traditional risk factors, baseline serum NGAL could be considered a predictor of the occurrence of CI-AKI.

Serum creatinine and urine output are the most frequently monitored parameters of kidney injury in practice. However, they have several limitations, such as a slow rate of change, low sensitivity and specificity, and appearing relatively normal in early diabetic nephropathy [24]. A biomarker that could be validated to predict CI-AKI would be very useful for guiding treatment. For these reasons, there have been many efforts to find a biomarker that can detect CI-AKI occurrence earlier. Serum or urinary NGAL, cystatin C, beta-2 microglobulin, kidney injury molecule-1, and calprotectin have been widely investigated [25,26]. Of these biomarkers, NGAL is known to reflect renal tubular injury [6]. Creatinine cannot be used for the early detection of CI-AKI since it increases 3 to 5 days after contrast use; it can monitor only the occurrence of AKI. On the other hand, NGAL is known to be increased within 1 day after contrast use. Studies have shown that NGAL is helpful for predicting CI-AKI in patients undergoing PCI [7–9,27]. Liao et al. showed an increase in serum NGAL after PCI associated with contrast-induced nephropathy. Using small registry data, Nusca et al. found that changes in serum NGAL at baseline and post-PCI hastened the diagnosis and treatment of CI-AKI. However, there are no studies showing an association of baseline serum NGAL with CI-AKI and clinical outcomes. In the present study, we showed that the baseline serum NGAL level, not the change in NGAL, could be used to predict the occurrence of CI-AKI. Even if the baseline creatinine, eGFR, and contrast volume values were the same, it was confirmed that the higher the baseline NGAL was, the more likely CI-AKI was to occur. This allows us to predict CI-AKI before PCI and prepare preemptive treatment in advance. Medical interventions to prevent CI-AKI may be necessary for patients with elevated baseline serum NGAL.

Notably, 30–40% of patients with coronary artery disease undergoing PCI were reported to have concomitant CKD [28,29]. Cardiovascular mortality has been shown to be inversely proportional to the estimated glomerular filtration rate, with impaired renal function being an independent predictor of cardiovascular risk [30]. Myocardial revascularization guidelines recommend evaluating renal function and the risk of contrast-induced nephropathy [12,31]. The progression to heart failure or renal failure was associated with poor clinical outcomes in ischemic heart disease. In addition, NGAL could be considered a marker of inflammation and vascular injury in patients with heart failure or renal failure because NGAL is secreted and expressed by neutrophils, epithelial cells, renal tubular cells, and hepatic cells. In coronary artery disease, Zahler et al. reported that elevated NGAL levels were associated with adverse renal and cardiovascular outcomes in 267 STEMI patients [17]. Bulluck et al. showed that a higher preoperative serum NGAL was associated with an increased risk of postoperative AKI and 1-year mortality after coronary artery bypass graft surgery [32]. Our study showed the association between baseline serum NGAL levels and MACCEs. To our knowledge, this study is the first analysis of baseline serum NGAL as a prognostic biomarker in all-comer PCI populations in a real-world registry. Measurement of baseline serum NGAL may help to identify CI-AKI early, and there might be a role for this biomarker in guiding treatment to improve cardiovascular outcomes. It seems beneficial that early interventions to protect renal function lead to better clinical outcomes because renal dysfunction affects the prognosis in CAD patients. Therefore, serum NGAL could be considered a stratification tool for identifying patients at risk for CI-AKI prior to coronary intervention.

Our study has some limitations. First, the possibility of unmeasurable confounders and selection bias should be considered because this study used a retrospective, observational, and nonrandomized study design. Second, we did not measure urinary NGAL or serial serum NGAL after the index procedure. If the urinary NGAL and serial serum NGAL levels were measured together, we could have better identified their associations with clinical outcomes. The relationship between changes in NGAL and outcomes has already been discussed in previous studies. We believe that showing the role of baseline serum NGAL as a predictor of CI-AKI and prognosis in post-PCI patients has clinical implications. Third, the incidence of CI-AKI was higher than that in previous large-scale studies; nonetheless, there were no patients who required dialysis. The criteria for defining AKI vary from study to study. It is possible that our broader definition of acute kidney injury (absolute change in creatinine of $\geq$0.3 mg/dL or of $\geq$1.5 times from baseline or oliguria) than that in other studies was responsible for the differences in CI-AKI incidence.

5. Conclusions

The measurement of serum NGAL before PCI is helpful in predicting the development of contrast-induced acute kidney injury. High serum NGAL is independently associated with an increased risk for long-term clinical outcomes in patients with CAD treated by PCI. Baseline serum NGAL could be used as a stratifying biomarker to identify patients at risk for CI-AKI prior to PCI and long-term prognosis.

Supplementary Materials: The following supporting information can be downloaded at: https://www.mdpi.com/article/10.3390/jcm11195971/s1, Table S1: Baseline clinical and angiographic characteristics.

Author Contributions: Conceptualization, I.J.C., M.-J.K. and D.S.J.; Data curation, I.J.C. and D.L.; Formal analysis, J.B.; Investigation, J.B., I.J.C. and D.L.; Methodology, I.J.C. and M.-J.K.; Project administration, M.-J.K.; Resources, D.L. and M.-J.K.; Software, Y.A.; Supervision, D.S.J.; Validation, Y.A. and D.S.J.; Visualization, J.B.; Writing—original draft, J.B.; Writing—review & editing, I.J.C. and D.S.J. All authors have read and agreed to the published version of the manuscript.

Funding: D.S.J. has received research grants from YUHAN.

Institutional Review Board Statement: The study protocol conformed to the Declaration of Helsinki regarding investigations in humans and was approved by the Incheon St. Mary Hospital Institutional Review Board (IRB No. OC15OISI0084).

Informed Consent Statement: Informed consent was obtained from all subjects involved in the study.

Data Availability Statement: The data presented in the current study are available on reasonable request from the corresponding author.

Conflicts of Interest: The authors declare no conflict of interest.

References

1. Tsai, T.T.; Patel, U.D.; Chang, T.I.; Kennedy, K.F.; Masoudi, F.A.; Matheny, M.E.; Kosiborod, M.; Amin, A.P.; Messenger, J.C.; Rumsfeld, J.S.; et al. Contemporary incidence, predictors, and outcomes of acute kidney injury in patients undergoing percutaneous coronary interventions: Insights from the NCDR Cath-PCI registry. *JACC Cardiovasc. Interv.* **2014**, *7*, 1–9. [CrossRef] [PubMed]
2. Bartholomew, B.A.; Harjai, K.J.; Dukkipati, S.; Boura, J.A.; Yerkey, M.W.; Glazier, S.; Grines, C.L.; O'Neill, W.W. Impact of nephropathy after percutaneous coronary intervention and a method for risk stratification. *Am. J. Cardiol.* **2004**, *93*, 1515–1519. [CrossRef] [PubMed]
3. Ng, A.K.; Ng, P.Y.; Ip, A.; Lam, L.T.; Ling, I.W.; Wong, A.S.; Yap, D.Y.; Siu, C.W. Impact of contrast-induced acute kidney injury on long-term major adverse cardiovascular events and kidney function after percutaneous coronary intervention: Insights from a territory-wide cohort study in Hong Kong. *Clin. Kidney J.* **2022**, *15*, 338–346. [CrossRef] [PubMed]
4. Bucaloiu, I.D.; Kirchner, H.L.; Norfolk, E.R.; Hartle, J.E., 2nd; Perkins, R.M. Increased risk of death and de novo chronic kidney disease following reversible acute kidney injury. *Kidney Int.* **2012**, *81*, 477–485. [CrossRef] [PubMed]
5. Mehran, R.; Dangas, G.D.; Weisbord, S.D. Contrast-Associated Acute Kidney Injury. *N. Engl. J. Med.* **2019**, *380*, 2146–2155. [CrossRef] [PubMed]
6. Haase-Fielitz, A.; Haase, M.; Devarajan, P. Neutrophil gelatinase-associated lipocalin as a biomarker of acute kidney injury: A critical evaluation of current status. *Ann. Clin. Biochem.* **2014**, *51*, 335–351. [CrossRef] [PubMed]
7. Liao, B.; Nian, W.; Xi, A.; Zheng, M. Evaluation of a Diagnostic Test of Serum Neutrophil Gelatinase-Associated Lipocalin (NGAL) and Urine KIM-1 in Contrast-Induced Nephropathy (CIN). *Med. Sci. Monit.* **2019**, *25*, 565–570. [CrossRef] [PubMed]
8. Nusca, A.; Miglionico, M.; Proscia, C.; Ragni, L.; Carassiti, M.; Lassandro Pepe, F.; Di Sciascio, G. Early prediction of contrast-induced acute kidney injury by a "bedside" assessment of Neutrophil Gelatinase-Associated Lipocalin during elective percutaneous coronary interventions. *PLoS ONE* **2018**, *13*, e0197833. [CrossRef]
9. Li, H.; Yu, Z.; Gan, L.; Peng, L.; Zhou, Q. Serum NGAL and FGF23 may have certain value in early diagnosis of CIN. *Ren. Fail.* **2018**, *40*, 547–553. [CrossRef]
10. Quintavalle, C.; Anselmi, C.V.; De Micco, F.; Roscigno, G.; Visconti, G.; Golia, B.; Focaccio, A.; Ricciardelli, B.; Perna, E.; Papa, L.; et al. Neutrophil Gelatinase-Associated Lipocalin and Contrast-Induced Acute Kidney Injury. *Circ. Cardiovasc. Interv.* **2015**, *8*, e002673. [CrossRef]
11. Levine, G.N.; Bates, E.R.; Blankenship, J.C.; Bailey, S.R.; Bittl, J.A.; Cercek, B.; Chambers, C.E.; Ellis, S.G.; Guyton, R.A.; Hollenberg, S.M.; et al. 2011 ACCF/AHA/SCAI Guideline for Percutaneous Coronary Intervention: A report of the American College of Cardiology Foundation/American Heart Association Task Force on Practice Guidelines and the Society for Cardiovascular Angiography and Interventions. *Circulation* **2011**, *124*, e574–e651.
12. Neumann, F.J.; Sousa-Uva, M.; Ahlsson, A.; Alfonso, F.; Banning, A.P.; Benedetto, U.; Byrne, R.A.; Collet, J.P.; Falk, V.; Head, S.J.; et al. 2018 ESC/EACTS Guidelines on myocardial revascularization. *Eur. Heart J.* **2019**, *40*, 87–165. [CrossRef]
13. Khwaja, A. KDIGO clinical practice guidelines for acute kidney injury. *Nephron. Clin. Pract.* **2012**, *120*, c179–c184. [CrossRef]
14. Devarajan, P. Neutrophil gelatinase-associated lipocalin–an emerging troponin for kidney injury. *Nephrol. Dial. Transplant.* **2008**, *23*, 3737–3743. [CrossRef]
15. Schmidt-Ott, K.M.; Mori, K.; Li, J.Y.; Kalandadze, A.; Cohen, D.J.; Devarajan, P.; Barasch, J. Dual action of neutrophil gelatinase-associated lipocalin. *J. Am. Soc. Nephrol.* **2007**, *18*, 407–413. [CrossRef]

16. Cruz, D.N.; Gaiao, S.; Maisel, A.; Ronco, C.; Devarajan, P. Neutrophil gelatinase-associated lipocalin as a biomarker of cardiovascular disease: A systematic review. *Clin. Chem. Lab. Med.* **2012**, *50*, 1533–1545. [CrossRef]
17. Zahler, D.; Merdler, I.; Banai, A.; Shusterman, E.; Feder, O.; Itach, T.; Robb, L.; Banai, S.; Shacham, Y. Predictive Value of Elevated Neutrophil Gelatinase-Associated Lipocalin (NGAL) Levels for Assessment of Cardio-Renal Interactions among ST-Segment Elevation Myocardial Infarction Patients. *J. Clin. Med.* **2022**, *11*, 2162. [CrossRef]
18. Barbarash, O.L.; Bykova, I.S.; Kashtalap, V.V.; Zykov, M.V.; Hryachkova, O.N.; Kalaeva, V.V.; Shafranskaya, K.S.; Karetnikova, V.N.; Kutikhin, A.G. Serum neutrophil gelatinase-associated lipocalin has an advantage over serum cystatin C and glomerular filtration rate in prediction of adverse cardiovascular outcome in patients with ST-segment elevation myocardial infarction. *BMC Cardiovasc. Disord.* **2017**, *17*, 81. [CrossRef]
19. Rihal, C.S.; Textor, S.C.; Grill, D.E.; Berger, P.B.; Ting, H.H.; Best, P.J.; Singh, M.; Bell, M.R.; Barsness, G.W.; Mathew, V.; et al. Incidence and prognostic importance of acute renal failure after percutaneous coronary intervention. *Circulation* **2002**, *105*, 2259–2264. [CrossRef]
20. Weisbord, S.D.; Gallagher, M.; Jneid, H.; Garcia, S.; Cass, A.; Thwin, S.S.; Conner, T.A.; Chertow, G.M.; Bhatt, D.L.; Shunk, K.; et al. Outcomes after Angiography with Sodium Bicarbonate and Acetylcysteine. *N. Engl. J. Med.* **2018**, *378*, 603–614. [CrossRef]
21. Chen, Y.L.; Fu, N.K.; Xu, J.; Yang, S.C.; Li, S.; Liu, Y.Y.; Cong, H.L. A simple preprocedural score for risk of contrast-induced acute kidney injury after percutaneous coronary intervention. *Catheter. Cardiovasc. Interv.* **2014**, *83*, E8–E16. [CrossRef]
22. Sadat, U. N-acetylcysteine in contrast-induced acute kidney injury: Clinical use against principles of evidence-based clinical medicine! *Expert Rev. Cardiovasc. Ther.* **2014**, *12*, 1–3. [CrossRef]
23. NICE. National Institute for Health and Care Excellence: Guidelines. In *Acute Kidney Injury: Prevention, Detection and Management*; National Institute for Health and Care Excellence (NICE): London, UK, 2019.
24. Herget-Rosenthal, S.; Marggraf, G.; Hüsing, J.; Göring, F.; Pietruck, F.; Janssen, O.; Philipp, T.; Kribben, A. Early detection of acute renal failure by serum cystatin C. *Kidney Int.* **2004**, *66*, 1115–1122. [CrossRef]
25. Seibert, F.S.; Heringhaus, A.; Pagonas, N.; Rudolf, H.; Rohn, B.; Bauer, F.; Timmesfeld, N.; Trappe, H.J.; Babel, N.; Westhoff, T.H. Biomarkers in the prediction of contrast media induced nephropathy—The BITCOIN study. *PLoS ONE* **2020**, *15*, e0234921. [CrossRef]
26. Banda, J.; Duarte, R.; Dix-Peek, T.; Dickens, C.; Manga, P.; Naicker, S. Biomarkers for Diagnosis and Prediction of Outcomes in Contrast-Induced Nephropathy. *Int. J. Nephrol.* **2020**, *2020*, 8568139. [CrossRef]
27. Wang, K.; Duan, C.Y.; Wu, J.; Liu, Y.; Bei, W.J.; Chen, J.Y.; He, P.C.; Liu, Y.H.; Tan, N. Predictive Value of Neutrophil Gelatinase-Associated Lipocalin for Contrast-Induced Acute Kidney Injury After Cardiac Catheterization: A Meta-analysis. *Can. J. Cardiol.* **2016**, *32*, e19–e29. [CrossRef]
28. Tsai, T.T.; Messenger, J.C.; Brennan, J.M.; Patel, U.D.; Dai, D.; Piana, R.N.; Anstrom, K.J.; Eisenstein, E.L.; Dokholyan, R.S.; Peterson, E.D.; et al. Safety and efficacy of drug-eluting stents in older patients with chronic kidney disease: A report from the linked CathPCI Registry-CMS claims database. *J. Am. Coll. Cardiol.* **2011**, *58*, 1859–1869. [CrossRef]
29. Dehmer, G.J.; Weaver, D.; Roe, M.T.; Milford-Beland, S.; Fitzgerald, S.; Hermann, A.; Messenger, J.; Moussa, I.; Garratt, K.; Rumsfeld, J.; et al. A contemporary view of diagnostic cardiac catheterization and percutaneous coronary intervention in the United States: A report from the CathPCI Registry of the National Cardiovascular Data Registry, 2010 through June 2011. *J. Am. Coll. Cardiol.* **2012**, *60*, 2017–2031. [CrossRef]
30. Matsushita, K.; van der Velde, M.; Astor, B.C.; Woodward, M.; Levey, A.S.; de Jong, P.E.; Coresh, J.; Gansevoort, R.T. Association of estimated glomerular filtration rate and albuminuria with all-cause and cardiovascular mortality in general population cohorts: A collaborative meta-analysis. *Lancet* **2010**, *375*, 2073–2081.
31. Lawton, J.S.; Tamis-Holland, J.E.; Bangalore, S.; Bates, E.R.; Beckie, T.M.; Bischoff, J.M.; Bittl, J.A.; Cohen, M.G.; DiMaio, J.M.; Don, C.W.; et al. 2021 ACC/AHA/SCAI Guideline for Coronary Artery Revascularization: A Report of the American College of Cardiology/American Heart Association Joint Committee on Clinical Practice Guidelines. *Circulation* **2022**, *145*, e18–e114. [CrossRef]
32. Bulluck, H.; Maiti, R.; Chakraborty, B.; Candilio, L.; Clayton, T.; Evans, R.; Jenkins, D.P.; Kolvekar, S.; Kunst, G.; Laing, C.; et al. Neutrophil gelatinase-associated lipocalin prior to cardiac surgery predicts acute kidney injury and mortality. *Heart* **2017**, *104*, 313–317. [CrossRef] [PubMed]

MDPI
St. Alban-Anlage 66
4052 Basel
Switzerland
Tel. +41 61 683 77 34
Fax +41 61 302 89 18
www.mdpi.com

Journal of Clinical Medicine Editorial Office
E-mail: jcm@mdpi.com
www.mdpi.com/journal/jcm

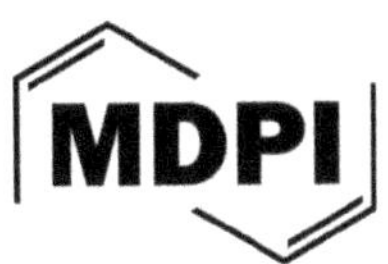